# Milk and Dairy Foods

## Nutrition, Processing and Healthy Aging

A. K. M. Humayun Kober

CRC Press
Taylor & Francis Group
Boca Raton London New York

CRC Press is an imprint of the
Taylor & Francis Group, an **informa** business

First edition published 2025
by CRC Press
2385 NW Executive Center Drive, Suite 320, Boca Raton FL 33431

and by CRC Press
4 Park Square, Milton Park, Abingdon, Oxon, OX14 4RN

*CRC Press is an imprint of Taylor & Francis Group, LLC*



ISBN: 978-1-032-50098-0 (hbk)
ISBN: 978-1-032-50290-8 (pbk)
ISBN: 978-1-003-39778-6 (ebk)

DOI: 10.1201/9781003397786

Typeset in Times
by Apex CoVantage, LLC

# Contents

# About the Author

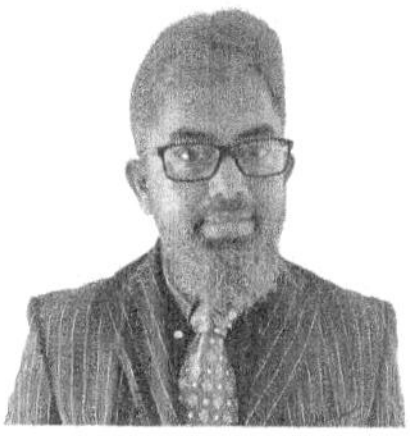

**Dr. A. K. M. Humayun Kober** is a professor in the Department of Dairy and Poultry Science at Chattogram Veterinary and Animal Sciences University (CVASU), Bangladesh. Dr. Kober earned his B.Sc. (Animal Husbandry) and M.S. (Dairy Science) degrees from the Bangladesh Agriculture University in 1999 and 2001, respectively, and his Ph.D. from the Tokyo University of Agriculture and Technology, Japan (through a MEXT Fellowship) in 2011. He completed a JSPS post-doc (2015–2017) and JSPS Invitational Research Fellow (2022–2023) program on Food Immunology at Tohoku University, Japan. He was a visiting researcher (2014) at the Norwegian University of Life Sciences, Norway. He served as head of the department. Dr. Kober has published more than 50 refereed journal articles, more than 40 conference proceedings/talks, and more than 13 popular articles published in leading national dailies such as *Prothom Alo* and *Ittefaq*.

He has supervised 15 master's students and is now supervising five master's students. He received many research grants and fellowships as a recognition of his good impact on research from home and abroad. He received several prestigious national and international awards during his academic career, including the Best Researcher Award 2019–2020 for CVASU researchers and holding national consultant (Department of Livestock Services, Government of Bangladesh) positions. Dr. Kober has chaired scientific meetings and served as Guest Editor/Review Editor/Associate Editor on the editorial boards of scientific publications such as *Microorganisms* and *Frontiers in Microbiology*. He is actively engaged in professional societies. Furthermore, he presented his research works in reputed societies such as the Japanese Society of Dairy Science/ Food Immunology, the Federation of European Microbiological Societies, and the Canadian Society of Microbiologists etc. His current research interests include developing functional dairy foods, probiotics, antimicrobial resistance, and food safety concerns for healthy human and animal growth strategies.

# Preface

Milk and dairy foods can be termed as *nature's gift, crafted with tradition and savored with delight.* Milk and dairy foods (also referred to as superfoods) offer all the nutrients required for a healthy existence. Milk is nature's most complete food, and dairy foods are considered the most nutritious foods of all. Milk components are multifunctional. Milk products possess a natural "cluster" of nutrients that protect health and enhance the immune system. Milk includes biologically active substances besides its primary proteins, which have crucial physiological and biochemical functions with a significant influence on human health. Consumers who introduce milk and dairy foods into their diet early will reap the benefits. The consumption of whey protein beginning at a young age can assist in maintaining and growing muscle mass, which is advantageous to consumers at an older age. According to recent research published in the *American Journal of Clinical Nutrition*, eating whole and low-fat dairy products such as milk, cheese, and yogurt was not linked to an increased risk of cardiovascular disease-related incidence and may even improve human health. Various dairy functional ingredients, including α-lactalbumin, β-lactoglobulin, lactoferrin, immunoglobulins, oligosaccharides, whey protein concentrates, bovine serum albumin, peptides, sphingolipids, butyric acid, modified whey protein concentrate, lactoperoxidase, kappa casein glycomacropeptide, and conjugated linoleic acid, have beneficial health effects on humans. Examples of those effects consist of antimicrobial/antiviral, anti-inflammatory, biostatic, antihypertensive, angiotensin-converting enzyme-inhibitory, antithrombic activity, anti-adhesion, antidiabetic, anti-cholesterol, anticarcinogenic, immunomodulatory, anticariogenic, anti-obesity, toxin-binding, probiotic, and prebiotic activities. Among the various valuable ingredients in milk and dairy foods, the high level of calcium plays a very significant role in the growth, strength, and density of bones in youngsters, as well as the prevention of osteoporosis in elderly people. Furthermore, calcium also aids in reducing cholesterol levels, controlling weight, and managing blood pressure.

This book, *Milk and Dairy Foods: Nutrition, Processing and Healthy Aging*, is up-to-date and properly referenced for the convenience of all readers. This book covers the definition, types, nutritional facts, global production and consumption trends, manufacturing process, physicochemical properties, factors influencing the quality, quality judging, defects, health benefits, and innovations from production to nutritional and health attributes of major value-added dairy foods such as yogurt, cheese, cream, butter, ghee, dried milk, condensed milk, ice cream, and traditional dairy foods. To the best of my knowledge, there have been few books written on milk and dairy foods that are relevant to human health benefits and the immunomodulation potential of dairy components.

This is a comprehensive book; I strongly believe that this book will be useful to readers all over the world, especially students, scientists, and health-conscious consumers. This book is unique in that it discusses the various dairy foods that people consume today that greatly impact their survival and well-being. This book will provide the most current information and the finest accessible expertise from international authorities and scientists in the field of food and dairy science. For this book, a wide range of readers may be expected. My hope is that this book will be utilized in classrooms at colleges/universities, libraries, and government organizations for subjects such as dairy science, food science, nutrition, and technology-related courses, where it can be used as a textbook or a reference book. The intended audience for this book mainly consists of students specializing in dairy and food sciences and nutrition, as well as professionals such as food scientists, dairy producers, nutritionists, and healthcare providers. Health-conscious consumers may also be interested in reading it. I also believe that more comprehensive audiences would include the dairy industry, producers, dairy processors, dairy marketers (retail and wholesale), veterinarians, libraries, agricultural schools and colleges, consumers, and connoisseurs. More importantly, I expect this book's most significant audience should include the consumer, end users, health-food lovers, and dietary specialists. The book provides exceptional and extremely useful information specifically targeted toward individuals working in food/dairy science and related fields, in both industry and academia.

I hope that this detailed and unique information source, along with its inclusive coverage of the scientific literature, will have a long-term impact on the understanding of manufacturing methods of different dairy foods and the food value, quality control, and health benefits of different dairy foods, including traditional dairy foods. In recent days, dried milk and fermented dairy foods are expected to become the fastest-growing dairy products.

This book is divided into 12 chapters. Nutritional components, different types of milk (particularly A1 and A2), dairy foods, healthy aging, and the health benefits of milk and dairy foods are all highlighted at the start of this book (Chapter 1). Heat treatments used during milk processing ensure the safety and stability of the milk. The antioxidant activity of dairy products may increase during storage due to the formation of bioactive peptides. As a result, an efficient processing and storage system may improve milk quality, as discussed in Chapter 2. From Chapter 3 to Chapter 10, nutritional attributes, types, production and processing, biochemical and microbiological aspects, quality evaluation and quality control, defects with possible remedies, functional properties, and advances from production to nutritional and health attributes of value-added major dairy foods such as yogurt, cheese, cream, butter, ghee, dried milk, condensed milk, and ice cream are discussed. The utilization of functional probiotics in yogurt acts as a supplement, resulting in the improvement of health status. So, the criteria for the selection of functional probiotics have also been discussed in Chapter 3. Cheese Analogues, cheese alternatives made from plant sources (vegetable proteins and fats) and produced with the desired nutritional, functional, and storage qualities, have also been discussed in Chapter 4.

Uniquely, this book covers the production procedure along with the health benefits of traditional or indigenous dairy foods of various regions, especially South Asian countries (Chapter 11). Traditional or indigenous dairy food has been produced and marketed in these countries for centuries. The manufacture and trading of these indigenous dairy foods are largely confined to confectionery and sweet manufacturers. This work will serve as a valuable and in-depth reference guide for these traditional dairy products including rasgulla (syrup cheese ball), chomchom (sweetmeats), kheer (rice pudding), gulabjamun (rose berry dipped in sugar syrup), kachagolla (ricotta cheese sweets), peda (sweet made with full-fat milk and sugar), barfi (sweet confectionery), sandesh (sweet), rasmalai (cottage cheese balls), buttermilk, laban (fermented milk), and lassi (yogurt drink).

The unique contents of this book could be correlated or contribute to the United Nations (UN)'s sustainable development goals (SDGs); dairy sector is closely connected to 4 out of the 17 goals including SDG1 (poverty reduction), SDG2 (no hunger), SDG3 (good health), and SDG5 (gender equality). The focus of Chapter 12 is on examining the role of the dairy industry in supporting the achievement of the UN's sustainable development goals (SDGs). Moreover, it will provide insight into the current obstacles faced by the dairy industry and explore future possibilities. In conclusion, I hope this book will be well received across the world.

Working on this book has been a thrilling experience. Without the helpful suggestions from several people, it would not have been achievable. I would like to convey my deep appreciation to my mentor, Professor Dr. Haruki Kitazawa (lab of animal food function), Dean, Graduate School of Agricultural Science, Tohoku University, Japan, for his guidance, valuable suggestions, constructive criticism, and insightful feedback, which greatly contributed to the successful completion of this book. I am grateful and appreciative of his support. I would especially like to thank CRC Press/Taylor & Francis Group, the publisher, in particular for offering the editors an opportunity to publish this extensive work in the discipline, as well as all the staff members, Bhavik Sawhney and Neha Bhatt, who have contributed significantly to making this project a reality. I am also thankful to the teams responsible for editing and typesetting this publication, as well as the independent project manager for their outstanding job and empathetic approach toward the difficulties encountered in the editing of this book's 12 chapters to achieve clear and comprehensible language, coherence, and well-organized tables and figures. Last but not least, I owe huge gratitude to my students, Umme

Salma Amin and, Md. Ridoy Chowdhury; my wife Shamima Akter, my son Farhan Kabir Rhaad, my daughter Ruqayyah Bint Kabir, my nephew Rafi, and my father Md Ekin Ali and mother Rohima Khanom, and others (Zhou, Tahalil, Fahim, Nakib, Safa, Akib, Tanzina, Marzia and Dola) for their continuous support, dedication, and effort throughout this project. This book is therefore dedicated to my respected parents, from whom I have learned so much, and my beloved family members.

I would like to appeal to all readers for critical analysis and suggestions for further improvement of this book.

**A. K. M. Humayun Kober**

# 1 Introduction to Milk and Dairy Foods

## 1.1 LEARNING OBJECTIVES

By the end of the chapter, the reader will be able to:

- Gain knowledge of terms and definitions of different types of milk and dairy foods
- Identify foods in the dairy group and understand their needs
- Learn about worldwide milk production and dairy food consumption patterns
- Gain knowledge of recent advancements in milk and dairy food technologies
- Learn about the nutritional properties of milk and dairy food
- Understand the role of milk and dairy foods in healthy aging

Milk and dairy foods are vital sources of nutrients for fortifying human health. It is a historically significant and strategically important sector of the global economy. Dairy foods help preserve muscle health, beat against certain physiological processes, function to delay the onset of sarcopenia, and balance the flora in the gut. Adding dairy items to a usual diet may be a promising dietary improvement strategy. Ultimately, such a strategy can prevent muscle reduction in the elderly population.

## 1.2 TERMS AND DEFINITIONS

**Milk**: Milk may be defined as the whole, fresh, clean, lacteal secretion obtained by the complete milking of one or more healthy cows, excluding that obtained within 15 days before or 5 days after calving, that is practically free from colostrum and contains the minimum prescribed percentage of milk fat (usually ≥3.25%) and solids-not-fat (SNF) (usually ≥8.25%).

Excluding that obtained 15 days before or 5 days after or such periods as may be necessary to render the milk practically free of colostrum. Milk is a complete food for the newborn (**Figure 1.1**). Cow milk is pale yellow to yellowish white in color due to its richness in carotene, whereas buffalo milk is snow white, as there is less carotene present. In general, milk means cow milk; in the case of other milk, we can include the species name such as goat milk, sheep milk, and human milk.

**Market milk:** Market milk refers to fluid whole milk that is sold to individuals, usually for direct consumption (pasteurized). It excludes milk consumed on the farm and that used for the manufacture of dairy foods.

**Dairy science:** Dairy science refers to milk production on farms for dairy production and the processing and distribution of milk and milk products in dairy plants.

Dairy science includes the study of milk and milk-derived food products, examining the biological, chemical, physical, and microbiological aspects of milk itself, as well as the technological (processing) aspects of the transformation of milk into its various consumer products, including beverages, fermented products, concentrated and dried products, butter, and ice cream (Fuquay et al., 2011).

DOI: 10.1201/9781003397786-1

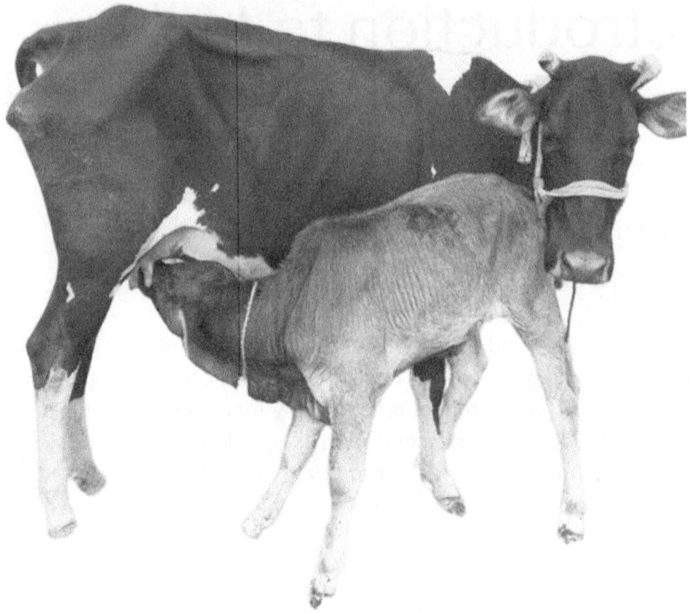

**FIGURE 1.1 Direct consumption of milk by a newborn calf.** Milk feeding has a long-term positive influence on calves' growth and productive performance.

Dairy science is a comprehensive term for several sciences concerned with milk in its raw state and the processes to which it is subjected such as chemistry, physics, biology, engineering, animal and human health, and nutrition and their application in the dairy industry. Knowledge of the fundamental principles of these sciences is essential for the efficient performance of various processes and the expansion of the industry.

**Dairy technology:** Dairy technology is the application of dairy science to the manufacturing, processing, and preservation of dairy foods.

## 1.3 MILK COMPOSITION

Milk is one of the most significant foods derived from animals which is nature's most complete food with essential nutrients (**Figure 1.2**). It improves the quality of the human diet and provides all the nutrients—including fats, proteins, lipids, calcium, and vitamins—necessary to support the survival of the newborn and early infant. Fat and solids-not-fat (SNF) contents in milk are the two important constituents. SNF (also known as non-fat milk solids, milk solids not-fat, solids no-fat, etc.) is that nutrient portion present in milk other than milk fat and water. When SNF is combined with milk fat, then it is called total solids (TS). Dairy products, which frequently have an even higher biological value, are substantially impacted by the composition of milk. Milk composition varies depending on different factors including the species (cow, goat, and sheep) (**Table 1.1**), breed (Holstein, Jersey), feed, breeding factors (e.g., genetic potential, nutrition, breeding methods, etc.), factors of animal health, physiological factors (e.g., stage and order of lactation, the individuality of the animal, etc.), and external environmental factors (e.g., climatic conditions) (Islam et al., 2002; Kober et al., 2015; Debnath et al., 2014).

**Bovine colostrum:** Colostrum is the secretion of the mammary gland during the first 3 to 5 days after calving. The composition of colostrum differs from that of normal milk (**Table 1.2**). It changes

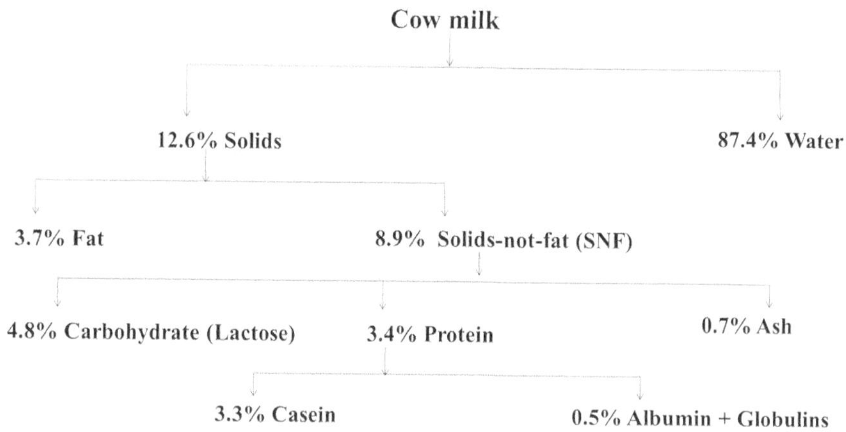


**FIGURE 1.2 Gross composition of milk.** Milk composition varies according to species (cow, goat, sheep), breed (Jersey, Holstein), diet of animals, lactation stage, and so on.

**TABLE 1.1**
**Nutritional Composition of Milk from Different Mammalian Species (%)**

| Species | Water | Solids | Fat | Proteins | Lactose | Minerals |
|---|---|---|---|---|---|---|
| Cow | 87.5 | 12.5 | 3.7 | 3.3 | 4.7 | 0.8 |
| Sheep | 80.7 | 19.3 | 8 | 5.6 | 4.8 | 0.9 |
| Goat | 87 | 13 | 4 | 3.6 | 4.5 | 0.9 |
| Buffalo | 82 | 18 | 7.9 | 4.5 | 4.8 | 0.8 |
| Horse | 89 | 11 | 1.9 | 2.5 | 6.3 | 0.3 |
| Human | 87.6 | 12.4 | 4 | 1.2 | 7 | 0.2 |

*Source:* Kober et al., 2015; Rebouillat & Ortega-Requena, 2015; Webb et al., 1974

**TABLE 1.2**
**Nutritional Composition of Colostrum Compared to Milk**

| Ingredients | Colostrum day 1 | Colostrum day 3 | Milk |
|---|---|---|---|
| Total solids (%) | 21.0 | 13.0 | 12.9 |
| Fat (%) | 6.3 | 4.3 | 4.0 |
| Protein (%) | 11.4 | 4.1 | 4.0 |
| Lactose (%) | 3.3 | 4.7 | 5.0 |
| Minerals (%) | 1.03 | 0.81 | 0.74 |
| Immunoglobulins (%) | 5.1 | 1.0 | 0.09 |
| Vitamin A, µg/100 ml | 240 | 74 | 34 |
| Vitamin E, µg/g | 80 | 31 | 15 |

rapidly upon successive milking and becomes normal in about 5 days after calving. Colostrum is rich in globulins, which serve as the carriers of antibodies to protect the calves against diseases. Physicochemical characteristics of milk and colostrum are varied (**Table 1.3**).

**TABLE 1.3**
**Comparative Physicochemical Characteristics of Milk and Colostrum**

| Parameter | Milk | Colostrum |
|---|---|---|
| Color | Yellowish white to white | Deep yellow to pale yellow |
| Taste | Sweet | Bitter |
| Acidity (%) | 0.12 to 0.14 | 0.2 to 0.4 |
| Freezing point (°C) | –0.52 to (–0.56) | –0.605 |
| Chloride (%) | 0.14 | 0.149 to 0.156 |
| Specific gravity | 1.028 to 1.032 | 1.048 to 1.08 |
| Refractive index at 20°C | 1.344 to 1.348 | More than milk |
| Electrical conductivity | 0.005 ohm | More than milk |
| Viscosity at 20°C | 1.5 to 2.0 centipoise | More than milk |
| Total solids (%) | 12.7 | 24.71 |
| Protein (%) | 3.7 | 16.42 |
| Casein (%) | 3.2 | 5.08 |
| Albumin and globulin (%) | 0.5 | 11.34 |
| Fat (%) | 3.8 | 5.1 |
| Lactose (%) | 4.5 | 2.19 |

### 1.3.1 Health Benefits of Colostrum

It contains immunoglobulins, lactoferrins, lysozymes, lactoperoxidase, growth factors, and bioactive peptides. Colostrum has greater levels of protein, fat, vitamins, and minerals than milk (**Table 1.2**) (Wadud et al., 2002). This compositional singularity of colostrum enables full development of the newborn calf and also ensures immunity to a number of diseases (**Figure 1.3**) (Kober et al., 2022). Bovine colostrum is considered safe for human consumption.

## 1.4 TYPES/FORMS OF MILK AND DAIRY FOODS

### 1.4.1 Types/Forms of Milk

**Raw milk or whole milk:** Raw milk or whole milk is milk just as it comes from the cow. It is not changed in any way. When whole milk is allowed to stand, the butterfat rises, making cream at the top. This cream is sometimes called "top milk."

**Pasteurized milk:** Pasteurized milk is either whole milk or skim milk that has been heated to kill all harmful bacteria and make it safe for use.

**Homogenized milk:** Homogenized milk is pasteurized milk. The fat has been so finely divided that it remains mixed with the milk and does not rise to the top as cream.

**Vitamin D milk:** Vitamin D milk is pasteurized milk that has been enriched with vitamin D. This is done by exposing it to ultraviolet rays, by adding cod liver oil, or, by including vitamin D in the feed given to cows.

**Buttermilk:** Buttermilk is the liquid left from the cream after butter is made from it.

**Chocolate milk or chocolate-flavored milk:** Chocolate milk or chocolate-flavored milk is a milk drink made by adding cocoa or chocolate syrup to whole or skim milk.

**Canned milk:** There are two kinds of canned milk.

**Evaporated milk:** Evaporated milk is whole milk that has been heated before canning to remove more than half the water content. When used just as it comes from the can,

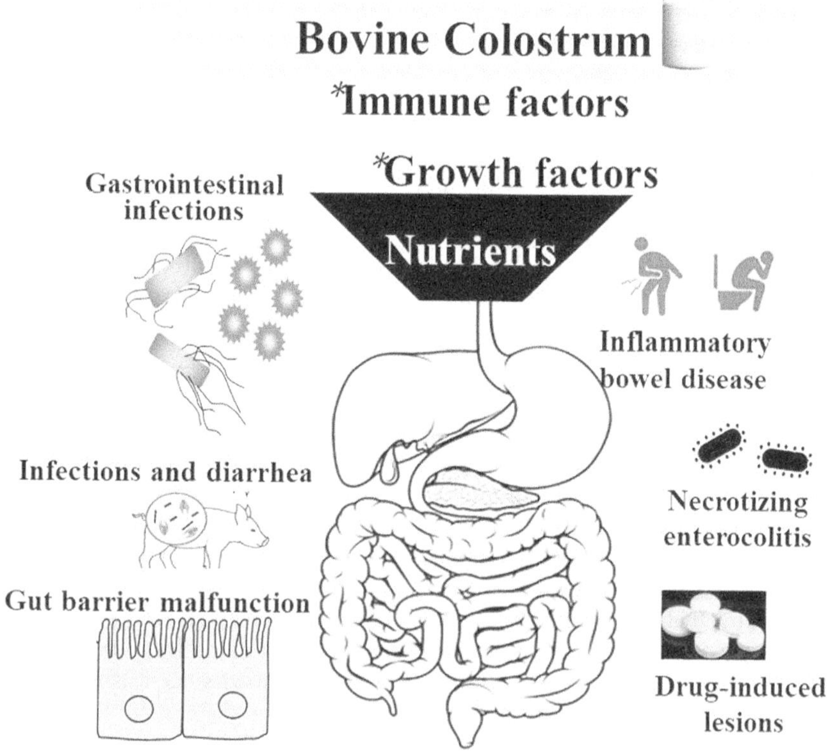


**FIGURE 1.3 Health benefits of colostrum.** Functional components of bovine colostrum, particularly immune and growth factors, are related to beneficial effects on the gastrointestinal tract under different altered conditions.

evaporated milk is referred to in recipes as undiluted milk. When mixed with an equal amount of water, it is referred to as diluted milk. Diluted evaporated milk has almost the same food value as whole milk.

**Sweetened condensed milk:** Sweetened condensed milk is evaporated milk to which about 50% sugar has been added.

**Non-fat dry milk solids or dried skim milk:** Non-fat dry milk solids, or dried skim milk, are made from fresh milk by the removal of fat and water. Non-fat milk has the same food value as skim milk or buttermilk.

**Dried whole milk:** Dried whole milk is whole milk from which only the water has been removed. It has the same food value as fresh whole milk.

**Standardized milk:** This is made by combining buffalo milk and skimmed milk. The fat percentage is maintained at 4.5%, while the non-fat solids percentage is 8.5%.

**Whole milk:** This refers to milk that must contain at least 3.25% milk fat and 8.25% milk solids by weight, which means it derives about 50% of its calories from fat.

**Reduced-fat milk (2%):** This refers to milk where the milkfat is 2% of the total weight of the milk.

**Low-fat milk (1%):** 1% means that the milk contains approximately 1% milkfat by weight. Many people find low-fat milk more appealing and a good compromise.

**Skim milk/non-fat milk:** There is an extremely low-fat content in this milk. It may not contain more than 0.5% milk fat by weight and usually contains less than 0.5 g of fat per cup, deriving just 5% of its calories from fat. The calorie content of skimmed milk is only half that of whole milk. It is the most optimal choice for adults and the sole type of milk suitable for individuals adhering to strict low-fat diets. Sadly, skim milk doesn't have much taste and looks unattractive, with a blue tint.

**Flavored milk:** Milk to which some flavors are added is termed as flavored milk. It is a ready-to-drink product that is produced from skim milk, added sugar, and natural flavors (e.g., banana, pineapple, orange, chocolate, etc.).

**Toned milk:** Toned milk (also called single-toned milk) refers to milk that is obtained by the addition of water and skim milk powder to whole milk. Usually, it contains fat 1–3%, non-fat solids 8.5–10.5%, total solids (TS) 11.5%, and water 88.5%.

**Sterilized milk:** Sterilized milk refers to milk that has undergone heating at or above 100°C for a designated period of time. This particular process ensures that milk remains suitable for drinking at room temperature for a duration of at least 7 days. Commercially sterilized milk is rarely sterile in the strictest bacteriological sense. Sterilized milk must (i) keep without deterioration, i.e., remain stable and have good commercial value for a sufficient period to satisfy commercial requirements; (ii) be free of microorganisms that are harmful to consumer health, i.e., pathogens, toxic germs, and toxins; and (iii) be free of any microorganism liable to proliferate, i.e., should not show sign of bacterial growth.

**Reconstituted/rehydrated milk:** This refers to milk prepared by dispersing whole milk powder (also called dried whole milk) in water approximately in the proportion of 1 part powder to 7–8 parts water. (Usually, spray-dried powder is used since it is more soluble and produces less sediment.)

**A1 and A2:** A1 and A2 milk are two varieties of milk classified based on the type of beta-casein present in the milk. Because A1 milk includes A1 beta-casein and A2 milk has A2 beta-casein protein, this is the primary distinction between A1 and A2 milk (Fernández-Rico et al., 2022) (**Figure 1.4**). Furthermore, A1 beta-casein produces beta-casomorphin-7 (BCM-7) during digestion, which can cause alterations in gastrointestinal function and increase inflammation in the gut. However, upon digestion, A2 beta-casein does not generate BCM-7.

A new variety of cow's milk known as "A2 milk" has recently been released on the market. Since its initial commercialization in New Zealand, this kind of milk has been making inroads into the market throughout the world. The absence of the A1 variant of β-casein, a protein that makes up around 30% of the caseins in cow's milk, is what distinguishes A2 milk from other varieties. One can create a dairy farm that only produces A2-type milk by genotyping dairy cows and using the sperm from chosen bulls, or by genotyping and only choosing A2 calves as replacements. The coding gene in β-casein synthesis is the *CNS2* gene, for which 13 different allelic variants have been described (A1, A2, A3, B, C, D, E, F, G, H1, H2, I and J) (Fernández-Rico et al., 2022). While the A1 version is only found in cows, the A2 form is found in the milk of various species, including humans, goats, sheep, and cows (Fernández-Rico et al., 2022).

### 1.4.2 Dairy Foods

Dairy foods or dairy products or milk products, often known as lacticinia, are milk-based foods. Cows, water buffalo, goats, and ewes are the most prevalent dairy animals. Dairy foods include familiar grocery store foods such as yogurt, cheese, butter, and so on throughout the world. (**Figure 1.5**).

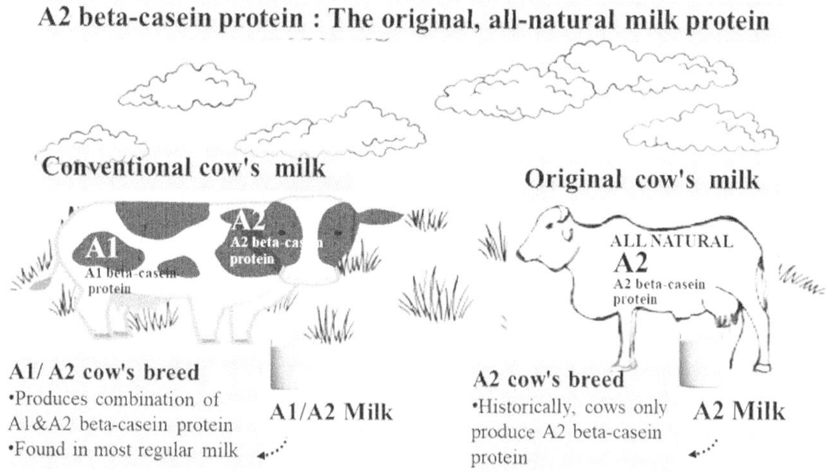


FIGURE 1.4 **Features of A1 and A2 milk.** In general, favorable results found in experimental animal studies about the health effects of A2 milk have not always been supported by clinical trials in people. However, there appears to be a substantial consensus on the favorable benefits of A2 milk for a decrease in digestive intolerance linked with the use of A1 milk. Despite the contradicting results to date, there have not been enough clinical studies conducted for the conclusions gained to be final, and it would be quite fascinating to further the study in this regard.

#### 1.4.2.1 Types of Dairy Foods

**Fermented dairy foods:** Dairy foods prepared by bacterial fermentation (e.g., yogurt) or a combination of this and yeast fermentation (e.g., kefir) are called fermented dairy foods (**Figure 1.6**). Fermented milk products or fermented dairy foods are also known as cultured dairy foods. As fresh products, they have a limited shelf life and should preferably be kept refrigerated throughout distribution. Fermented milk products such as cheese, yogurt, kefir, and soured milk are the primary varieties available; however, there are numerous regional cultured dairy foods as well. Fermented dairy foods contain, for example, bacteria that are used in fermentation and bioactive peptides that are produced in the fermentation process. These things can reduce inflammation in the body by changing the bacteria in our gut or working with our immune system cells (Bordoni et al., 2017). Studies show that fermented dairy products, namely cheese and yogurt, might be able to reduce inflammation in the body (Hess et al., 2021).

**Non-fermented dairy foods:** Non-fermented dairy foods are prepared from milk and or milk products without fermentation (**Figure 1.7**). Whey protein concentrate, skim milk, evaporated milk, sweetened condensed milk, milk powder, and ice cream are the main varieties of non-fermented dairy foods.

**Traditional dairy foods:** Traditional or indigenous dairy foods can be defined as all milk products which are native to any region/country and which were evolved over ages utilizing locally available fuels and cooking ware (**Figure 1.8**). Examples—Buttermilk, laban (fermented milk), lassi (yogurt drink), rasgulla (sweet syrup cheese ball), chomchom (sweetmeats), kheer (rice pudding), gulabjamun (rose water berry), kachagolla (ricotta cheese sweets), peda (sweet made with full-fat milk and sugar), barfi (sweet confectionery), sweet sandesh, rasmalai (cottage cheese balls), etc.

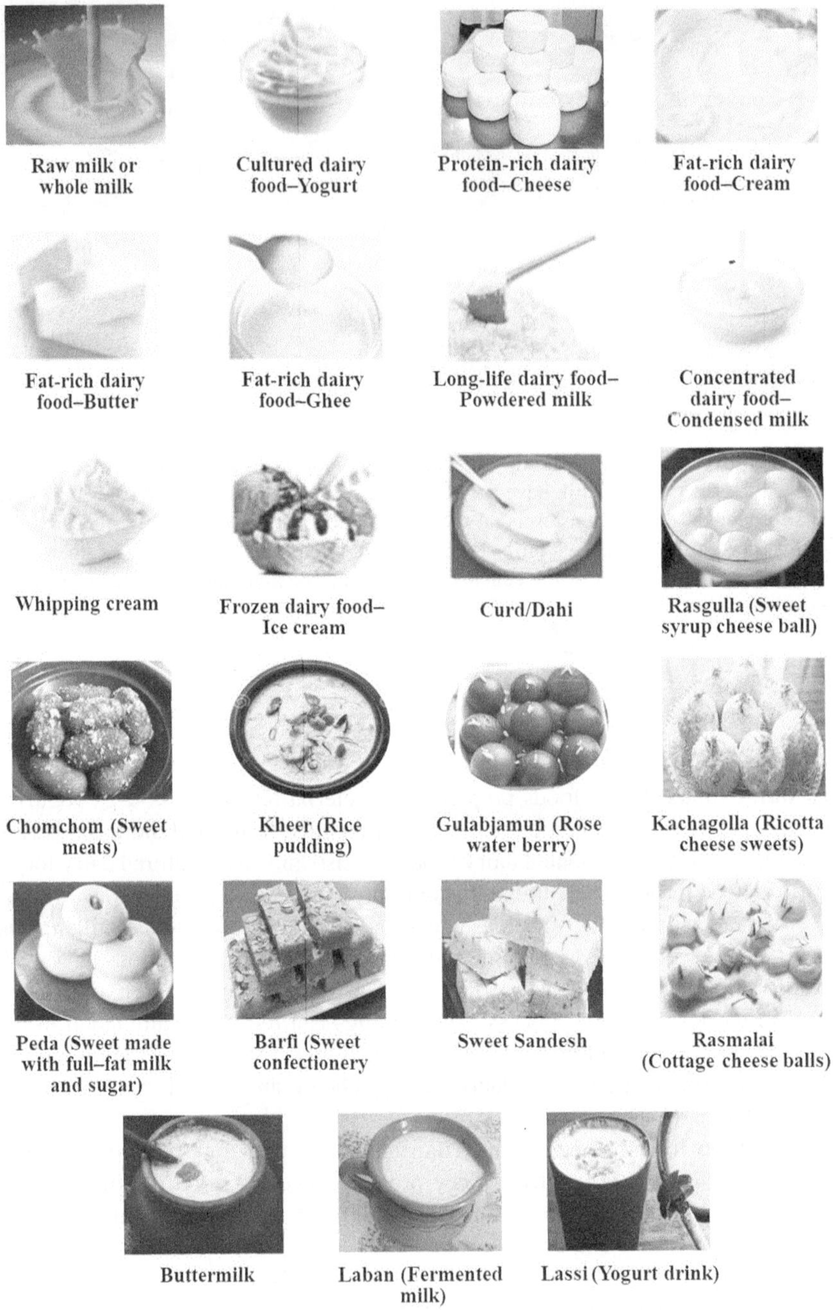


**FIGURE 1.5 Milk and major dairy foods, including traditional dairy foods.** Dairy foods include common grocery store staples such as yogurt, cheese, milk, and butter across the world. The world's most popular dairy foods: Kiselo mlyako, Bulgaria; Greek yogurt, Greece; ghee/malai, India; clotted cream, England; Twaróg (cheese), Poland; cheese, USA; dahi/sweetmeat, Bangladesh.

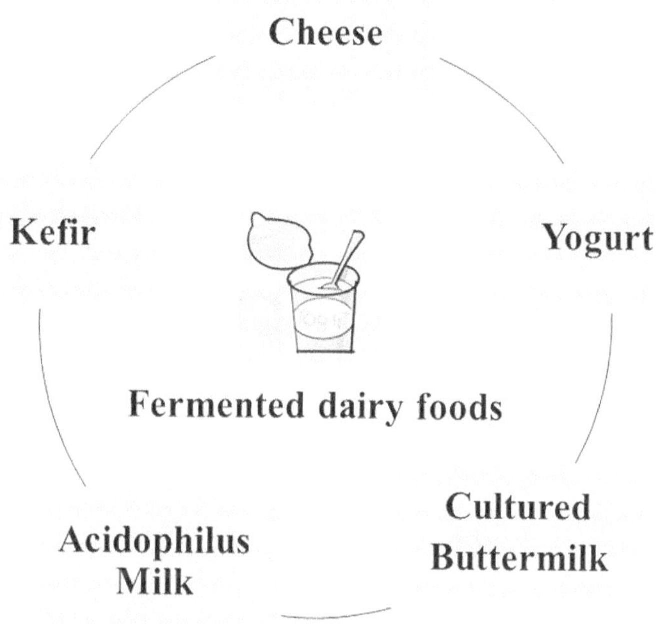


**FIGURE 1.6 Fermented dairy foods.** Yogurt, koumiss, dahi, labneh, and kefir are examples of fermented foods.

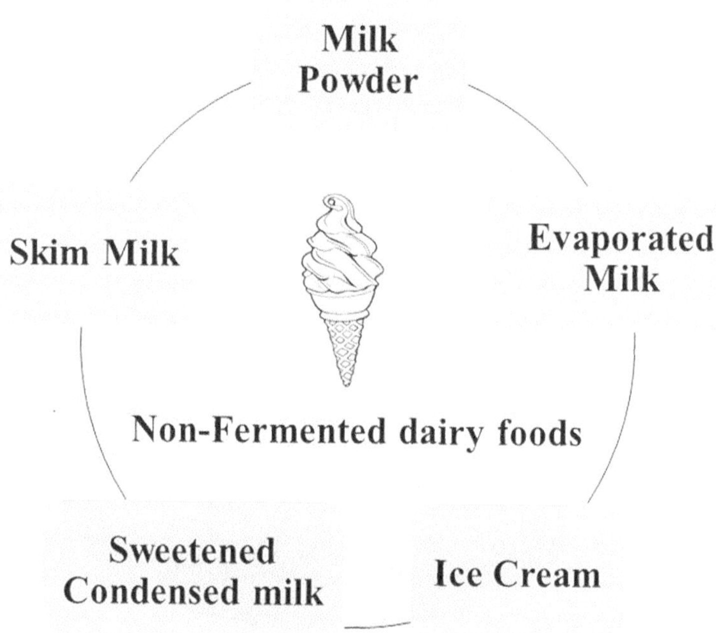


**FIGURE 1.7 Non-fermented dairy foods.** Whey protein concentrate, skim milk, evaporated milk, sweetened condensed milk, milk powder, khoa, and ice cream are examples of non-fermented dairy foods.

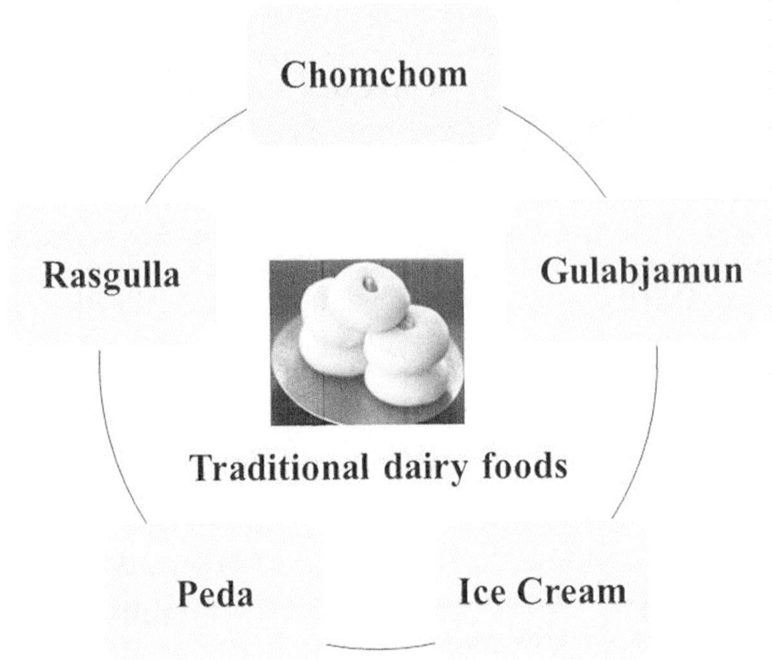


**FIGURE 1.8 Traditional dairy foods (traditional dairy foods that customers consume instead of the original dairy foods).** Different types of sweets, rabri, kulfi, srikhand, lassi, ghee, paneer, chhana, kheer, makkhan, and dahi are examples of traditional dairy foods. Nutritional attributes of traditional dairy foods would be quite fascinating to study further.

## 1.5 WORLDWIDE MILK PRODUCTION AND DAIRY FOOD CONSUMPTION PATTERNS

World cow milk production increased from 441.97 million tons (MT) in 2010 to 524.41 MT in 2019, an 18.65% increase (USDA, 2020). The year 2019 saw a 1.3% increase in global milk output, which reached 852 MT (81% cow milk, 15% buffalo milk, and 4% goat, sheep, and camel milk combined). In 2019, the biggest producing countries were in the EU (155.2 MT), with the leading share of 33.1 MT in Germany, in addition to the USA (99.06 MT), and India (92 MT) (USDA, 2020). According

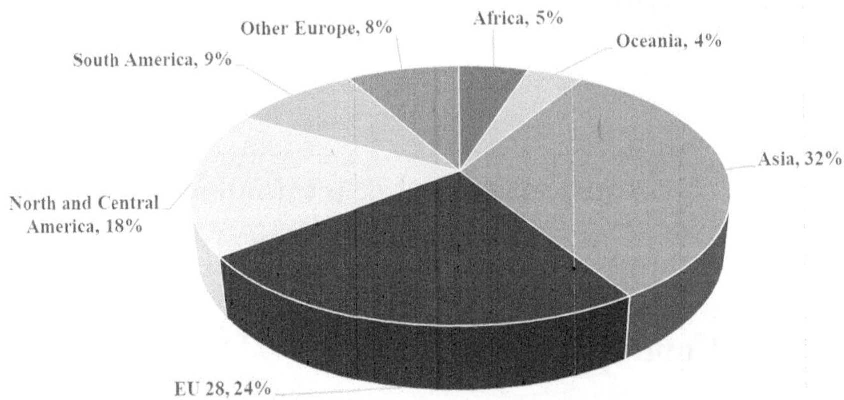


**FIGURE 1.9 Worldwide milk production (IDF, 2020).** Global milk production reached almost 906 million tons in 2020, a 2% rise over 2019, driven by gains in all geographical areas except Africa, where output remained steady. Asia (32%), the EU (28.24%), and North and Central America (18%) were the leading milk-producing areas in 2020. In terms of specific nations, the greatest milk producers remain India (141 MT) and the United States (93 MT).

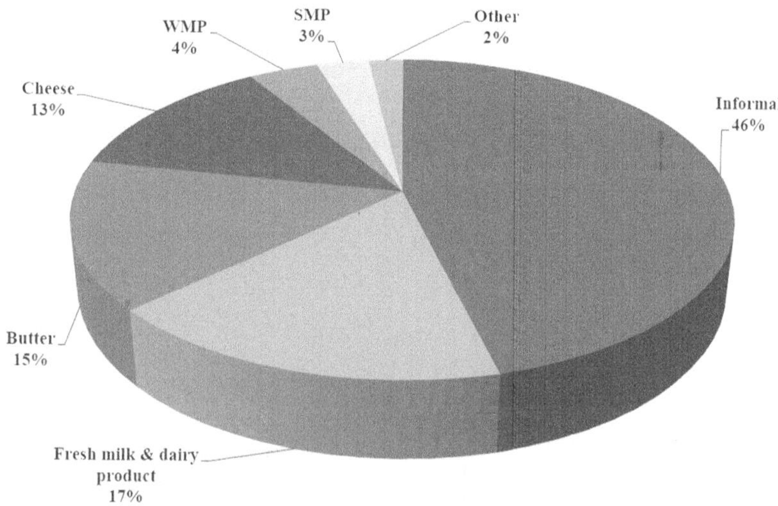


**FIGURE 1.10 Worldwide dairy food consumption (IDF, 2015).** Despite the expansion of organized dairy (particularly in developing countries of the world), informal trading accounts for a considerable portion (46%) of dairy consumption. Fresh milk and dairy products account for 17% of the remaining 54%, including butter (15%), cheese (13%), whole-milk powder (WMP) (4%), skim milk powder (SMP) (3%), and others (2%).

to the International Dairy Federation (IDF), worldwide cow milk production patterns in terms of regions are illustrated in **Figure 1.9**. Globally, the average amount of milk consumed per person, including milk equivalents of dairy products without butter, grew from 78.24 kg in 2000 to 111.6 kg in 2019, a rise of 29.9% over this time (FAO, 2020). In addition, the United States, Canada, and World Health Organization dietary guidelines recommend a regular intake of milk and dairy products. Dairy items like cheese and yogurt are believed to contribute to healthy aging. Worldwide dairy food consumption patterns are illustrated in **Figure 1.10.**

## 1.6 HEALTHY AGING WITH MILK AND DAIRY FOODS

The term "healthy aging" describes the "process of developing and maintaining the functional ability that enables well-being in older age" and has recently become a source of concern (WHO, 2015). Functional abilities comprise physiological, cognitive, metabolic, and immunological functions in the elder stages of human life.

The world economy is significantly impacted by the aging population. Milk and dairy foods like cheese and yogurt are ideally positioned as healthy aging products. Functional dairy ingredients (**Figure 1.11**) are already perceived by many as being healthy, functional, and effective for the health of elderly individuals (Clare & Swaisgood, 2000; Thorning et al., 2016). Different healthy aging functions of milk and dairy foods are as follows:

### 1.6.1 Improving Muscle Aging

The process of acquiring and preserving the functional capacity that promotes well-being as people age is known as healthy aging. Protein, calcium (Ca), phosphate (P), and vitamin D are essential nutrients for the human body and have an impact on muscle mass and quality. These nutrients are abundant in milk and dairy products, suggesting that they may be particularly beneficial for the aged population (Du et al., 2019). Dairy products give older people essential nutrients, preserve the health of their muscles, fight against certain physiological processes, and work with skeletal muscle bulk and function to delay the onset of sarcopenia (a key issue in the aging process) (Drewnowski, 2011). Therefore, taking the right nutritional measures as an aged person can reduce the risk of

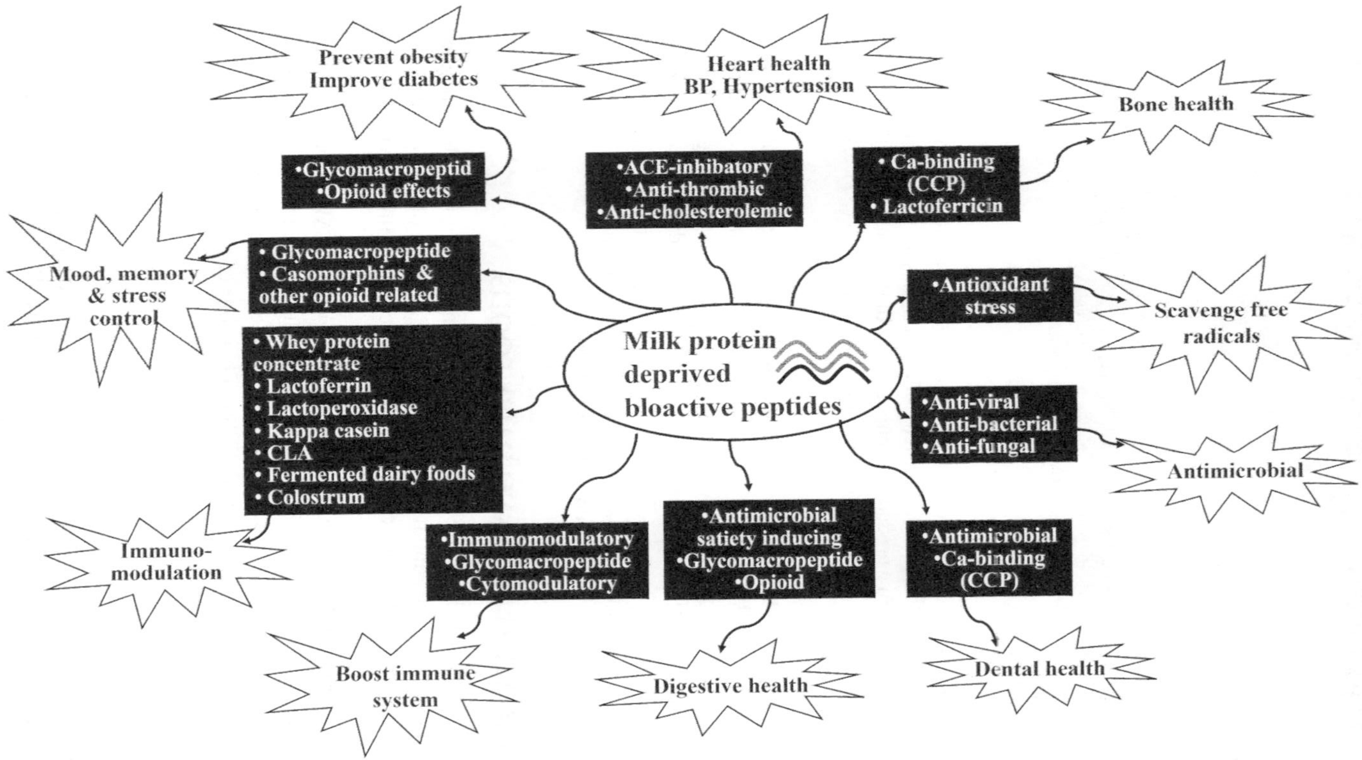


**FIGURE 1.11 Healthy aging functions of milk protein-derived bioactive peptides.** Milk protein is a rich source of bioactive peptides that may help as modulators of several regulatory mechanisms in the body, including neurological, gastrointestinal, cardiovascular, and immunological systems. Milk protein-derived bioactive peptides have been demonstrated to have antihypertensive, antibacterial, immunomodulatory, antioxidative, mineral-binding, and other activities. The food industry is particularly interested in bioactive peptides generated from milk proteins due to their possible functional and physiclogical significance.

**ABBREVIATIONS:** BP; blood pressure, CLA; conjugated linoleic acid, ACE; angiotensin-converting enzyme

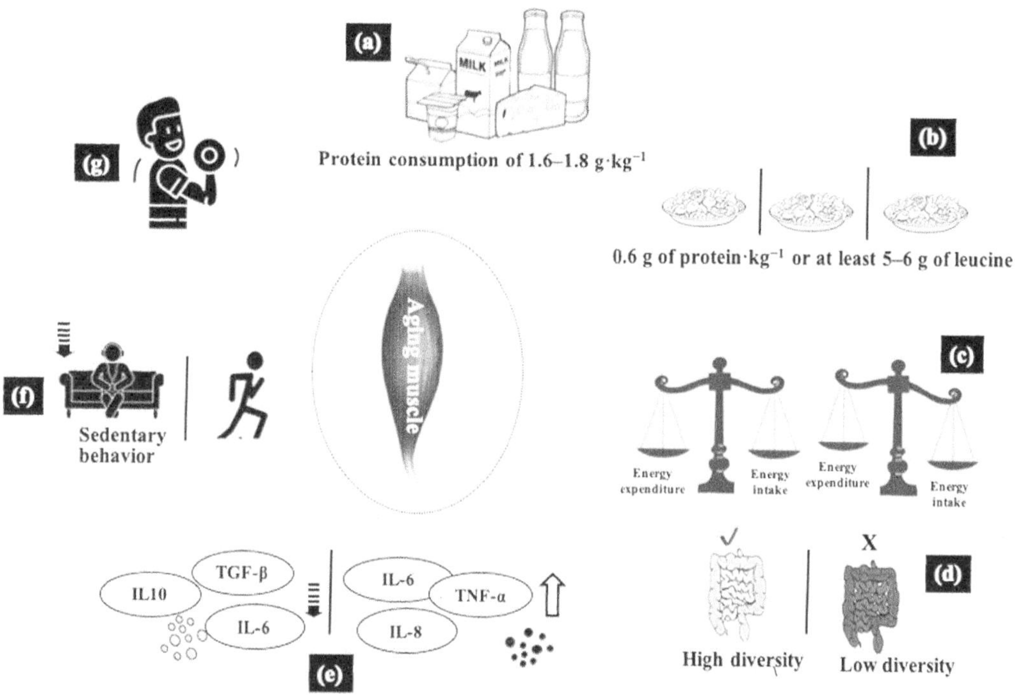


**FIGURE 1.12 Advantage of dairy foods for improving aging muscle/skeletal muscle.** A minimum of 0.6 g/kg/meal of protein, equally distributed over three main meals, with a minimum of 5–6 g of leucine, is necessary to improve aging muscle. Therefore, the risk of sarcopenia can be alleviated by appropriate nutrition measures in the elderly. (**a**) A total of 1.6 to 1.8 g of protein per kilogram of body weight per day, with emphasis on dietary or supplemental sources of high-biological-value protein. (**b**) Three protein-rich meals per day with 0.6 g of protein per kg or at least 5–6 g of leucine. (**c**) A daily energy balance that is positive or neutral. (**d**) Keeping intestinal diversity active. (**e**) Higher concentration of anti-inflammatory markers (muscular IL-6, IL-10, and TGF-β) with a reduced or controlled pro-inflammatory state compared to pro-inflammatory cytokines (adipocyte IL-6, IL-8, and TNFα). (**f**) Reduced sedentary behavior. (**g**) At least twice a week, perform resistance training.

**Abbreviations:** IL; interleukin, TNF; tumor necrosis factor, TGF; transforming growth factor

developing sarcopenia. Increased consumption of dairy products, in particular, enhances muscles and slows down the loss of muscle mass. It also has no negative effects on kidney function or the development of metabolic or chronic disorders. Yang et al. suggest that adding dairy products to a usual diet may be a promising dietary improvement strategy. Ultimately, such a food strategy can prevent muscle reduction in the elderly population (**Figure 1.12**) (Yang et al., 2019).

### 1.6.2 Improving Heart Health and Blood Pressure

The high-biological-value protein found in milk and dairy products is particularly rich in essential and branched-chain amino acids. Dairy products that are low in fat and contain calcium and magnesium are thought to help reduce high blood pressure. According to the available data, consuming 200–300 ml of milk and dairy products per day does not raise the risk of cardiovascular disease. In particular, the risk of hypertension and stroke are inversely related. A meta-analysis by Soedamah-Muthu et al. found no consistent link between milk or dairy consumption and stroke, coronary heart disease, or cardiovascular disease (Soedamah-Muthu et al., 2011). Protein metabolites, such as small peptides (small peptides derived from milk protein, primarily casein and whey protein), have been shown to have bioactive properties (Ricci et al., 2010; Savica et al., 2010; Jauhiainen &

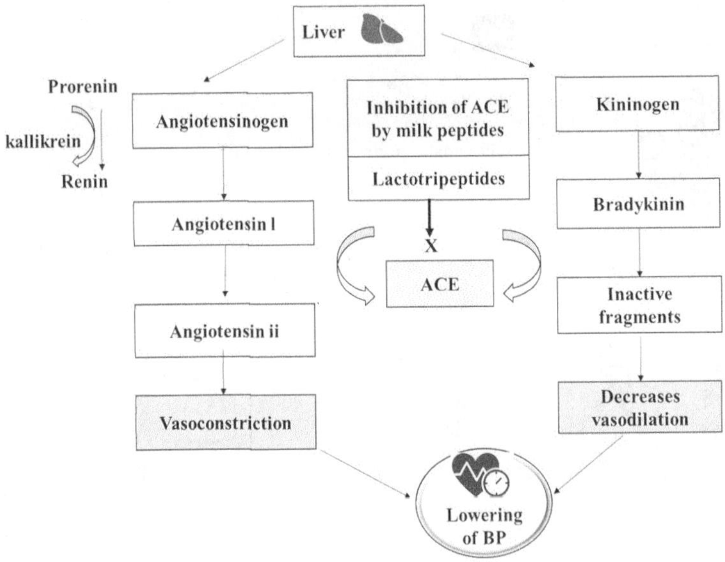


**FIGURE 1.13 Effects of dairy food consumption on cardiovascular health and blood pressure.** Angiotensin II is created by ACE by removing the C-terminal dipeptide from the decapeptide angiotensin I. Angiotensin II is a vasoconstrictor that also increases the secretion of aldosterone, which causes the kidneys to retain salt and water as well as increase blood volume. Further raising blood pressure, ACE also deactivates the vasodilator bradykinin by cleaving the C-terminal dipeptide and releasing inactive fragments. The competitive binding of lactotripeptides to the ACE active site results in ACE activity inhibition (Ricci et al., 2010; Savica et al., 2010).

Korpela, 2007). The primary substrate for the creation of bioactive peptides is casein, which enhances calcium and phosphate absorption in the small intestine. Small dairy peptides are either the result of lactobacilli fermenting milk or human small intestine digestion of milk protein, with the peptides absorbed intact. Some of these bioactive molecules are referred to as lactotripeptides. These lactotripeptides are thought to decrease blood pressure through the following mechanism because they block angiotensin-converting enzyme (ACE) in vitro (**Figure 1.13**) (Ricci et al., 2010; Savica et al., 2010).

### 1.6.3 Improving Obesity

Obesity is a growing health problem in developed countries and is arousing concern in developing countries (Tada et al., 2020). It is estimated that today's predominance of obesity will affect 573 million people worldwide in 2030 (Kelly et al., 2008). In the global population overall, about 13% of adults (11% of males and 15% of females) suffer from obesity (Kober et al., 2024). In this sense, bioactive milk peptides, some probiotic strains, and fermented dairy foods that have shown anti-obesity effects may be used as potential strategies.

New evidence indicates that probiotics may restore gut microbiota dysbiosis that is associated with obesity. Thus, the evaluation of gut microbiota in animal and clinical studies administered with fermented dairy products with anti-obesity effects may be of utmost importance. Also, the potential anti-obesity effects of metabolites produced by probiotics in fermented dairy foods, such as dairy bioactive peptides and exopolysaccharides, postbiotics, and their effect on microbiota need to be addressed by in vivo studies (Manzanarez-Quín et al., 2021). Lactoferrin is a multifunctional protein found in milk. Ono et al. reported the anti-obesity effects of lactoferrin (Ono et al., 2010, 2018) (**Figure 1.14**). Overall, most research linked the probiotic strains present to the anti-obesity

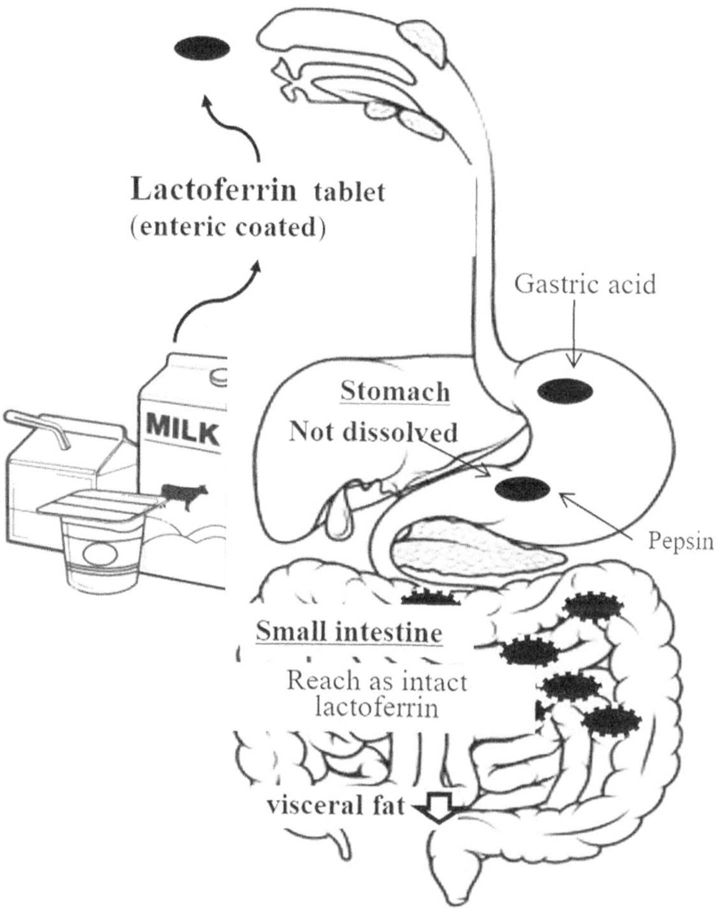


**FIGURE 1.14 Effects of dairy food consumption on the prevention of obesity.** Enteric-coated lactoferrin has a powerful anti-obesity effect: a reduction in visceral fat accumulation in Japanese men and women with abdominal obesity was observed following an 8-week course of enteric-coated lactoferrin tablets.

effects of fermented dairy diets; however, this effect could also be brought on by bioactive peptides that are generated during milk fermentation.

Lactic acid bacteria (LAB) promote anti-obesity effects by suppressing the differentiation of pre-adipocytes through immune cell activation and the production of Th1 cytokines as well as changing the composition of intestinal microbiota and modulating energy metabolism (**Figure 1.15**) (Manzanarez-Quín et al., 2021).

### 1.6.4 Improving Diabetes

Around 40% of people (about 537 million) are living with diabetes globally. Alihosseini et al. reported that compared to those who received conventional fermented milk, diabetic individuals who drank probiotic fermented milk (kefir) had reduced fasting blood glucose and HbA1C levels (Alihosseini et al., 2017). In another study, fermented milk containing the *Lactobacillus casei* strain AP was as effective as the conventional diabetes medication metformin when given orally to 8-week-old diabetic male rats (Alihosseini et al., 2017). Another study found that consuming

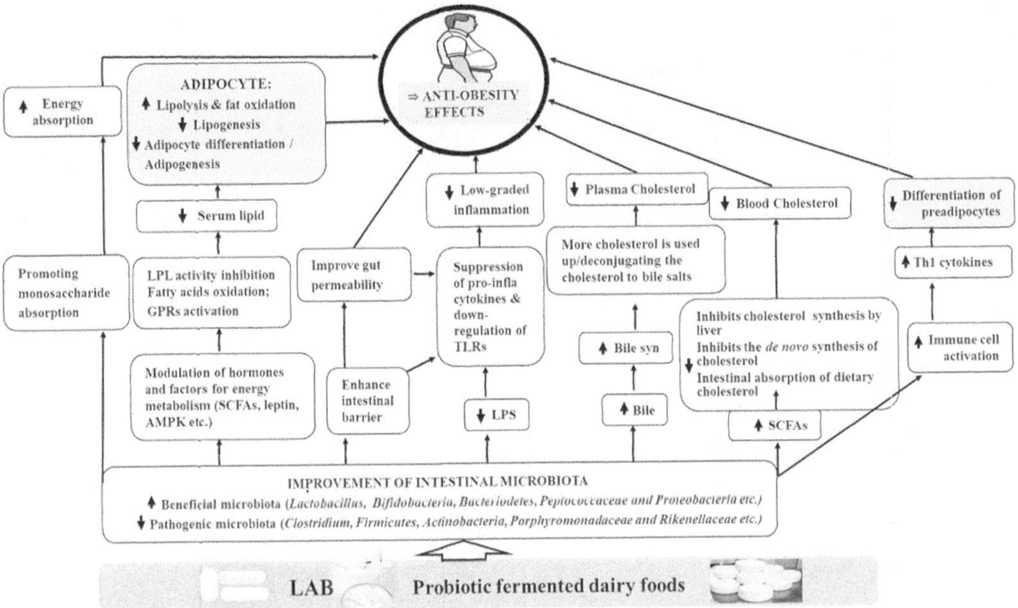


**FIGURE 1.15 Effects of probiotic fermented dairy food consumption on obesity.** Oral administration of probiotics promotes anti-obesity effects by changing the composition of intestinal microbiota; modulating energy metabolism; altering intestinal barrier function, bile salts, and LPS; and suppressing the differentiation of pre-adipocytes through immune cell activation and production of Th1 cytokines. Also, probiotics containing LAB may reduce the release of LPS from intestinal epithelial cells and downregulate the expression of pro-inflammatory cytokines, chemokines, and TLRs in adipose tissues. Decreases in the translocation of bacteria may occur as a result of the ability of probiotics to tighten the mucosal barrier. Probiotics disallow colonization by disease-provoking bacteria through competition for nutrients, immune system upregulation, production of antitoxins, and upregulation of intestinal mucin genes.

**Abbreviations:** ↑, increased; ↓, decreased; TG, triacylglycerol. SCF, short-chain fatty acids; LPS, lipopolysaccharide; TLRs, toll-like receptors; AMPK, AMP-activated protein kinase; LPL, lipoprotein lipase; Syn, synthesis; Th1, Type 1 T helper; LAB, lactic acid bacteria.

probiotic fermented milk with *L. rhamnosus* (MTCC 5897), *L. fermentum* (MTCC 5898), and *L. rhamnosus* (MTCC 5957) had antidiabetic effects both separately and collectively by controlling glucose metabolism, inflammation status, and serum lipid profile in diabetic rats in comparison to the control group (Widodo et al., 2019).

### 1.6.5 Improving Nutrition in Older Adults

Healthy practices, such as wellness and proper diet, are the foundation of healthy aging. As humans get older, it's critical to safeguard against diseases like osteoporosis and sarcopenia that are linked to changes in bone and muscle mass. Dairy products that are nutrient rich offer high-quality protein to assist in maintaining muscle mass as well as nutrients crucial for bone growth during the postmenopausal bone remodeling process. Elderly people are looking for ways to balance the demands of life while retaining energy and preventing chronic diseases, whether they are working, retiring gradually, caring for elderly parents, helping friends, or keeping up with the kids and grandkids. Healthy nutrition and regular strength training are crucial and don't have to be difficult. For instance, adopting healthy dietary habits that include three servings of dairy each day, plenty of fruits and vegetables, lean protein sources, and healthy fats like nuts and olive oil might help elderly people succeed. The daily dairy guidelines given by the World Health Organization, Canadian, and American Dietary

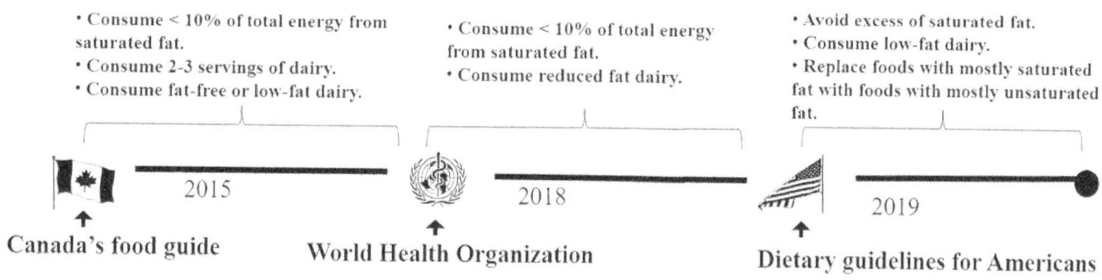


**FIGURE 1.16 Dietary recommendations of dairy fat intake from the United States, Canada, and the World Health Organization.** The risk of sarcopenia rises with aging. Malnutrition in the older population is a significant risk factor for sarcopenia. Calcium (Ca), phosphate (P), vitamin D, and protein are essential nutrients for the human body that impact muscle mass and quality. Dairy products are high in several nutrients, suggesting that they may be beneficial to the elderly. Low-fat dairy, when consumed in three servings per day, can help meet several of the specific dietary demands for healthy aging.

Guidelines are not met by older persons (**Figure 1.16**). Increasing dairy to three servings per day can assist in meeting several of the specific nutritional requirements for healthy aging.

### 1.6.6 Improving Cancer

Approximately 6% of people (about 18.1 million) living with cancer globally. Dairy foods contain a variety of bioactive compounds that could exert both protective and occasionally harmful effects. Breast cancer, bladder cancer, stomach cancer, and colorectal cancer may all be prevented by consuming milk and dairy products. There is no evidence suggesting that drinking milk raises the likelihood of acquiring pancreatic cancer, ovarian cancer, or lung cancer. However, there isn't a clear agreement among experts about whether milk affects the risk of prostate cancer (Thorning et al., 2016). Dairy consumption among women lowers the risk of both serious and common colorectal cancer and may also lower the risk of breast cancer. It is determined that the preventive impact of milk and dairy products on both serious and common colorectal cancers beats any potential increase

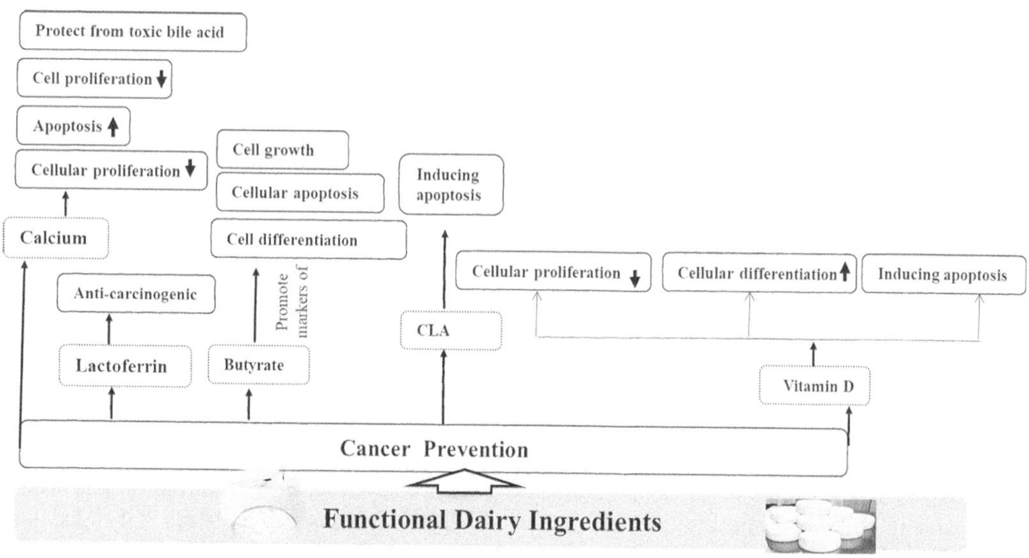


**FIGURE 1.17 Effects of dairy food consumption on preventing cancer.** The Cancer Council and the USDA suggest three servings of milk and milk products each day. Consumption of more than a glass of milk (250 ml) per day was associated with a 15% lower risk of getting colorectal cancer. Dairy foods (either indigenous or exogenous components) have been shown to reduce the risk of many cancers.

in prostate cancer risk in men (Thorning et al., 2016). Three servings of milk and milk products per day are advised by the Cancer Council and the United States Department of Agriculture (USDA). Davoodi et al. reported the capacity of milk and milk products (their natural or exogenous constituents) to reduce various cancer risks (**Figure 1.17**) (Davoodi et al., 2013).

### 1.6.7 Improving Bone and Oral Health

Milk and dairy food not only provide highly bioavailable calcium, but are also good suppliers of vitamins and proteins. Protein, calcium, and vitamins (**Figure 1.18**) included in milk and dairy products may be good for bone health (Tunick & Van Hekken, 2015). Drinking milk at a young age helps protect against osteoporosis later in life.

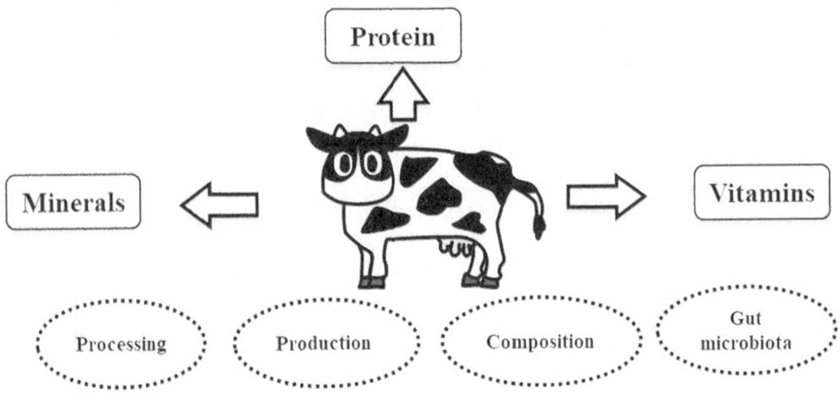


**FIGURE 1.18 Effects of dairy food consumption on bone health.** Calcium and protein, among other nutrients, are critical for bone health. Dairy products supply these nutrients. The latter help to fulfill nutritional requirements. Dairy products have been proven in intervention trials to improve bone mass accretion in children and adolescents, as well as bone turnover in young and older people. The consumption of dairy products, particularly fermented ones that include probiotics in addition to calcium, phosphorus, and protein, appears to be connected with a decreased risk of hip fracture.

### 1.6.8 Enhancing Healthy Growth Strategies

Almost all milk constituents, including proteins, peptides, lipids, carbohydrates, minerals, and vitamins, may offer potential health advantages. Although the number of calories in milk varies depending on the amount of fat, it is an energy source. The majority of studies have been on calcium and insulin-like growth factor-1 (IGF-1), two nutrients in milk that are particularly crucial for bone formation, even though many of the minerals in milk are believed to contribute in specific ways to the overall growth process (Wiley, 2011). IGF-1 increases the intake of amino acids in the skeleton, which leads to the synthesis of new proteins and the lengthening of bones (Wiley, 2011). Adding milk to a child's diet can help them grow and get the important nutrients they need if their diet is lacking nutrition (Hoppe et al., 2006). In healthy youngsters, milk's effect on linear development is probably due to its stimulation of IGF-1 rather than its ability to make up for dietary shortages (Hoppe et al., 2006). Growth hormones and diet both influence IGF-1 synthesis, but nutritional control over IGF-1 is probably more significant during infancy when IGF-1 concentrations are low than later in childhood and maturity (Hoppe et al., 2006). Increased circulating IGF-1 has been linked to milk intervention trials in kids (Cadogan et al., 1997). Although IGF-1 is present in cow milk, it is not absorbed when taken orally (Larsson et al., 2005). IGFs are thought to be stimulated by bioactive peptides, milk IGF-1, amino acids (particularly the branched-chain amino acids leucine, isoleucine, and valine), or milk minerals (particularly calcium and zinc) (Hoppe et al., 2006).

IGF-1 levels may be associated (both positively and negatively) with mortality and risk of numerous noncommunicable diseases (NCDs), including cancer; therefore, understanding the intricate interactions between IGF and milk is of importance (Hoppe et al., 2006; van der Pols et al., 2009). A longitudinal study of the Boyd Orr cohort examined the potential "programming effects" of calcium and dairy consumption throughout childhood on adult cardiovascular diseases (CVDs) mortality (van der Pols et al., 2009). A total of 88% of the original children were found through the study. Although childhood calcium consumption was negatively associated with stroke mortality, the investigators could not find compelling evidence linking a diet high in dairy products to coronary heart disease (CHD) or stroke mortality. Regardless of how tall a child is, eating a diet high in dairy or calcium was linked to a lower risk of dying from any cause as an adult. This means that the way the body produces and uses a hormone called IGF (Insulin-like growth factor) did not play a role in this relationship. It concludes that childhood meals may have programmed adult IGF-1 levels in ways that are not necessarily represented by childhood height.

### 1.6.9 Improving Immune Health Status

#### 1.6.9.1 Immunomodulation of Cytokines and Immunoglobulin by Probiotic Fermented Dairy Foods

Yogurt consumption slowed tumor growth in a mouse colon cancer model by enhancing IL-10-secreting cells, decreasing procarcinogen enzyme levels, and reducing inflammation (Raheem et al., 2021).

#### 1.6.9.2 Immunomodulation of Toll-Like Receptors (TLRs) by Probiotic Fermented Dairy Foods

The TLR-2/TLR-6 signaling pathways can be activated by probiotic dairy foods, and 16 different LAB strains with food and human-derived origins were described and examined for their interactions with various TLRs (Karaffová et al., 2021). In the presence of *E. coli*, the probiotic *L. fermentum* (MTCC-5898) suppresses immune function by reducing the production of pro-inflammatory cytokines and increasing the expression of anti-inflammatory cytokines via the TLR-2/TLR-4 and NF-B signaling pathways (Hoarau et al., 2006).

#### 1.6.9.3 Immunomodulation of Dendritic Cells (DCs) by Probiotic Fermented Dairy Foods

Numerous studies have shown that probiotics that are fermented have a good effect on the cells that make up the lining of the intestine—intestinal epithelial cells (IEC) (Miller et al., 2019; Kaur et al., 2019). IECs are crucial for promoting tolerance because they prevent DC activation, which in turn regulates the suppressive activity of T regulatory cells (Tregs). IECs have also been designated to stimulate the development of CD103+ DCs. This Forkhead box P3 (FOXP3)$^+$ Treg cell-inducing population of tolerogenic DCs is reliant on TGF-β (**Figure 1.19**) (Miller et al., 2019; Kaur et al., 2019).

#### 1.6.9.4 Immunomodulation of Natural Killer Cells by Probiotic Fermented Dairy Foods

Natural killer cells (NKs) play an important role in the immune response and regulation of homeostasis. With altered or missing histocompatibility complex class I molecules, they can discriminate between normal and diseased cells. According to Kaur et al., certain LAB may efficiently trigger NK contacts, enhancing the cytolytic capability of NK cells in mucosal immunity. NK cell function in healthy older people is improved by probiotic *Lactobacillus* interventions, alone or in combination with *Bifidobacterium*, according to a recent study (Gui et al., 2020; Kaur et al., 2019; Frank & Paust, 2020)

#### 1.6.9.5 Immunomodulation of Neutrophils by Probiotic Fermented Dairy Foods

By inhibiting neutrophil-associated immunological responses, Li et al. recently showed that oral treatment with the microbial metabolite butyrate significantly reduced mucosal inflammation in

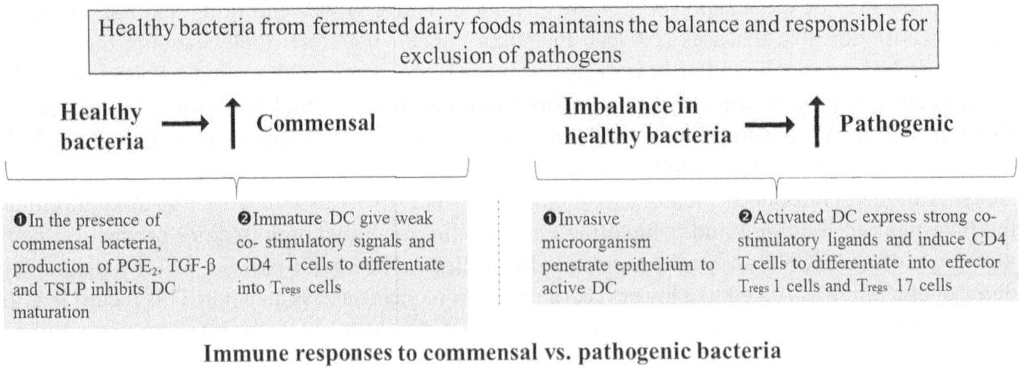


**FIGURE 1.19 Effects of dairy food consumption on immune health status.** Dairy products containing probiotic bacteria offer more help to boost the immune system and support the body to fight illnesses. Healthy probiotic bacteria from fermented dairy foods prevent illnesses and maintain the immune system's balance.

**Abbreviations:** $T_{regs}$, T regulatory cells; PGE2, prostaglandin E2; TSLP, thymic stromal lymphopoietin

dextran sulfate sodium (DSS)-induced mouse colitis (Li et al., 2021). Butyrate inhibited neutrophil migration and neutrophil extracellular trap (NET) formation in sample from patients with Crohn's disease (CD) and ulcerative colitis (UC), according to in vitro investigations. It has been demonstrated that the *L. rhamnosus* GG and *B. animalis* MB5 strains restrict neutrophil transmigration by blocking enterotoxigenic *E. coli* K88 activation of the nuclear factor kappa B (NF-κB)-dependent inflammatory mediators TNF, IL-1, IL-8, and so on (Aprea et al., 2023).

#### 1.6.9.6 Immunomodulation by Biologically Active Dairy Peptides/Components

Immunomodulatory bioactive peptides are defined as those that mediate the humoral and cell-mediated immune systems of the body. These include glycopeptides, hormones, and peptide fragments produced from immunoglobulins (Igs). Components of dairy that may exhibit immunomodulation are whey protein concentrate, lactoferrin, lactoperoxidase, kappa casein glycomacropeptide, CLA, and colostrum. Numerous bovine β-casein peptides were later found to cause phagocytic reactions in people and prevent the transfer of *K. pneumoniae* to mice when used in vivo. Casein and whey peptides may have been produced for immunomodulatory peptides, according to cytochemical investigations. Human lymphocyte synthesis, antibody production, macrophage phagocytic participation, and cytokine modulation are all correlated with protein activation and proliferation (Clare et al., 2003; Gill et al., 2000). Through the activation and stimulation of capable immune system cells, casein-derived peptides can prevent the proliferation of cancer cells (Meisel & FitzGerald, 2003). Glycomacropeptides' immuno-suppressive effects on the production of IgG antibodies and their derivatives have been proven to be crucial immunological co-modulatory actions (Meisel & FitzGerald, 2003). Lactoferricin B, which interacts with neutrophils and behaves like opsonin, is released after lactoferrin digestion. Other bovine peptides, such as β-casein f (residues 63–680), (Monnai et al., 1998) and β-casein f (residues 191–193), may have an impact on human in vitro phagocytic medicines used in immunotherapy for human immunodeficiency disorder, which may entail viral infections involving j-casein and α-lactalbumin peptides. The casino-macro peptide (CMP) promotes the growth of bifidobacteria and/or lactobacilli that suppress enteroinfection.

#### 1.6.9.7 Reinforcement of Gut Barrier Function by Probiotic Fermented Dairy Foods

Consuming probiotic bacteria through fermented milk is another fantastic method for balancing the flora in the gut and maintaining the function of the epithelial barrier (Kaur & Ali, 2022; Marco et al., 2017). Probiotics and released metabolites enhance barrier function by promoting the

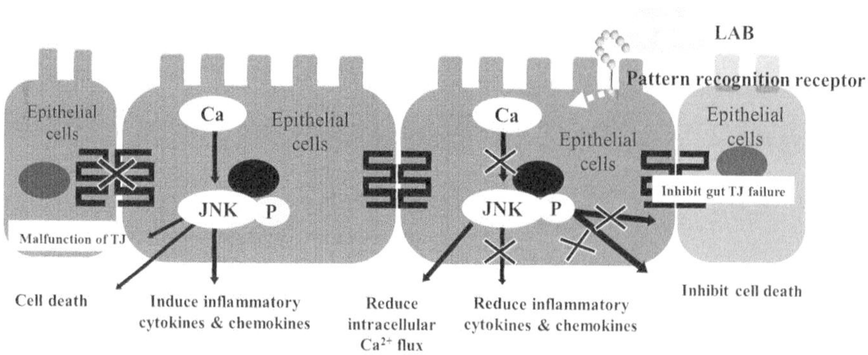


**FIGURE 1.20** **Reinforcement of gut barrier function by probiotic fermented dairy foods.** LAB are able to remarkably reduce the phosphorylation of JNK and intracellular $Ca^{2+}$ flux, decrease the expression of inflammatory cytokines and chemokines, increase TER, inhibit gut TJ failure, and inhibit cell death (Hemarajata & Versalovic, 2013).

**Abbreviations**: LAB, lactic acid bacteria; TJ, tight junction; TER, transepithelial electrical resistance; JNK, c-jun N-terminal kinase.

generation and assembly of tight junction proteins. They also protect against inflammatory stimuli's ability to damage tight junctions. They also stimulate several cell signaling pathways, strengthening tight junctions and promoting the barrier function (**Figure 1.20**) (Hemarajata & Versalovic, 2013).

### 1.6.10 Improving Antioxidant Status

The presence of antioxidant components (i.e., proteins), which are rich sources of sulfur amino acids; vitamins A, E, and C; and carotene, is primarily responsible for milk and dairy products' antioxidant potential. Additionally, cheese biopeptides produced during the fermentation process have antioxidant properties. Dairy products' antioxidant potential depends on the type of heat treatment, bacterial starter cultures, and natural plant additions employed during processing, in addition to the caliber of the raw material. The highest antioxidant status is found in fermented foods, particularly when they are utilized as probiotic starter cultures. Probiotics create bioactive peptides that act as powerful antioxidants and may lessen the consequences of free radical damage. By lowering malondialdehyde (MDA) and lipofuscin levels and monoamine oxidase activity in older animals, probiotics increased antioxidant enzymatic effectiveness and decreased lipid oxidation (Liu et al., 2017). According to Wang et al., *Bacillus amyloliquefaciens* SC06 reduces reactive oxygen species (ROS) and controls the nuclear factor erythroid 2–related factor 2 (Nrf-2) and Kelch-like ECH-associated protein 1 (Keap-1) pathways in intestinal porcine epithelial cells (Wang et al., 2017). Garcia-Gonzalez et al. isolated *L. plantarum* DM5 from fermented drinks and demonstrated its anti-oxidative action by reducing hydroxyl radical levels to prevent ascorbate auto-oxidation and the production of amino butyric acid (Garcia-Gonzalez et al., 2021). According to Wang et al., eating fermented goat milk for 21 days increased antiatherogenicity in healthy humans; decreased levels of oxidized LDL, oxidized lipoproteins, and 8-isoprostanes; and increased glutathione redox ratio (**Figure 1.21**) (Wang et al., 2017; Kaur et al., 2022).

### 1.6.11 Enhancing Sleep Quality

Dairy foods, particularly milk, are frequently referred to as "sleep-promoting" foods. For years, people have been told to drink a glass of warm milk before bed, and research has been conducted to uncover the science underlying the long-standing link between dairy and sleep. People

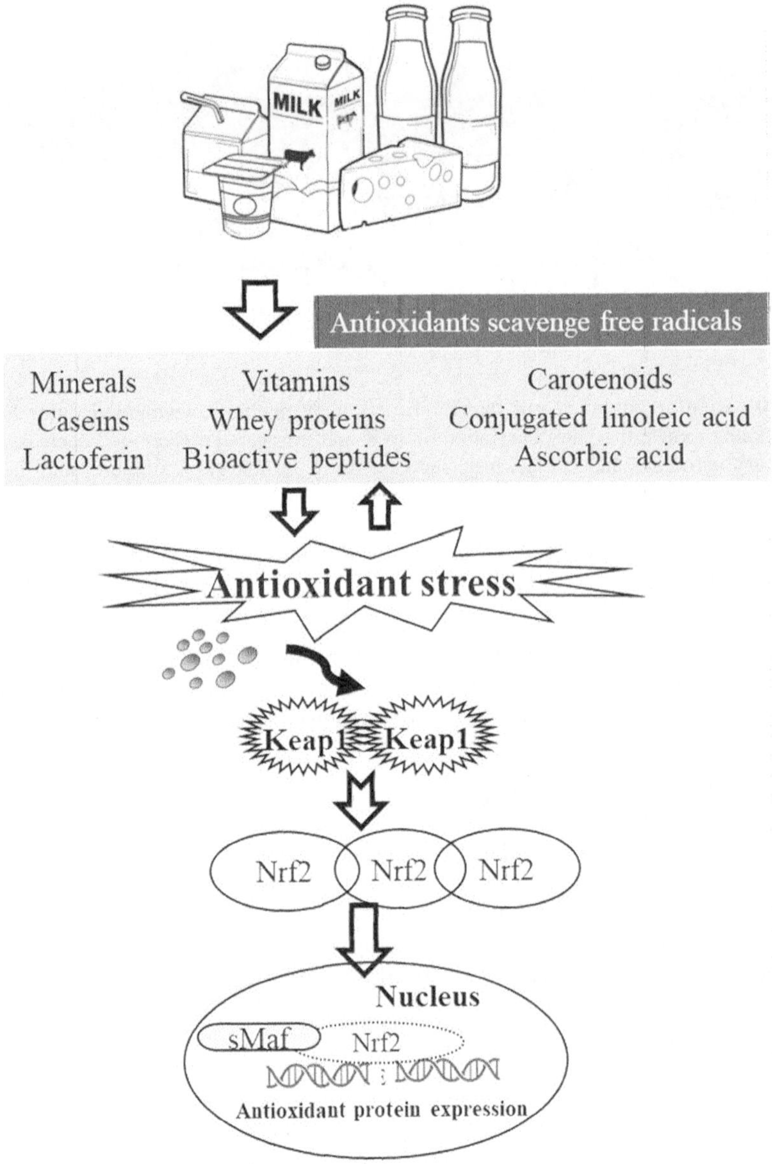


**FIGURE 1.21 Antioxidant properties of milk and dairy foods.** The diagram illustrates the elements required to neutralize free radicals and deliver antioxidants found in fermented dairy products. Free radicals are neutralized by these antioxidants in a variety of ways. Important cellular stress and anti-oxidative stress signaling pathways are conceptually represented in diagrams.

**Abbreviations:** Nrf-2, nuclear factor erythroid 2–related factor 2; Keap-1, Kelch-like ECH-associated protein 1

who consume adequate amounts of milk and dairy products meet the recommended daily calcium intake requirements and tend to have high health literacy and better sleep habits. Milk and dairy product intake in the diet may be an indicator of sleep quality (Komada et al., 2020). Dairy foods contain a greater tryptophan level, and fermented dairy contains gamma-aminobutyric acid (GABA) and numerous chemicals that may interact with the microbiome (brain–gut–microbiome axis) (Komada et al., 2020) (**Figure 1.22**). Alpha-lactalbumin, a protein found in milk, includes

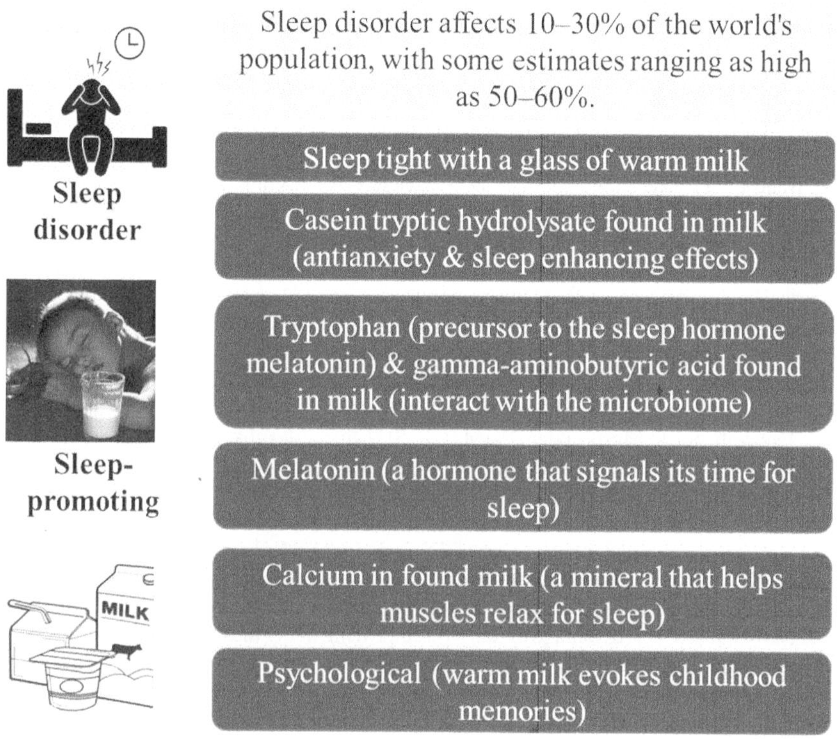


**FIGURE 1.22 Sleep-promoting properties of milk and dairy foods.** Milk and dairy products are widely thought to improve sleep quality and have a favorable impact on physical and mental health.

large quantities of tryptophan, an amino acid and precursor to the sleep hormone melatonin (Layman et al., 2018). According to research, taking alpha-lactalbumin before bed may assist in enhancing sleep quality (Ong et al., 2017; Layman et al., 2018). The consumption of milk and dairy products in the diet may be an indicator of sleep quality. However, more research is needed to understand this association.

## 1.7 CONCLUSIONS

Humans have traditionally consumed milk and dairy foods. Dairy foods are among the most varied food groups because they come in both liquid and powder form, as well as everything in between. Some dairy products, like probiotic yogurt, not only provide consumers with necessary nutrients but also possibly useful ingredients. New research suggests that dairy products may have an impact on human health. The function of specific dairy ingredients, such as fat, protein, and other bioactive ingredients, is becoming more and more interesting. Despite being a source of saturated fat, dairy fat may have a neutral or positive impact on gastrointestinal and cardiometabolic health. Dairy proteins, especially those consumed after exercise, may help preserve muscle mass in the elderly by delaying the onset of sarcopenia. While there is still much to learn about each dairy component, there may also be advantages to the total dairy food matrix. For instance, the fermentation process used in the manufacture of cheese and yogurt may improve the nutritive and functional qualities of these foods. As new processing innovations emerge and are commercialized, more dairy foods (novel dairy-based functional foods) need to be develop for the consumer markets.

## REFERENCES


Alihosseini, N., Moahboob, S. A., Farrin, N., Mobasseri, M., Taghizadeh, A., & Ostadrahimi, A. R. (2017). Effect of probiotic fermented milk (kefir) on serum level of insulin and homocysteine in type 2 diabetes patients. *Acta Endocrinologica* (Buchar), *13*(4), 431–436.

Aprea, G., Del Matto, I., Tucci, P., Marino, L., Scattolini, S., & Rossi, F. (2023). In vivo functional properties of dairy bacteria. *Microorganisms*, *11*(7), 1787.

Bordoni, A., Danesi, F., Dardevet, D., Dupont, D., Fernandez, A. S., Gille, D., Nunes Dos Santos, C., Pinto, P., Re, R., Rémond, D., Shahar, D. R., & Vergères, G. (2017). Dairy products and inflammation: A review of the clinical evidence. *Critical Reviews in Food Science and Nutrition*, *57*(12), 2497–2525.

Cadogan, J., Eastell, R., Jones, N., & Barker, M. E. (1997). Milk intake and bone mineral acquisition in adolescent girls: Randomised, controlled intervention trial. *British Medical Journal*, *315*, 1255–1260.

Clare, D. A., Catignani, G. L., & Swaisgood, H. E. (2003). Biodefense properties of milk: The role of antimicrobial proteins and peptides. *Current Pharmaceutical Design*, *9*, 1239–1255.

Clare, D. A., & Swaisgood, H. E. (2000). Bioactive milk peptides: A prospectus. *Journal of Dairy Science*, *83*(6), 1187–1195.

Davoodi, H., Esmaeili, S., & Mortazavian, A. M. (2013). Effects of milk and milk products consumption on cancer: A review. *Comprehensive Reviews in Food Science and Food Safety*, *12*(3), 249–264.

Debnath, G. K., Kober, A. K. M. H., Chanda, T., Chanda, G. C., & Bari, M. S. (2014). Comparative study on the quality of available brand and nonbrand fluid milk consumed by the people of Chittagong City of Bangladesh. *International Journal of Natural Science*, *4*(1), 16–20.

Drewnowski, A. (2011). The contribution of milk and milk products to micronutrient density and affordability of the US diet. *Journal of the American College of Nutrition*, *30*(Suppl. 5), 422S–428S.

Du, Y., Oh, C., & No, J. (2019). Advantage of dairy for improving aging muscle. *Journal of Obesity & Metabolic Syndrome*, *28*(3), 167–174.

Fernández-Rico, S., Mondragón, A. D. C., López-Santamarina, A., Cardelle-Cobas, A., Regal, P., Lamas, A., Ibarra, I. S., Cepeda, A., & Miranda, J. M. (2022). A2 milk: New perspectives for food technology and human health. *Foods (Basel, Switzerland)*, *11*(16), 2387.

Food and Agriculture Organization of the United Nations (FAO). (2020). *Food outlook. Biannual report on global food markets* (p. 8). Food and Agriculture Organization of the United Nations.

Frank, K., & Paust, S. (2020). Dynamic natural killer cell and T cell responses to influenza infection. *Frontiers in Cellular and Infection Microbiology*, *10*, 425.

Fuquay, J. W., McSweeney, P. L., & Fox, P. F. (2011). *Encyclopedia of dairy sciences*. Academic Press.

Garcia-Gonzalez, N., Battista, N., Prete, R., & Corsetti, A. (2021). Health-promoting role of Lactiplantibacillus plantarum isolated from fermented foods. *Microorganisms*, *9*(2), 349.

Gill, H. S., Doull, F., Rutherfurd, K. J., & Cross, M. L. (2000). Immunoregulatory peptides in bovine milk. *The British Journal of Nutrition*, *84*(Suppl. 1), S111–S117.

Gui, Q., Wang, A., Zhao, X., Huang, S., Tan, Z., Xiao, C., & Yang, Y. (2020). Effects of probiotic supplementation on natural killer cell function in healthy elderly individuals: A meta-analysis of randomized controlled trials. *European Journal of Clinical Nutrition*, *74*(12), 1630–1637.

Hemarajata, P., & Versalovic, J. (2013). Effects of probiotics on gut microbiota: Mechanisms of intestinal immunomodulation and neuromodulation. *Therapeutic Advances in Gastroenterology*, *6*(1), 39–51.

Hess, J. M., Stephensen, C. B., Kratz, M., & Bolling, B. W. (2021). Exploring the links between diet and inflammation: Dairy foods as case studies. *Advances in Nutrition (Bethesda, Md.)*, *12*(Suppl. 1), 1S–13S.

Hoarau, C., Lagaraine, C., Martin, L., Velge-Roussel, F., & Lebranchu, Y. (2006). Supernatant of Bifidobacterium breve induces dendritic cell maturation, activation, and survival through a Toll-like receptor 2 pathway. *The Journal of Allergy and Clinical Immunology*, *117*(3), 696–702.

Hoppe, C., Mølgaard, C., & Michaelsen, K. F. (2006). Cow's milk and linear growth in industrialized and developing countries. *Annual Review of Nutrition*, *26*, 131–173.

International Dairy Federation (IDF) (2015). The world dairy situation 2015. *Bulletin of the international dairy federation*. www.fil-idf.org/.

International Dairy Federation (IDF) (2020). *The global impact of dairy*. https://fil-idf.org/dairys-global-impact/.

Islam, M. N., Kober, A. K. M. H., & Amin, M. R. (2002). Quality of milk consumed by residential people of Bangladesh Agricultural University campus, Mymensingh. *The Bangladesh Veterinarian*, *19*, 29–33.

Jauhiainen, T., & Korpela, R. (2007). Milk peptides and blood pressure. *The Journal of Nutrition*, *137*(3 Suppl. 2), 825S–829S.

Karaffová, V., Mudroňová, D., Mad'ar, M., Hrčková, G., Faixová, D., Gancarčíková, S., Ševčíková, Z., & Nemcová, R. (2021). Differences in immune response and biochemical parameters of mice fed by kefir milk and *Lacticaseibacillus paracasei* Isolated from the Kefir Grains. *Microorganisms*, *9*(4), 831.

Kaur, H., & Ali, S. A. (2022). Probiotics and gut microbiota: Mechanistic insights into gut immune homeostasis through TLR pathway regulation. *Food & Function*, *13*(14), 7423–7447.

Kaur, H., Kaur, G., & Ali, S. A. (2022). Dairy-based probiotic-fermented functional foods: An update on their health-promoting properties. *Fermentation*, *8*(9), 425.

Kaur, K., Kozlowska, A. K., Topchyan, P., Ko, M. W., Ohanian, N., Chiang, J., Cook, J., Maung, P. O., Park, S. H., Cacalano, N., Fang, C., & Jewett, A. (2019). Probiotic-treated super-charged NK cells efficiently clear poorly differentiated pancreatic tumors in hu-blt mice. *Cancers*, *12*(1), 63.

Kelly, T., Yang, W., Chen, C. S., Reynolds, K., & He, J. (2008). Global burden of obesity in 2005 and projections to 2030. *International Journal of Obesity*, *32*(9), 1431–1437.

Kober, A. K. M. H., Bari, M. S., Morshed, S., & Momin, M. M. (2015). Evaluation of nutritional quality, contamination, adulteration and preservative quality of different sources of milk. *Bangladesh Journal of Veterinary and Animal Sciences*, *3*(1), 25–29.

Kober, A. K. M. H., Saha, S., Mutamed, A., Namai, F., Nishiyama, K., Yoda, K., Villena, J., Kitazawa, H. (2024). Insights into the anti-adipogenic and anti-inflammatory potentialities of probiotics: A perspective on addressing the risk of obesity and overweight in humans. *Nutrients* (Under review).

Kober, A. K. M. H., Villena, J., Kitazawa, H., & Saha, S. (2022). Immunomodulatory effects of probiotics: A novel preventive approach for the control of bovine mastitis. *Microorganisms*, *10*(11), 1–17, Article number 2255.

Komada, Y., Okajima, I., & Kuwata, T. (2020). The effects of milk and dairy products on sleep: A systematic review. *International Journal of Environmental Research and Public Health*, *17*(24), 9440.

Larsson, S. C., Bergkvist, L., & Wolk, A. (2005). High-fat dairy food and conjugated linoleic acid intakes in relation to colorectal cancer incidence in the Swedish Mammography Cohort. *The American Journal of Clinical Nutrition*, *82*, 894–900.

Layman, D. K., Lönnerdal, B., & Fernstrom, J. D. (2018). Applications for α-lactalbumin in human nutrition. *Nutrition Reviews*, *76*(6), 444–460.

Li, G., Lin, J., Zhang, C., Gao, H., Lu, H., Gao, X., Zhu, R., Li, Z., Li, M., & Liu, Z. (2021). Microbiota metabolite butyrate constrains neutrophil functions and ameliorates mucosal inflammation in inflammatory bowel disease. *Gut Microbes*, *13*(1), 1968257.

Liu, M. Y., Yang, Z. Y., Dai, W. K., Huang, J. Q., Li, Y. H., Zhang, J., Qiu, C. Z., Wei, C., Zhou, Q., Sun, X., Feng, X., Li, D. F., Wang, H. P., & Zheng, Y. J. (2017). Protective effect of *Bifidobacterium infantis* CGMCC313-2 on ovalbumin-induced airway asthma and β-lactoglobulin-induced intestinal food allergy mouse models. *World Journal of Gastroenterology*, *23*(12), 2149–2158.

Manzanarez-Quín, C. G., Beltrán-Barrientos, L. M., Hernández-Mendoza, A., González-Córdova, A. F., & Vallejo-Cordoba, B. (2021). Invited review: Potential antiobesity effect of fermented dairy products. *Journal of Dairy Science*, *104*(4), 3766–3778.

Marco, M. L., Heeney, D., Binda, S., Cifelli, C. J., Cotter, P. D., Foligné, B., Gänzle, M., Kort, R., Pasin, G., Pihlanto, A., Smid, E. J., & Hutkins, R. (2017). Health benefits of fermented foods: Microbiota and beyond. *Current Opinion in Biotechnology*, *44*, 94–102.

Meisel, H., & FitzGerald, R. J. (2003). Biofunctional peptides from milk proteins: Mineral binding and cytomodulatory effects. *Current Pharmaceutical Design*, *9*(16), 1289–1295.

Miller, L. E., Lehtoranta, L., & Lehtinen, M. J. (2019). Short-term probiotic supplementation enhances cellular immune function in healthy elderly: Systematic review and meta-analysis of controlled studies. *Nutrition Research*, *64*, 1–8.

Monnai, M., Horimoto, Y., & Otani, H. (1998). Immunomodificatory effect of dietary bovine kappa-caseinoglycopeptide on serum antibody levels and proliferative responses of lymphocytes in mice. *Milchwissenschaft*, *53*, 129–132.

Ong, J. N., Hackett, D. A., & Chow, C. M. (2017). Sleep quality and duration following evening intake of alpha-lactalbumin: A pilot study. *Biological Rhythm Research*, *48*(4), 507–517.

Ono, T., Murakoshi, M., Suzuki, N., Iida, N., Ohdera, M., Iigo, M., Yoshida, T., Sugiyama, K., & Nishino, H. (2010). Potent anti-obesity effect of enteric-coated lactoferrin: Decrease in visceral fat accumulation in Japanese men and women with abdominal obesity after 8-week administration of enteric-coated lactoferrin tablets. *The British Journal of Nutrition*, *104*(11), 1688–1695.

Ono, T., Murakoshi, M., & Uchiyama, A. (2018). Anti-Obesity effect of lactoferrin; subgroup analysis excluding subjects with obese and/or hyper-ldl cholesterolemia. *Immunology, Endocrine & Metabolic Agents in Medicinal Chemistry*, *18*(1), 105–109.

Raheem, A., Liang, L., Zhang, G., & Cui, S. (2021). Modulatory effects of probiotics during pathogenic infections with emphasis on immune regulation. *Frontiers in Immunology*, *12*, 616713.

Rebouillat, S., & Ortega-Requena, S. (2015). Potential applications of milk fractions and valorization of dairy by-products: A review of the state-of-the-art available data, outlining the innovation potential from a bigger data standpoint. *Journal of Biomaterials and Nanobiotechnology*, *6*(03), 176.

Ricci, I., Artacho, R., & Olalla, M. (2010). Milk protein peptides with angiotensin I-converting enzyme inhibitory (ACEI) activity. *Critical Reviews in Food Science and Nutrition*, *50*(5), 390–402.

Savica, V., Bellinghieri, G., & Kopple, J. D. (2010). The effect of nutrition on blood pressure. *Annual Review of Nutrition*, *30*, 365–401.

Soedamah-Muthu, S. S., Ding, E. L., Al-Delaimy, W. K., Hu, F. B., Engberink, M. F., Willett, W. C., & Geleijnse, J. M. (2011). Milk and dairy consumption and incidence of cardiovascular diseases and all-cause mortality: Dose-response meta-analysis of prospective cohort studies. *The American Journal of Clinical Nutrition*, *93*(1), 158–171.

Tada, A., Kober, A. K. M. H., Islam, M. A., Igata, M., Takagi, M., Suzuki, M., Aso, H., Ikeda-Ohtsubo, W., Yoda, K., Miyazawa, K., He, F., Takahashi, H., Villena, J., & Kitazawa, H. (2020). Evaluation of fat accumulation and adipokine production during the long-term adipogenic differentiation of porcine intramuscular preadipocytes and study of the influence of immunobiotics. *Cells*, *9*(7), 1715.

Thorning, T. K., Raben, A., Tholstrup, T., Soedamah-Muthu, S. S., Givens, I., & Astrup, A. (2016). Milk and dairy products: Good or bad for human health? An assessment of the totality of scientific evidence. *Food & Nutrition Research*, *60*, 32527.

Tunick, M. H., & Van Hekken, D. L. (2015). Dairy products and health: Recent insights. *Journal of Agricultural and Food Chemistry*, *63*(43), 9381–9388.

U.S. Department of Agriculture (USDA) and U.S. Department of health and human services. (2020). *Dietary guidelines for Americans, 2020–2025* (9th ed.). Washington, DC: US Government Publishing Office.

Van der Pols, J. C., Gunnell, D., Williams, G. M., Holly, J. M., Bain, C., & Martin, R. M. (2009). Childhood dairy and calcium intake and cardiovascular mortality in adulthood: 65-year follow-up of the Boyd Orr cohort. *Heart (British Cardiac Society)*, *95*(19), 1600–1606.

Wadud, A., Ali, M. K., Kober, A. K. H. M., Islam, M. N., & Debnath, G. K. (2002). Physical, chemical and microbiological qualities of buffaloes milk. *Bangladesh Journal of Animal Science*, *31*, 91–98.

Wang, Y., Wu, Y., Wang, Y., Fu, A., Gong, L., Li, W., & Li, Y. (2017). Bacillus amyloliquefaciens SC06 alleviates the oxidative stress of IPEC-1 via modulating Nrf2/Keap1 signaling pathway and decreasing ROS production. *Applied Microbiology and Biotechnology*, *101*(7), 3015–3026.

Webb, B. H., Johnson, A. H., & Alford, J. A. (1974). *Fundamentals of dairy chemistry* (2nd ed.). AVI Publishing Co., Chap. 1.

Widodo, W., Harsita, P. A., Sukarno, A. S., & Nurrochmad, A. (2019). Antidiabetic effect of milk fermented using intestinal probiotics. *Nutrition & Food Science*, *49*(6), 1063–1074.

Wiley, A. S. (2011). Cow milk consumption, insulin-like growth factor-I, and human biology: A life history approach. *American Journal of Human Biology*, *24*(2), 130–138. https://doi.org/10.1002/ajhb.22201

World Health Organization (WHO). (2015). *World report on ageing and health.* WHO.

Yang, L. J., Wu, G. H., Yang, Y. L., Wu, Y. H., Zhang, L., Wang, M. H., Mo, L. Y., Xue, G., Wang, C. Z., & Weng, X. F. (2019). Nutrition, physical exercise, and the prevalence of sarcopenia in elderly residents in nursing homes in china. *Medical Science Monitor: International Medical Journal of Experimental and Clinical Research*, *25*, 4390–4399.

# 2 Overview of Milk Science and Processing

## 2.1 LEARNING OBJECTIVES

By the end of the chapter, the reader will be able to:

- Understand the recent evolutions of milk science and processing
- Learn about integrating the knowledge of milk chemistry/engineering/microbiology and the physical properties of milk to understand the production of dairy foods
- Gain knowledge of the biochemical processes that convert milk triglycerides and fatty acids into taste and flavor compound

Milk's ingredients and their processing system can affect the quality of the milk by reducing antioxidants and producing compounds that cause oxidation. The processing methods ensure that the milk becomes safe and remains stable. However, the ability of dairy products to fight harmful substances in the body may get better over time because of certain substances that are produced.

## 2.2 DAIRY CHEMISTRY

### 2.2.1 Introduction

Dairy chemistry may be defined as the branch of dairy science that deals with the chemistry of milk and milk products. The knowledge of dairy chemistry in the field of dairy science is very important (**Figure 2.1**). The following points will give an idea about the importance of dairy chemistry:

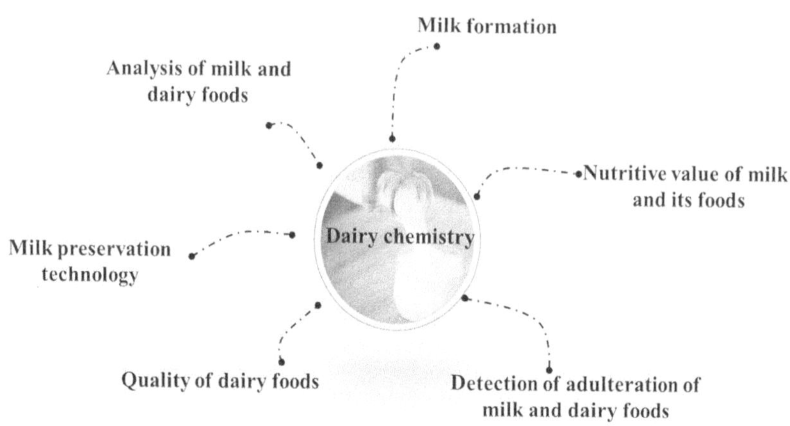


**FIGURE 2.1 Importance of dairy chemistry.** It helps in determining the quality and adulteration of milk foods and so on.

DOI: 10.1201/9781003397786-2

#### 2.2.1.1 Examining Milk and Dairy Foods

To know the chemical composition of milk and different dairy products, we need to analyze them in the laboratory. Different types of tests have been developed by dairy chemists for this purpose. So, practical knowledge of this subject is very much helpful for analytical purposes.

#### 2.2.1.2 Mechanism of Milk Formation and Synthesis of Milk

Milk forms in the mammary gland, and several theories have been given by different scientists about milk formation. None of the theories is complete. A lot of things are yet to be understood. Similarly, the synthesis of milk components involves complex chemistry. To understand these things, knowledge of dairy chemistry will certainly help.

#### 2.2.1.3 Evaluation of the Nutritive Value of Milk and Dairy Foods

Dairy chemistry also helps to evaluate the nutritive value of milk and its products. For example, to know the energy value of milk, the biological value of milk protein, or the digestibility of individual nutrients, some tests need to be done. All these tests regarding the evaluation of the nutritive value of milk and milk products have been developed by dairy chemists. So, knowledge of dairy chemistry is very helpful in this connection.

#### 2.2.1.4 Detection of Adulteration of Milk and Dairy Foods

Sometimes, milk vendors (mostly developing countries) try to adulterate milk by adding water or other substances like sodium bicarbonate, formalin, flour, etc. In some cases, they withdraw a portion of fat from the milk and sell the remaining low-quality milk in local markets. Some sweetmeat makers used to adulterate butter and ghee by adding vegetable or animal fat to them. All these adulteration techniques can be detected by using some specific tests that have been developed by dairy chemists.

#### 2.2.1.5 Quality Control of Milk and Dairy Foods

The nutritive value and market value of milk and dairy foods depend on their quality. For this reason, in the receiving plant, a dairy chemist always checks the quality of incoming milk with the help of different tests. These are routine activities of a dairy plant, and the tests conducted to check the quality of milk are commonly known as platform tests. Quality control also contributes to measuring rancidity and milk preservation.

### 2.2.2 Biochemical Ingredients

With over 100,000 distinct molecular species present in milk, it is also a relatively complex meal. When examining milk under a microscope, low magnification (5×) reveals a homogeneous yet turbid liquid. The fat globules, or spherical droplets of fat, are visible at a 500× magnification. The casein micelles can be seen at even greater magnification (50,000×). Later on, a more thorough analysis of the primary structural elements of milk, fat globules, and casein micelles will take place.

The main constituents of milk include lactose (milk sugar), fat, proteins, water, and minerals (salt) (**Table 2.1**). Milk also contains small amounts of other substances like pigments, enzymes, vitamins, phospholipids (similar to fat), and gases.

#### 2.2.2.1 Lactose

Lactose, also known as milk sugar, is usually only found in milk. Lactose is the principal milk sugar, and glucose and galactose are the two sugars (monosaccharides) that make up the disaccharide known as lactose (**Figure 2.2**). There are two isomers of lactose: beta, in which the hydroxyl on the anomeric carbon points up on the ring structure, and alpha (Misselwitz et al., 2019).

It is a reducing disaccharide that, upon hydrolysis, yields one molecule of glucose and one molecule of galactose. It has the same molecular formula ($C_{12}H_{24}O_{11}$) as ordinary cane sugar or sucrose.

**TABLE 2.1**
**Precursors of Milk Components**

| Milk components | | Precursors |
|---|---|---|
| Lactose | | Blood D-glucose |
| Fat | SFA | Acetate and β-hydroxy butyrate |
| | LFA | Blood plasma triglyceride (TG) |
| Protein | Caseins (α, β, γ), lactoglobulin | Free amino acid |
| | Immunoglobulin | Blood immunoglobulin |
| | Milk serum albumin | Blood serum albumin |
| Vitamins | Vitamin A | β-carotene |
| | Vitamin D | Cholecalciferol |
| | Vitamin C | D-glucose |
| Minerals | | – |

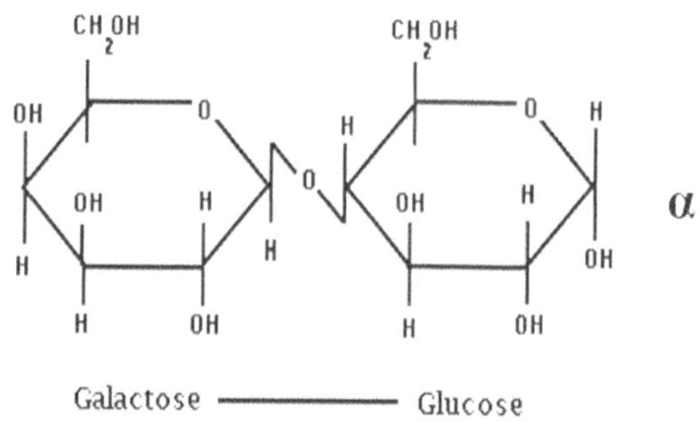


**FIGURE 2.2 Biochemical structure of lactose.** Mammalian milk is the sole natural source of lactose. Lactose is a disaccharide made up of galactose and glucose.

In terms of molecule arrangement, taste, sweetness, dissolution rate, and chemical reactions, sucrose differs significantly. Sucrose is about six times sweeter than lactose. Lactose is present in milk in true solution in milk serum. Its solubility is 1/3rd that of sucrose at 100°C and 1/14th at 0°C.

Although it is believed that lactose is present only in milk, recently, it was observed that a low percentage also appears in blood and urine, especially during pregnancy and lactation. At that moment, the mammary gland can occasionally escape. About 9% of healthy people with a typical diet have lactosuria, a condition marked by the presence of lactose in the urine. It most likely has an alimentary origin. Milk contains about 4.4–5.2% lactose with an average of 4.8%. This makes up 50–52% of the total solids (TS) in skim milk on average. Human milk contains about 6.3% lactose, and for this reason, in modifying cow's milk for infant feeding, it becomes necessary to add lactose or some other CHO to cow milk.

#### *2.2.2.1.1 Nutritive Value*

The nutritional value of lactose is distinct in many ways. Like other CHOs, it provides energy and has a caloric value of 2 to 4 kcal/g. However, compared to the majority of the other dietary CHOs, lactose does not seem to be used for this function as well. In the gut, lactose mostly remains unaltered. Galactose and lactose both withstand the digestive process longer than other sugars. Due to stronger resistance to hydrolysis and its comparatively sluggish rate of absorption, lactose accumulates at these higher levels in the intestine.

Some people with lactose intolerance may consume small quantities of milk throughout the day, and hence they may be able to eat modest amounts of yogurt.

The favoring of an acid type of fermentation, which in turn supports greater utilization of Ca and P, is one of its important effects on the intestine. Additionally, putrefactive organism growth is typically inhibited by lactic acid formation. In general, lactose's nutritional benefits are most significant for young children and newborns. Apart from this property, lactose tends to produce diarrhea in some people who have a shortage of lactase enzymes in the digestive system. This condition is known as lactose intolerance syndrome. Regarding the rising public awareness of lactose intolerance (LI), there is a growing market for lactose-free (LF) goods, and as a result, the food and pharmaceutical industries are using new technologies to create LF solutions that cater to the needs of those who are sensitive to lactose. The majority of individuals on earth appear to have LI, a clinical condition that prevents people from properly digesting lactose and, consequently, the goods that contain this sugar. There is a lack of thorough scientific research on lactose's use and replacement in food and medication. To offer relevant LF goods to people with LI in this situation, a greater understanding is needed. Given the importance of these goods in satisfying a particular nutritional need, it is crucial to immediately and clearly identify them. In this regard, the Lfree® certification mark may be a valuable labeling tool for LF goods that have less than 10 mg/kg of lactose residue (Ségurel & Bon, 2017).

In addition to these nutritional properties, there is some proof of the other benefits of lactose listed here:

i. When milk fat and lactose are supplied together as part of the diet, certain species grow more satisfactorily than when milk fat alone is fed.
ii. In some species, lactose may help with intestinal vitamin production.
iii. Due to its less effective utilization compared to other CHOs, propensity to promote gastrointestinal motility, and ability to prevent fat accumulation in the body, lactose may be useful in minimizing diets.
iv. Lactose appears to make calcium (Ca) absorption easier, probably by converting to the easily absorbed calcium–lactose in the colon.
v. In the developing brain (in case of young individuals), galactose produced from lactose can be used to create cerebrosides, significant brain structural components, and the medullary sheaths of nerves.

*2.2.2.1.2 Uses*

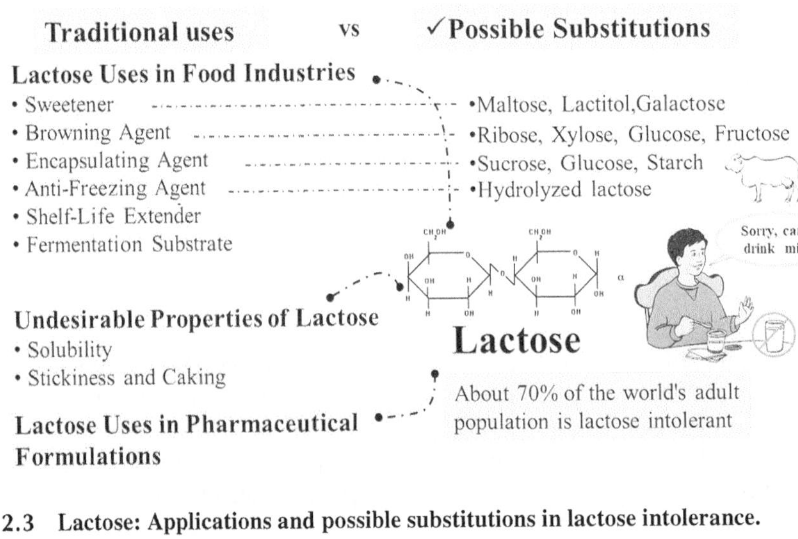


**FIGURE 2.3 Lactose: Applications and possible substitutions in lactose intolerance.**

The following are the main applications for lactose (**Figure 2.3**):

i. As a component of baby food and goods for people on special diets.
ii. When pharmaceutical tablets and pills are manufactured and standardized.
iii. In the mold substrate, it is used to make penicillin.
iv. In the production of caramel color.
v. As a seed material for promoting the production of fine crystals in specific dairy products.
vi. For the production of certain lactose derivatives.

##### *2.2.2.1.3 Negative Effects of Lactose on Health (Lactose Intolerance)*

Lactose intolerance is the inability to digest lactose, the sugar in milk. According to estimates, the lactase enzyme is only expressed to a limited extent in roughly 70% of adult humans globally, with significant regional and national diversity (Storhaug et al., 2017). Different factors, such as genetically determined lactase non-persistence (LNP) or the presence of other gastrointestinal illnesses that harm the gut brush boundary where lactase-phlorizin hydrolase (LPH) is found can contribute to this problem (Fassio et al., 2018). In both situations, lactose cannot be absorbed (lactose malabsorption) or digested (lactose maldigestion), which causes the intestinal bacteria to ferment it. A clinical condition known as LI, which is primarily characterized by the presence of gastrointestinal symptoms, may eventually result from lactose maldigestion and lactose malabsorption (Facioni et al., 2020). An excess of short-chain fatty acids induces acidification and irritation of the gastrointestinal mucosa, which results in discomfort and diarrhea or constipation; this situation creates gas and therefore flatulence, meteorism, and abdominal distention (Di Stefano, 2022).

#### 2.2.2.2 Milk Fat

Milk fat (also known as butterfat) contains about 400 distinct fatty acids, making it one of the most complex fat fractions found in nature. It contains all the essential fatty acids (linoleic, linolenic, and arachidonic acids). Milk fat is a complex mixture of several glycerides rather than a single chemical substance. Each glyceride is generated when glycerol and one or more organic fatty acids come together. Thus, it can be said that fats are esters of fatty acids with glycerol (Jensen, 2002). In milk fat, 12.5% glycerol and 85% fatty acids are usually present. During ester formation, the carboxyl group of fatty acids is bound with one of the three alcohol groups of the glycerol by reaction and liberation water, thus forming glycerides (Jensen, 2002).

Milk fats are mostly triglycerides (**Figure 2.4**), but about 3% of the glycerides are di- or monoglycerides. Compared to milk fat, animal fats are much simpler. Glycerides of palmitic, stearic, and oleic acids comprise beef fat. Glycerides of oleic acid constitute the majority of mutton tallow. More fatty acids are likely present in milk fat than any other natural fat. It is therefore one of the most complex fats found in nature. The presence of butyric, caproic, caprylic, capric, lauric, myristic, palmitic, stearic, and oleic acids in milk fat has been conclusively demonstrated (Spitsberg, 2005).

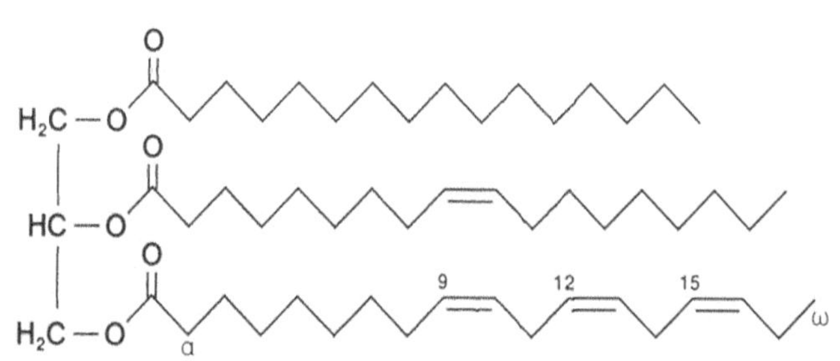


**FIGURE 2.4 Biochemical structure of milk fat (triglycerides).** Milk fat is mostly made up of triglycerides (98%). They are made up of three fatty acid chains that are joined together by a molecule called glycerol.

Scientists have identified at least an additional seven fatty acids, though it is debatable whether or not all of these are found in regular milk fat. Each dairy food has a unique fat content and composition due to several processes or factors, such as cow feed composition.

###### 2.2.2.2.1 Lipids of Milk

The lipids include a wide variety of organic compounds that are characteristically poorly soluble or not soluble in water but soluble in an organic solvent like ether, chloroform, benzene, etc. (Christie, 1995).

###### 2.2.2.2.2 Classification of Lipids of Milk

The lipids of milk may be classified as follows-

i. Fatty acids—They are long-chain aliphatic carboxylic acids.
ii. Neutral esters of glycerol and fatty acids—They are true milk fats.
iii. Ionic esters of glycerol, fatty acids, and phosphates—They are the phosphoglycerides.
iv. Lipids not containing glycerol– These include sphingolipids, waxes, cholesterol, terpenes, etc.
v. Lipids combined with other classes of compounds—Such as lipoprotein (combined with protein).

###### 2.2.2.2.3 Classes of Lipids with Percentage of Total Lipids

Classes of lipids with percentage of total lipids are as follows (**Table 2.2**):

**TABLE 2.2**
**Classes of Lipids with Percentage of Total Lipids**

| Classes of lipid of milk | Total lipids (%) |
|---|---|
| Triglycerides of fatty acids | 95–96 |
| Diglycerides of fatty acids | 1.2–1.59 |
| Monoglycerides of fatty acids | 0.016–0.038 |
| Keto acid glycerides | 0.85–1.28 |
| Ketogenic glycerides | 0.03–0.13 |
| Hydrogenic glycerides | 0.60–0.78 |
| Lactogenic glycerides | 0.60–0.70 |
| Phospholipids | 0.80–1.00 |
| Sphingolipids | 0.06–0.07 |
| Neutral plasmalogens | 0.10–0.44 |
| Steroids | 0.22–0.41 |
| Squalene | 0.007–0.008 |
| Carotenoids | Trace |
| Fat-soluble vitamins (A, D, E, K) | Trace |

###### 2.2.2.2.4 Principles of Cream/Fat Rising

The rise of cream/fat is based on the principle of milk fat because of its lower density than the skim milk portion. After the milk is drawn from the cow, normal milk will form a cream layer upon standing. In as few as 20 or 30 minutes, this layer can become visible. However, the layer can take at least a few hours to fully form. From the consumer's perspective, the presence of a cream layer in milk may be noteworthy. However, the phenomenon also involves features of fat globules, such as clustering, that are broadly significant in the behavior of milk and several of its products. The rate of rise of a spherical particle in a liquid medium is represented by an equation known as Stoke's law:

$$V = \frac{2G(d_s - d_f)r^2}{9\eta}$$

Where,

V = Rate of rise of fat globule in millimeters per second
r = Radius of fat globule
G = Force of gravity (981 dynes)
$\eta$ = Viscosity of skim milk
$d_s$ = Skim milk density
$d_f$ = Density of fat globule
*More details are discussed in Chapter 5.

##### 2.2.2.2.5 *Classification of Fatty Acids Found in Milk*

The fatty acids present in milk may be classified as follows:

i. Saturated and unsaturated fatty acids
ii. Volatile and non-volatile fatty acids
iii. Soluble and insoluble fatty acids

##### 2.2.2.2.6 *Saturated and Unsaturated Fatty Acids*

Fatty acids containing only a single bond are known as saturated fatty acids (**Table 2.3**). In contrast, unsaturated fatty acids (**Table 2.4**) refer to fatty acids that contain one or more double bonds (Christie, 1995).

**TABLE 2.3**
**Examples of Saturated Fatty Acids**

| Name | Carbon no | Structural formula | Wt % of total fatty acid content | Melting point (°C) |
|---|---|---|---|---|
| Butyric acid | $C_4$ | $CH_3$-$(CH_2)_2$-COOH | 3.1–4.4 | -8 |
| Caproic acid | $C_6$ | $CH_3$-$(CH_2)_4$-COOH | 1.8–2.7 | -4 |
| Caprylic acid | $C_8$ | $CH_3$-$(CH_2)_6$-COOH | 1.0–1.7 | 16 |
| Capric acid | $C_{10}$ | $CH_3$-$(CH_2)_8$-COOH | 2.2–3.8 | 31 |
| Lauric acid | $C_{12}$ | $CH_3$-$(CH_2)_{10}$-COOH | 2.6–4.2 | 44 |
| Myristic acid | $C_{14}$ | $CH_3$-$(CH_2)_{12}$-COOH | 9.1–11.9 | 54 |
| Palmitic acid | $C_{16}$ | $CH_3$-$(CH_2)_{14}$-COOH | 23.6–31.4 | 63 |
| Stearic acid | $C_{18}$ | $CH_3$-$(CH_2)_{16}$-COOH | 10.4–14.6 | 70 |
| Arachidic acid | $C_{20}$ | $CH_3$-$(CH_2)_{18}$-COOH | – | – |
| Behenic acid | $C_{22}$ | $CH_3$-$(CH_2)_{20}$-COOH | – | – |

**TABLE 2.4**
**Examples of Unsaturated Fatty Acids**

| Name | Carbon no. | Structural formula | Wt % of total fatty acid content | Melting point (°C) |
|---|---|---|---|---|
| Palmitoleic acid | $C_{16}$ | $CH_3$-$(CH_2)_5$-CH=CH-$(CH_2)_7$-COOH | – | – |
| Oleic acid | $C_{18}$ | $CH_3$-$(CH_2)_7$-CH=CH-$(CH_2)_7$-COOH | 14.9–22.0 | 16 |
| Linoleic acid | $C_{18}$ | $CH_3$-$(CH_2)_4$-CH=CH-$CH_2$-CH=CH-$(CH_2)_7$-COOH | 1.2–1.7 | –5 |
| Linolenic acid | $C_{18}$ | $CH_3$-$CH_2$-CH=CH-$CH_2$-CH=CH-$CH_2$-CH=CH-$(CH_2)_7$-COOH | 0.9–1.2 | –12 |
| Arachidonic acid | $C_{20}$ | $CH_3$-$(CH_2)_4$-(CH=CH-$CH_2)_4$-$(CH_2)_2$-COOH | – | – |

#### *2.2.2.2.7 Volatile and Non-Volatile Fatty Acids*

The volatile fatty acids are those that disappear quickly when they are kept at ordinary room temperature in a free state. On the other hand, the non-volatile fatty acids do not disappear when they are kept at room temperature in a free state. Fatty acids containing $C_4$–$C_{12}$ are volatile fatty acids, and the remaining fatty acids are non-volatile ($C_{14}$–$C_{22}$).

#### *2.2.2.2.8 Soluble and Insoluble Fatty Acids*

Fatty acids that are soluble in water are known as soluble fatty acids, and fatty acids that are insoluble in water are known as insoluble fatty acids. Fatty acids containing $C_4$–$C_{10}$ are soluble in water, and the remaining fatty acids ($C_{12}$–$C_{22}$) are insoluble in water.

#### *2.2.2.2.9 The Good and the Bad: Perceptions and Realities of Milk Fat*

- Milk fat is regarded as hypercholesterolemic, even if milk has a low cholesterol content (intake of unsaturated FA reduces the plasma cholesterol concentrations). This is primarily due to its high amount of saturated fatty acids (60 to 65%).
- Bovine milk fat has high levels of short-chain fatty acids and relatively low levels of $C_{18}$ fatty acids (Huot et al., 2010).
- Dietary long-chain fatty acid (LFAs), microbial synthesis of fatty acids, and body fat stores contribute to the production of some milk fatty acids; the remainder is created from scratch in the mammary gland. The balance between dietary long-chain fatty acids delivered to the mammary gland and short- and medium-chain fatty acids synthesized by the dairy cow's mammary gland can be significantly changed by manipulating the diet of the animal.

### 2.2.2.3 Milk Protein

Milk proteins (high-quality proteins) include all nine essential amino acids that humans require. Milk proteins are made in the mammary gland, but 60% of the amino acids used to build the proteins are obtained from the cow's feed. Proteins are polymers of amino acids united by peptide linkage and having a molecular weight of at least 5000. Proteins are made up of large molecules containing carbon, hydrogen, oxygen, nitrogen, sulfur, and sometimes phosphorus. Cow's milk contains approximately 3.5% protein, out of which 2.9% is casein (**Figure 2.5**) and 0.6% is whey protein (Medhammar et al., 2012).

#### *2.2.2.3.1 Milk Protein Fractionation*

Caseins make up about 76% of the nitrogen in milk, followed by whey proteins (19%) and non-protein nitrogen (NPN) (6%) (**Table 2.5**). The minor proteins linked to the fat globule membrane (FGM) are not included in this. The Rowland fractionation method can be used to determine this nitrogen distribution.

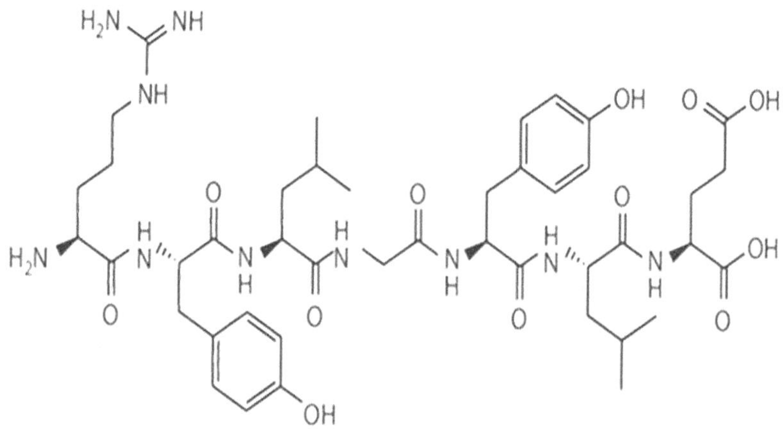

FIGURE 2.5 **Biochemical structure of milk protein (casein).** Casein (cow milk contains about 80%) micelles are complex macromolecular assemblies composed of four different caseins (αs1, αs2, β, and κ-caseins). These types of casein proteins do not have a clear and defined shape because they contain a high amount of propyl residues.

**TABLE 2.5**
**Concentrations of Proteins in Milk**

| | g/liter | Amount (%) |
|---|---|---|
| Total protein | 33 | 100 |
| Casein | 26 | 79.5 |
| Alpha S1 | 10 | 30.6 |
| Alpha S2 | 2.6 | 8.0 |
| Beta | 9.3 | 28.4 |
| Kappa | 3.3 | 10.1 |
| Whey protein | 6.3 | 19.3 |
| Alpha-lactalbumin | 1.2 | 3.7 |
| Beta lactoglobulin | 3.2 | 9.8 |
| BSA | 0.4 | 1.2 |
| Immunoglobulins | 0.7 | 2.1 |
| Proteose peptone | 0.8 | 2.4 |

1. Precipitation at pH 4.6 separates caseins from whey nitrogen.
2. Using acetic acid and sodium acetate precipitation, which has a pH of 5, total proteins are separated from whey NPN.

#### 2.2.2.3.2 *Classification of Milk Protein*

Milk protein may be classified as follows:

i. Casein
ii. Whey protein
iii. Protease-peptone fraction
iv. Non-protein nitrogenous substances

**Casein**: May be classified as follows:

- i. α-casein
  - a. $\alpha_s$-casein
    - 1. $\alpha_{s1}$-casein
    - 2. $\alpha_{s2}$-casein
  - b. κ-casein
- ii. β-casein
- iii. γ-casein

**Whey protein:** Whey protein may be classified as:

- i. Lactalbumin
  - a. α- lactalbumin
  - b. β- lactalbumin
- ii. Lactoglobulin
  - a. Euglobulin
  - b. Pseudo globulin
  - c. IgG (IgG5, IgG2)
  - d. IgM
  - e. IgA

**Non-protein nitrogenous substances:** They exist in very small amounts and are found in urine.

##### *2.2.2.3.3 Casein*

Casein is one of the few proteins containing phosphorus and exists in a state of suspension in milk. It is probably present in milk as calcium-caseinate and, like other proteins, is very complex, with colloidal properties and a high molecular weight believed to be about 93,000. Casein contains about 15.8% $N_2$. So, the factor for converting nitrogen percentage to casein by Kjeldahl is 6.38. It is a major portion of milk protein and is precipitated from milk at a pH of 4.6 at about 20°C (Potočnik et al., 2011).

##### *2.2.2.3.4 Preparation of Milk Casein*

Commercially, casein is prepared by using the following methods:

*i. Coagulation by rennin:* Fresh low-fat skim milk is warmed to 35.5°C and curdled with around 4 ounces of rennin extract for every 100 gallons of milk in the production of rennin. The coagulation should be completed within 15 to 20 minutes, after which the curd is broken up and gradually heated at 55–65°C. The curd is separated from the whey and repeatedly rinsed with water (at a temperature between 26 and 32°C) to eliminate the acid after it has settled for 10 minutes. It is shredded after an hour of pressing and then dried in thin layers at 43 to 46°C. If the product is to have a light hue, rapid drying at low temperatures is necessary. Casein prepared by this method is mainly used for the manufacture of plastics considered essential for this product.

*ii. Precipitation by acid/acidification method:* Lactic acid, which is produced by the bacterial fermentation of lactose into acid, is added to milk to precipitate the casein and bring the milk's acidity to the appropriate level. This method of acidification is known as the self-sour process. Various adjustments can be made based on the acid and temperature being utilized. A product with exceptional uniformity in composition, color, and adhesiveness is produced through a number of processes that use continuous precipitation, washing, and drying (Kaur et al., 2020).

The milk is mixed with lactic acid bacteria and let stand at a comfortable temperature until curdling occurs in the self-sour process. The curd at this acidity, at about pH 4.7, is soft and fine. Extremely high temperatures result in a rubbery curd that must first be chopped in order to be adequately washed.

After the draining of whey, the curd is washed several times, drained, pressed overnight, shredded, and dried at 55°C. This method of preparing casein is mostly utilized to produce sticky products.

#### *2.2.2.3.5 Uses of Casein*

The most extensive non-food use of casein is in coating paper of books and magazines. It is dissolved in an alkali for this purpose, together with mineral pigments, and the suspension is applied to the appropriate surfaces using rollers and brushes. Casein keeps the paper's surface smooth and non-absorptive while also holding the pigments on the surface in place, making it suited for fine printing. Formaldehyde may be bound to make the casein-bound coating waterproof, as on playing cards and wallpapers (Udenigwe & Aluko, 2012). It also has numerous traditional uses (**Figure 2.6**).

i. Casein glues are mostly utilized in the woodworking and construction sectors. They are made up of casein, a calcium compound, and an alkali solution as a solvent. When the calcium-caseinate is dried, it becomes insoluble and makes the glue waterproof.
ii. Casein is used for the preparation of plastic as well. Dried rennet casein, colors, and a trace amount of water are mixed into a thick dough to create plastic casein, which is then extruded. Under pressure, this dough dries out. As a hardening and insoluble agent, formaldehyde is employed.
iii. Casein is utilized in the textile industry for a variety of functions, including waterproofing, loading, softening, and fixing color.
iv. In the leather industry, casein is also widely used. In this instance, it is employed in a solution with a small amount of alkali to give light leather a glossy appearance. A mixture of lime and casein is used as an adhesive and sparkler in applying insecticides in the leather industry.
v. Casein may be converted into a fibrous form to produce wool-like substances for the manufacture of jackets. This fibrous casein was widely used during the Second World War as a substitute for wool.
vi. Casein is used for the preparation of plastic paint.
vii. The food sector makes extensive use of it as well. About 1/3 of the total casein produced in the United States (USA) is usually used for the manufacture of different types of fast food (Cui et al., 2011).

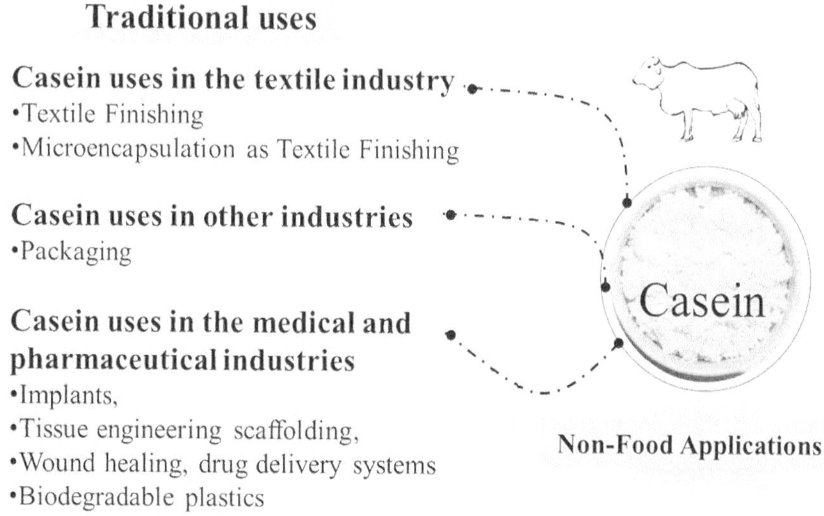


**FIGURE 2.6 Traditional uses of casein.** Casein can be utilized in foods, beverages, pharmaceuticals, health and personal care items, and agriculture/animal feed.

#### 2.2.2.4 Milk Enzymes

Enzymes are organic catalysts that enhance the rate of biological reactions from $10^6$ to $10^{12}$ times those of uncatalyzed reactions. They are all proteins and contain a functional site called an active site, where reactants are converted to products. Enzymes are highly specific and catalyze one or at least a few reactions.

Normal milk contains several enzymes (at least 70 indigenous enzymes). Milk enzymes are constituents and products of mammary tissue that gain entrance to the milk during the secretory process. It is not possible to classify the enzymes produced by milk bacteria as milk's typical ingredients (Mahony et al., 2013). None of these enzymes is absolutely necessary, although several of them are important for the nutrition and safety of the newborn. The technological significance of native milk enzymes has been extensively studied since some have a direct impact on the quality of dairy products (for example, through lipolysis or proteolysis) while others are used as markers of thermal history or product quality (Mahony et al., 2013).

Milk contains the following enzymes: lipase, phosphatase, xanthine oxidase, esterase, lactoperoxidase, catalase, protease, amylase, aldolase, salolase, lactase, ribonuclease, lysozyme, rhodonase, carbonic anhydrase (Fox & Kelly, 2006a, 2006b).

- **Lipase:** It is an enzyme that helps milk fat break down into glycerol and fatty acids. Due to hydrolysis, milk and milk products become rancid and produce a bitter taste. Despite having lipase enzymes, milk often does not spontaneously undergo lipolysis. The enzyme must first undergo some activation procedures before attacking fat globules. These include mixing, shaking, and a variety of temperature changes, including cooling to 5°C and then quickly rising to 30°C. These activities help to absorb the enzyme on the fat globule membrane, thus allowing the enzyme to properly activate.
- **Phosphatase:** Alkaline phosphomonoesterase, another name for this enzyme, catalyzes the hydrolysis of organic phosphates to produce phenol or alcohol and phosphoric acid ($H_3PO_4$). It is a naturally occurring enzyme found in milk. This enzyme is destroyed during pasteurization. For this reason, the presence or absence of milk gives an idea of whether the milk is pasteurized or not. The most popular phosphatase test is based on the enzyme. An acid phosphatase is also reported to be present in milk and cannot be destroyed during pasteurization.
- **Xanthine oxidase:** In milk, xanthine oxidase is a major enzyme. The enzyme contributes to the process of oxygenating a substance or dehydrogenating it.
- **Esterase:** An enzyme that catalyzes the hydrolysis of esters is known as an esterase. Esterase enzymes include lipase. In addition to lipase activity, milk also has significant esterase activity. There are three types of esterase are available in milk, A-esterase, B-esterase, and C-esterase.
- **Lactoperoxidase:** An enzyme called peroxidase catalyzes the oxygen transfer from peroxide, $H_2O_2$, to other molecules. All milk contains peroxidase enzymes. One of the most well-known sources of peroxidase is milk, but the quantity varies slightly. Milk per-oxidase is known as "Lactoperoxidase." Its optimum pH is 6.8, and pasteurization temperature does not inactivate the enzyme. It also indicates whether the pasteurization of milk is complete or not.
- **Catalase:** The function of catalase is to facilitate the decomposition of hydrogen peroxide into water and oxygen, thereby preventing any potential damage. The amount of catalase in milk varies depending on the breed of cow, the animal, and the interval between milking. The highest concentration of catalase is seen in the last fraction of milk taken. When green feeds are fed, the amount of catalase increases, and the milk's bacterial or leucocyte content also increases noticeably. For this reason, the catalase content of milk has been suggested as a way to measure its volume and identify milk from infected udders. Its optimum activity is at pH 6.8–7.0, and acidic media destroy its activity. This enzyme is destroyed by heating milk at 65 to 75°C for 30 minutes.
- **Protease:** An enzyme known as a protease catalyzes the breakdown of protein peptide bonds to create smaller protein fragments, i.e., peptones, proteoses, peptides, amino acids,

and ammonia ($NH_3$). This enzyme breaks down casein under neutral or slightly alkaline conditions; acidic conditions cause it to operate more slowly, and 1% chloroform or 15% NaCl can stop it in its tracks. Its optimum activity is at pH 8.5. This enzyme can be deactivated by heating at 75–80°C for about 10 minutes.

- **Amylase:** Amylase is an enzyme that catalyzes the hydrolysis of starch to dextrin or maltose. There are two principal kinds of amylase, namely α- and β-amylase. A-amylase is inactivated by heating milk at 55°C for 30 minutes. On the other hand, β-amylase stands at 65°C for 30 minutes without any loss of activity.
- **Aldolase:** The enzyme aldolase reversibly splits fructose 1,6-diphosphate into dihydroxy acetone phosphate and phosphoglyceraldehyde. It is present in milk at a lower concentration. It becomes unstable when it is in milk, but it becomes more stable when the milk starts to spoil. In milk, it is totally rendered inactive by 20 minutes of heating at 45°C.
- **Salolase:** Salolase is an enzyme that catalyzes the hydrolysis of phenyl salicylate to phenol and salicylic acid. The presence of this enzyme in milk had been reported by Vandevelde (1908).
- **Lactase:** The enzyme lactase, also known as β-galactosidase, catalyzes the hydrolysis of lactose to glucose and galactose. Some investigators reported that lactase is present in milk in low concentrations. On the other hand, some other scientists were not able to detect lactase in milk. The lactase enzyme present in milk is mainly of bacterial origin.
- **Ribonuclease:** This enzyme hydrolyzes nucleic acids to their component nucleotides. It can be found in milk at comparatively high concentrations. This enzyme is quite heat stable; when heated to 90°C for 20 minutes at pH 3.5, there is negligible loss. However, under the same condition at pH 7, all activity is lost.
- **Lysozyme:** This enzyme has natural antibacterial properties. The lysozyme content of milk varies from 0 to 260 micrograms/100 ml of milk. The average lysozyme content of Brown Swiss, Guernsey, Holstein Friesian, and Jersey milk is 21, 15, 11, and 5 micrograms/100 ml of milk, respectively (Shahani et al., 1962). Lysozyme secretion remains unaffected by the amount of milk produced during lactation. The lysozyme content of cow's milk is about 13 micrograms/100 ml of milk but for human milk is 40,000 micrograms/100 ml of milk.
- **Carbonic anhydrase:** This enzyme catalyzes the hydration of $CO_2$ and the reverse reaction, the dehydration of carbonic acid. It is a zinc (Zn)-containing protein associated with red blood cells (RBCs) and is an important enzyme in the animal body. It has been reported that cows, goats, and sheep contain little carbonic anhydrase, but its purpose or value in milk is unknown.
- **Rhodonase:** The conversion of cyanide into thiocyanide is facilitated by this enzyme. Rhodonase activity in cows' milk is higher than that of goat's and sheep's milk.

#### 2.2.2.5 Vitamins

Vitamins are organic compounds that are present in both plants and animals in very minute amounts. They are necessary for regular living functions, yet the body is unable to generate them. Although the chemical formula of vitamins is typically quite complex, formulae are now known for the majority of vitamins. Capital letters are used to denote vitamins, often with number subscripts, e.g. A, $B_1$, and $B_2$. Vitamins can be found in milk in variable concentrations (**Table 2.6**) and are a good source of nutrition. Among the most well-known vitamins are A, the vitamin B group, C, and D. While the other vitamins are soluble in water, vitamins A and D are soluble in fat or fat-based solvents. The two most significant fat-soluble vitamins are A and D. They impact the skin and eyesight. Low-fat milk products have fewer of these vitamins for physiological reasons. To make low-fat milk have the same vitamin content as whole milk, this vitamin shortage is often made up for by enriching the milk with vitamins A and D. Diseases linked to vitamin deficiency can happen (**Table 2.7**) (Cashman, 2016; Jayaratne et al., 2013). On the other hand, the reduction of vitamins is influenced by milk processing (both UHT and pasteurization milk) (**Table 2.8**).

**TABLE 2.6**
**Vitamin Content of Fresh Milk**

| Vitamin | Amount per liter |
|---|---|
| A (µg RE) | 400 |
| D (IU) | 40 |
| E (µg) | 1000 |
| K (µg) | 50 |
| $B_1$ (µg) | 450 |
| $B_2$ (µg) | 1750 |
| Niacin (µg) | 900 |
| $B_6$ (µg) | 500 |
| Pantothenic acid (µg) | 3500 |
| Biotin (µg) | 35 |
| Folic acid (µg) | 55 |
| $B_{12}$ (µg) | 4.5 |
| C (mg) | 20 |

* RE = Retinol Equivalent

**TABLE 2.7**
**Daily Requirements of Vitamins and Deficiency Diseases**

| Vitamin | Adult daily requirement (mg) | Deficiency diseases |
|---|---|---|
| A | 1–2 | Night blindness, impaired resistance to infectious diseases |
| $B_1$ | 1–2 | Stunted growth |
| $B_2$ | 1–4 | Loss of appetite, indigestion |
| C | 30–100 | Fatigue, pyorrhea, susceptibility to infection (scurvy) |
| D | 0.01 | Skeletal deformation (rickets) |

#### 2.2.2.6 Minerals

Milk contains all 22 minerals that are thought to be necessary for a human diet (Fantuz et al., 2022) (**Table 2.9**). These include three families of salts:

- **Sodium (Na), potassium (K), and chloride (Cl):** These charged particles that are free in milk have an inverse relationship to lactose in order to balance the water levels in milk with blood.
- **Calcium (Ca), magnesium (Mg), inorganic phosphorous (P(i)), and citrate:** In this group, 2/3 of the Ca, 1/3 of the Mg, ½ of the P(i), and less than 1/10 of the citrate exist in colloidal (non-diffusible) form and are present in the casein micelle.
- **Ca, Mg, citrate, and phosphate diffusible salts:** These salts are highly pH dependent and help maintain the overall acid–base equilibrium of milk.

**TABLE 2.8**
**Reduction in Important Vitamins in Milk Processed and Stored in Different Conditions**

| | Pasteurized milk | | UHT milk | |
|---|---|---|---|---|
| Vitamin | Heat treatment | Chilled storage | Heat treatment | Ambient storage |
| Ascorbic acid, C | 0–10% | 10 –100 % | 0–80% | up to 100% |
| Thiamin, $B_1$ | < 10% | Not investigated enough | < 10% | No further loss* |
| Riboflavin, $B_2$ | Insignificant | Insignificant* | < 10% | 10%* |
| Pyridoxine, $B_6$ | < 10% | Not investigated enough | 0–20% | 15–20% |
| Folic acid, $B_9$ | Insignificant | Not investigated enough | 10–20% | up to 100%** |
| Cobalamin, $B_{12}$ | < 10% | Insignificant | 0–30% | Up to 100% |
| Retinol, β-carotene, A | Insignificant | Insignificant*** | Insignificant*** | Insignificant*** |
| Calciferols, D | Insignificant | Insignificant | Insignificant | Insignificant |

* When not exposed to light; ** Dependent on oxygen content; *** If not fortified

**TABLE 2.9**
**Mineral Content of Fresh Milk**

| Mineral | Content per liter |
|---|---|
| Sodium (mg) | 250–640 |
| Potassium (mg) | 1100–1500 |
| Chloride (mg) | 800–1200 |
| Calcium (mg) | 1100–1300 |
| Magnesium (mg) | 70–140 |
| Phosphorus (mg) | 800–1000 |
| Iron (g) | 100–700 |
| Zinc (μg) | 2500–7000 |
| Copper (μg) | 100–350 |
| Manganese (μg) | 10–50 |
| Iodine (μg) | 50–600 |
| Fluoride (μg) | 20–80 |
| Selenium (μg) | 20–40 |
| Cobalt (μg) | 0.5–1.3 |
| Chromium (μg) | 0.5–20 |
| Molybdenum (μg) | 20–100 |
| Nickel (μg) | 0–50 |
| Arsenic (μg) | 20–60 |
| Aluminum (μg) | 50–1600 |
| Lead (μg) | 20 |

*Source:* Sola-Larrañaga & Navarro-Blasco, 2009

#### 2.2.2.7 Flavors and Off Flavors of Milk

##### *2.2.2.7.1 Nature of Flavor*

Milk flavor may be classified into two types. Natural, good, or normal tastes are desirable or necessary. Off-flavors are unwanted tastes that are not natural or typical. The main sources of aroma components of milk are illustrated in **Figure 2.7**. The perception of taste is one that can be experienced by using the nose, mouth, and other related organs as appropriate receptors. Olfactory, gustatory, and tactual stimuli, which are concerned with the odor, taste, and sensation of flavor, are the three fundamental components of flavor. Olfactory elements are odors, and as vapors travel up the back of the nose and into the olfactory area, the odor of food consumed in the mouth becomes notable. Gustatory elements deal with taste, which is focused on a small number of sensations found in the mouth and, more specifically, on the tongue. They are bitterness, saltiness, sourness, and sweetness. The third and possibly more frequently disregarded element of flavor is tactual, or how something feels in the mouth. Examples of tactual flavor responses include smoothness, graininess, softness, chalkiness, etc.

The volatile flavor and taste compounds in milk and milk products originate from the degradation of major milk constituents, namely:

i. Lactose
ii. Citrate
iii. Milk lipids
iv. Milk products (particularly the caseins)

To make sure the chemicals in the product are balanced correctly, certain methods need to be followed. These methods include controlling the temperature, acidity, moisture, and salt level and how long the product ages. The hydrolysis of triglycerides, which account for more than 98% of milk fat, is the primary biochemical change in fat, producing free fatty acids (FFAs), di- and monoglycerides, and perhaps glycerol (**Figure 2.8**). FFAs add to the cheese aroma.

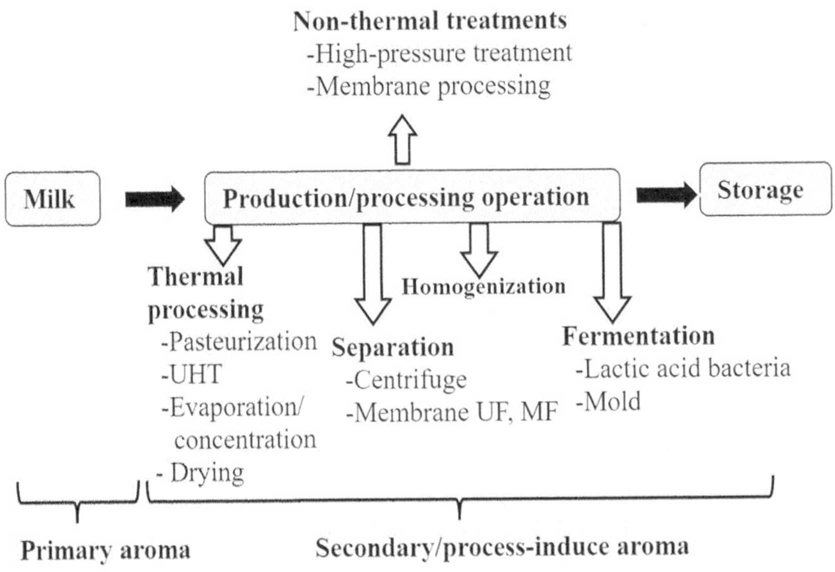


**FIGURE 2.7 Main sources of aroma components of milk foods.** Milk flavor may be classified into two types. Natural, good, or normal tastes are desirable or necessary. Off-flavors are unwanted tastes that are not natural or typical.

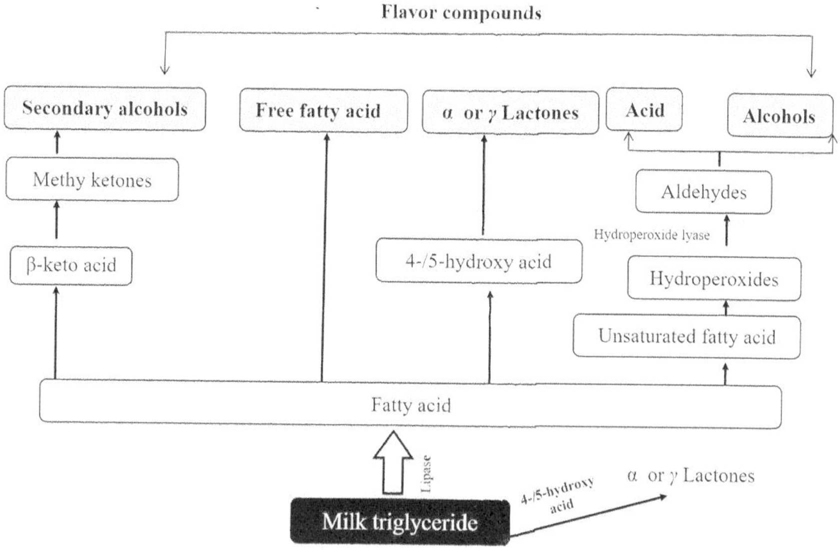


**FIGURE 2.8 The biochemical pathways for the metabolism of milk triglycerides and fatty acids.** Dairy taste and off-flavor molecules are formed by a coordinated set of chemical and biological interactions. Chemical and biological pathways are as follows: heat-induced alterations, lipid oxidation, glycolysis, lipolysis, and proteolysis.

## 2.3 MILK PROCESSING

The procedures involved in processing milk are as follows: stirring, mixing, and cooling at the farm; clarifying, separation, and standardization; pasteurization; homogenization; and packing, all of which are done in a sanitary manner (**Figure 2.9**).

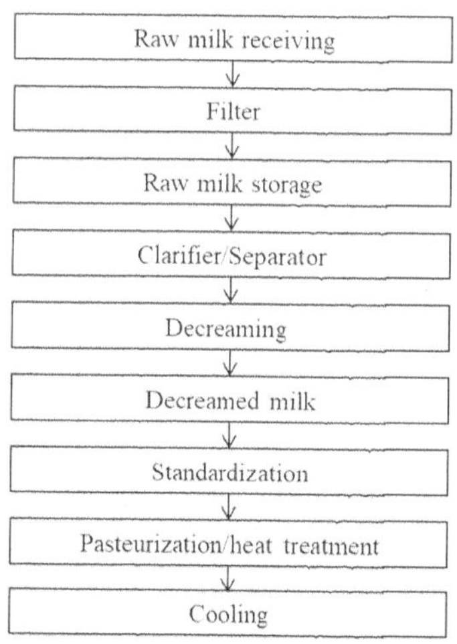


**FIGURE 2.9 Basic steps of milk processing.** This technique heats milk to 72°C for no less than 15 seconds, then promptly cools it to kill any hazardous germs and microorganisms.

### 2.3.1 Clarification and Standardization

#### 2.3.1.1 Centrifugation

In the dairy sector, centrifugal separation is a procedure that is frequently utilized. Some uses include clarification, skimming, standardizing, whey separation (separating fat from whey), quark separation (separation of quark curd from whey), bactofuge treatment (milk is filtered to remove microorganisms), and butter oil purification (segregation of the serum phase from the anhydrous milk fat).

##### *2.3.1.1.1 Principles of Centrifugation*

Centrifugation is based on Stoke's Law. The particle sedimentation velocity increases with:

- Increasing diameter
- Increasing differences between the densities of the two phases
- Decreasing viscosity of the continuous phase

If raw milk were left to stand, a process known as creaming would start to occur when the fat globules started to rise to the surface. Centrifugal forces also act on raw milk inside a spinning container. This enables the elimination of solid contaminants from the milk and the quick separation of milk fat from the fraction of skim milk.

#### 2.3.1.2 Clarification

In a single centrifuge, separation and clarification can both be accomplished simultaneously. Particles that are denser than the continuous milk phase are thrown back to the perimeter. The solids that assemble in the centrifuge consist of debris, epithelial cells, leucocytes, corpuscles, bacteria sediment, and sludge. The number of solids that are collected will vary; however, they must be removed from the centrifuge. The self-cleaning capabilities of the most recent centrifuges enable a continuous separation/clarification process. This kind of centrifuge comprises a bowl that has been specially made with discharge slots around the edges. These slots are kept closed under pressure. The contents of the sediment space are evacuated with a brief release of pressure that lasts for approximately 0.15 seconds. This could imply that 8 to 25 liters are evacuated every 60 minutes. For one dairy, self-cleaning results to a loss of 50 l/h of milk (**Figure 2.10a**).

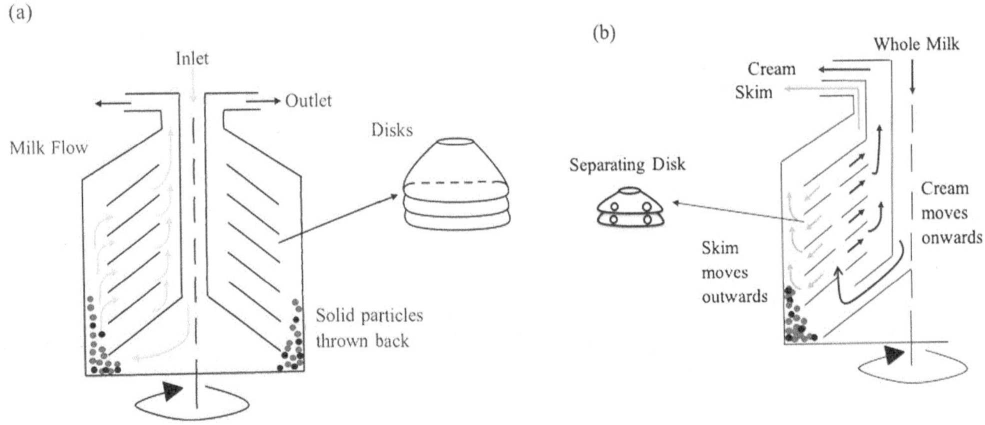


**FIGURE 2.10** (**a**) Schematic diagram of a clarification process; (**b**) schematic diagram of a self-cleaning separator.

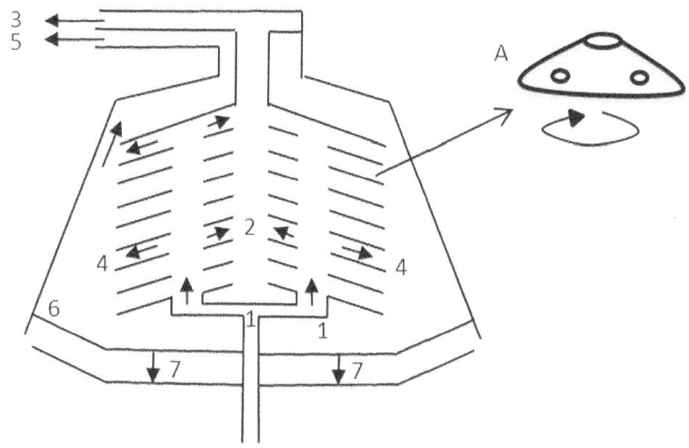


**FIGURE 2.11 Diagram of the centrifugal separation process.** A) Conical disk, from stack, showing top opening and milk distribution channels. Disk stack is rotating in separator. 1) Whole milk enters the disk distribution channel, from below, 2) Fat globules move inward, carried by some skim milk to form the cream, 3) Cream outlet port, 4) Skim milk devoid of fat globules moves outward and upward, over the solid disk at the top, 5) Skim outlet port, 6) Sediment collects, 7) Momentary periodic release of bowl pressure causes sediment cavity to open, releasing sediment.

### 2.3.1.3 Separation

To separate the cream from the milk, centrifuges can be employed (**Figure 2.10b**). The centrifuge is made up of up to 120 discs that are separated by a 0.4 to 2.0 mm separation channel and stacked together at a 45 to 60-degree angle. At the outermost edge of the disc stack, milk is added. The milk is poured into vertically aligned distribution holes in the stack of discs. The fat globules (cream), which are less dense than the skim milk, flow inward via the separation channels and toward the axis of rotation under the effect of centrifugal force. Skim milk will exit through a different outlet and flow outward (**Figure 2.11**)

### 2.3.1.4 Standardization

After separation, the streams of skim milk and cream must be blended again to a specific fat level. The cream outlet's throttling valve can be adjusted to change the flow of milk; the skim milk outlet will release entire milk if the valve is fully closed. Greater amounts of cream with decreasing fat contents are released from the cream outlet when the valve is gradually opened. Direct standardization automatically blends the cream and skim at the separator to get the correct fat content. Here are some illustrations of straightforward standardization problems, including mass balance and the Pearson square formula.

#### *2.3.1.4.1 Standardization Problems*

i. If a dairy has 160 kg of 40% cream and wishes to standardize it to 32% cream, how much skim milk must be added?

**Mass balance approach**

Let $x$ = kg skim milk

$y$ = kg of 32% cream

Mass balance (mass into the process = mass out of the process)

$160 + x = y$

Component balance for fat (fat into the process = fat out of the process)

$0.40(160) = 0.32y$ (which says 40% of 160 kg comes in and 32% of y goes out)

$0.40(160) = 0.32(160 + x)$ (substituting our equation for $y$)

$0.32x = 64 - 51.2$

$x = 40$ kg skim milk

ii. How much cream testing 35% fat must be added to 500 kg of milk testing 4% fat to obtain cream testing 10% fat?

**Mass balance approach**

Let $x$ = kg 35% cream
$y$ = kg of 10% cream
Mass balance (mass in = mass out)
$x + 500 = y$
Component balance for fat (fat in = fat out)
$x(0.35) + 500(0.04) = y(0.10)$
$x(0.35) + 20 = (x + 500)(0.10)$
$x(0.35) + 20 = x(0.10) + 50$
$0.25x = 30$
$x = 120$ kg of 35% cream

*2.3.1.4.2 Pearson Square Approach to Solve the Problem*

i. A shortcut for two-component mass balances.
ii. Place desired percentage in the center of a rectangle.
iii. Place percentage composition of two available streams in left corners of rectangle.
iv. Cross subtract lower from higher numbers for right corners of triangle (higher number – lower number).
v. Use right corners as ratios of two streams.

**Using the Earlier Problem**

| Component | | | Mass |
|---|---|---|---|
| 35 | | 6 | |
| | 10 | | |
| 4 | | 25 | 500 |
| | | ---- | ----- |
| | | 31 | |
| 35% cream | | = | 500 × 6 = 120 kg |
| | | | --------- |
| | | | 25 |

## 2.3.2 Pasteurization

The process of pasteurization was first developed in 1864 by Louis Pasteur. In the process of pasteurizing milk, raw milk is heated rapidly to the necessary temperature, held there for a predetermined amount of time, and then quickly cooled. Milk that has been pasteurized must be kept chilled to keep it fresh (**Figure 2.12**). According to Tay and Chua (2015), **Table 2.10** summarizes the various pasteurization temperatures and their related times.

### 2.3.2.1 Methods of Pasteurization

There are two fundamental techniques: batch and continuous.

*2.3.2.1.1 Batch Method*

Batch pasteurization, also known as low-temperature long-time (LTLT) pasteurization, is similar to heating raw milk in a pot on the kitchen stove. Milk is heated to 63°C in a large tank and maintained at 63°C for 30 minutes. A jacketed vat is encircled by either flowing water, steam, or heating coils of water or steam in the vat pasteurizer used in the batch process.

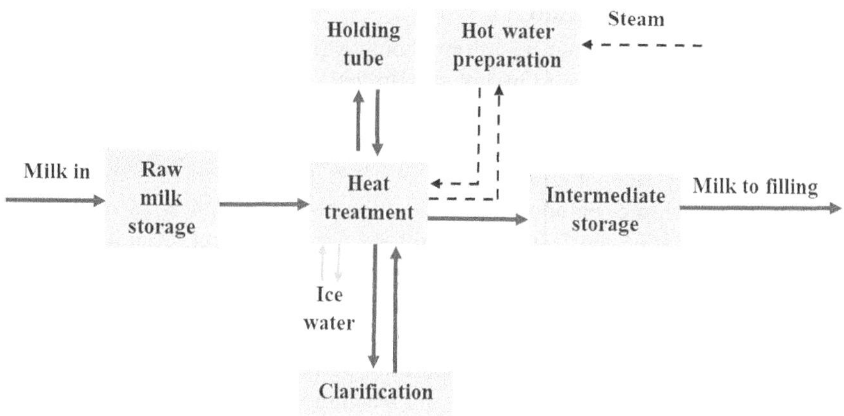


**FIGURE 2.12 Generalized block chart of the milk pasteurization process.** The figure depicts the heat treatment—pasteurization—of whole milk, e.g., market milk for sale to customers.

**TABLE 2.10**
**The Various Pasteurization Temperatures and Their Related Times**

| Temperature (°C) | Time |
|---|---|
| 63 | 30 minutes |
| 72 | 15 seconds |
| 89 | 1.0 seconds |
| 90 | 0.5 seconds |
| 94 | 0.1 seconds |
| 96 | 0.05 seconds |
| 100 | 0.01 seconds |

The milk is heated and kept in the vat while being stirred throughout the holding period. After the holding time for each particle has expired, the milk can either be chilled in the vat or withdrawn hot. To make a change, the milk can be warmed up a bit in a special heater before it goes into the container. The usage of milk in this process is quite limited, but it is employed for some milk byproducts (e.g., creams, chocolate) and special batches.

#### *2.3.2.1.2 Continuous Method*

The main benefits of the continuous process method over the vat method are time and energy savings. A high-temperature short-time (HTST) pasteurizer is used for the majority of continuous processing. HTST is the most commonly used way to pasteurize things in the industry. In 1933, the USA set a guideline for heating milk to 71.7°C for 15 seconds to kill harmful bacteria. This process has been very effective, resulting in a reduction of at least 99. 999% of the bacteria (Stabel, 2004).

A plate heat exchanger is used to carry out the heat treatment. A frame-mounted stack of corrugated stainless-steel plates makes up this piece of machinery. There are various flow patterns available. The primary function of gaskets is to create a seal at the edges of pipes so as to avoid any potential leakage. One can use hot water or vacuum steam for heating.

#### 2.3.2.2 HTST Milk Flow Overview

The regenerator portion of the pasteurizer draws cold raw milk that has been heated to 4°C from a constant-level tank. The heat released by hot pasteurized milk flowing in a counter-current direction on the opposite side of thin, stainless-steel plates warms the water to roughly 57–68°C. The raw milk travels via a positive displacement timing pump while still being delivered under suction to the rest of the HTST system (**Figure 2.13**). The heater part heats the raw milk to at least 72°C by forcing it through hot water on opposing sides of the plates. The milk goes through the holding tube under pressure and at pasteurization temperature, where it is kept for at least 16 seconds. The timing pump's speed, the holding tube's diameter and length, and the surface friction all influence the maximum velocity. Milk enters the flow diversion device (FDD) after passing the temperature sensors of an indicating thermometer and a recorder controller at the end of the holding tube. If the milk passes the recorder controller at the predetermined cut-in temperature (>72°C), the FDD takes a forward-flow configuration. If the milk does not reach the predetermined cut-in temperature, the FDD remains in its usual position with the flow diverted. The FDD's diverted flow line allows the milk that has been inadequately boiled to return to the raw milk constant-level tank. The forward-flow portion of the FDD transports properly heated milk to the pasteurized milk regenerator section, where it transfers heat to the raw product and is subsequently cooled from about 32°C to 9°C. The warm milk travels through the cooling portion, where it is cooled to 4°C or below by coolant on the opposing surfaces of the thin stainless-steel plates. The chilled, pasteurized milk is then sent to a storage tank filler for packing after passing through a vacuum breaker that is at least 12 inches above the highest raw milk in the HTST system.

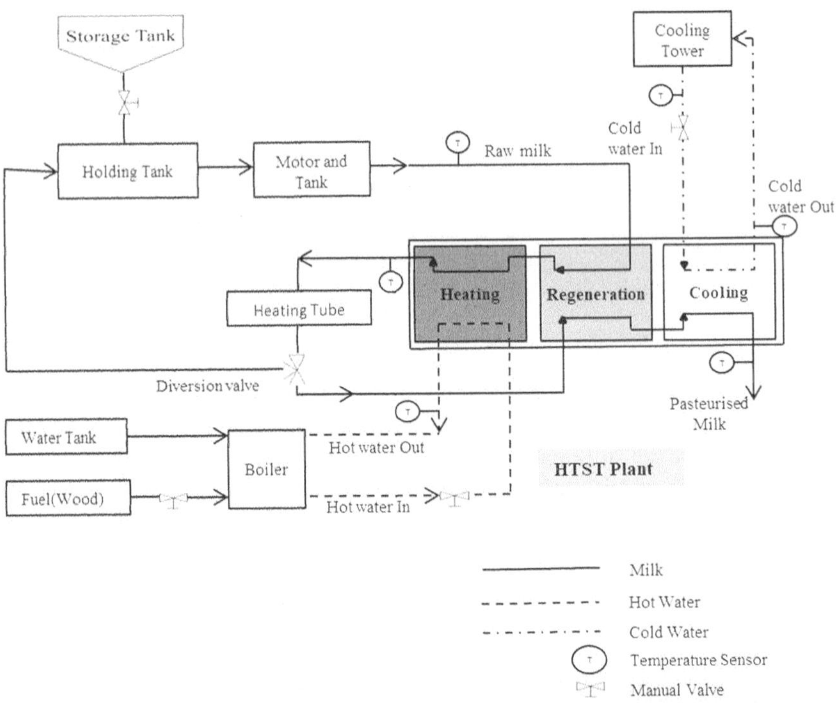


**FIGURE 2.13 Pasteurization machinery for milk using HTST and a milk flow diagram of a typical HTST pasteurizer.** HTST pasteurization is sometimes known as "continuous flow" or "flash" pasteurization. It is a contemporary technology for pasteurizing milk that is generally employed where significant volumes of milk are handled. This device provides a continuous flow of milk that is heated to 72°C for 15 seconds and then quickly cooled to 5°C or lower.

#### 2.3.2.2.1 Holding Time

A pipe can undergo one of two different types of flow while fluids are moving through it. The first type of flow is referred to as a turbulent flow, which is characterized by high velocity and the presence of eddies that move in all directions and at various angles to the usual path of flow. The second kind of flow is streamlined or laminar, which happens at low speeds and doesn't exhibit eddy currents. When determining whether a pipe will experience laminar or turbulent flow, the Reynolds number is used: Re > 4000 indicates a fully developed turbulent flow; Re < 2100 indicates laminar flow.

These flow patterns affect the estimation of holding times and the evaluation of appropriate holding tube lengths. The amount of time needed for a trace substance (salt) to pass through the holder is measured to establish the holding time. It is preferred that the milk particle moves at its fastest speed. Since a pump might not supply the same volume of milk as it does water, the findings obtained with water are transformed into the milk flow time by formulation.

#### 2.3.2.2.2 Pressure Differential

A higher pressure must be maintained on the pasteurized side of the heat exchanger for continuous pasteurization. In the case that a pin-hole leak occurs in the thin stainless-steel plates, contamination of the pasteurized milk with the raw milk is avoided by maintaining the pasteurized milk at least 1 psi higher than the raw milk in the regenerator. To maintain the pressure differential, basic systems use a timing pump; more complex systems use differential pressure controllers and back pressure flow regulators at the chilled pasteurization exit. The timing pump's position is essential for creating suction on the side of the raw regenerator and forcing milk under pressure through the pasteurized regenerator. The pressure differential is maintained by several other factors, including:

- The overflow level of the balance tank must be lower than the lowest milk passage in the regenerator.
- The only permissible connection between the balance tank and the raw regenerator is a properly mounted booster pump.
- After pasteurizing milk outlets to the vacuum breaker, there is no pump.
- The vacuum break must have a vertical rise of more than 12 inches.
- Upon shutdown, the raw regenerator drains freely into the balancing tank.

### 2.3.2.3 Basic Component of HTST Pasteurizers

#### 2.3.2.3.1 Balance Tank

A steady flow of milk is offered by the balance or constant-level tank. It has a float valve assembly that almost constantly regulates the liquid level to guarantee consistent head pressure on the product leaving the tank. The overflow level must always be below the level of the lowest milk passage in the regenerator. Thus, maintaining a higher pressure on the pasteurized side of the heat exchanger is beneficial. The exit pipe's top is set lower than the tank's lowest point, and there are downward slopes of at least 2% throughout the balance tank to prevent air from entering the pasteurizer. The balance tank (**Figure 2.14**) offers a way to recirculate milk that has been diverted or pasteurized.

#### 2.3.2.3.2 Regenerator

By using a regenerator that warms the incoming cold milk using the pasteurized milk's heat content, heating and cooling energy can be conserved. This formula can be used to determine its effectiveness:

% regeneration = temp. increase due to increasing regenerator/total temp.

For example, cold milk enters the system at 4°C after regeneration at 65°C, and a final temperature of 72°C would have 89.7% regeneration:

$$\frac{65-4}{72-4}=89.7$$

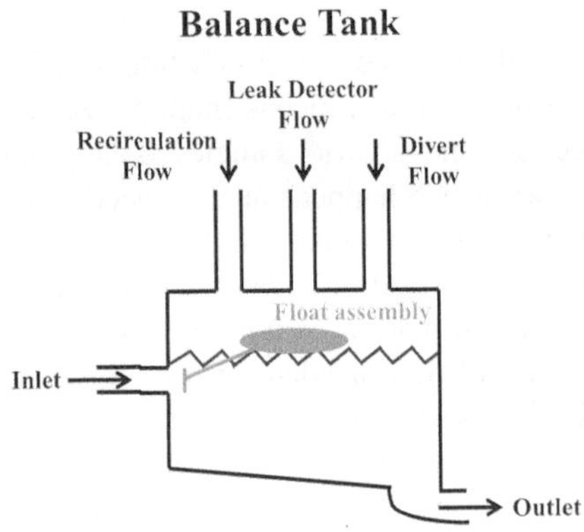


**FIGURE 2.14 Balance tank.** A balance tank is a container that keeps the product at the same level above a pump entrance and usually has a sensor to help keep the tank full.

#### 2.3.2.3.3 *Timing Pump*

The timing pump pushes milk under pressure through the pasteurized regenerator while drawing product through the raw regenerator. It controls how quickly fluid moves through the holding tube. To provide the shortest holding time in the holding tubes, there must be a positive displacement pump with a variable speed drive that can be legally sealed at the maximum rate. Additionally, it must be "fail-safe" and interwired to only function when the FDD is entirely forward or diverted. It is also possible to employ a centrifugal pump equipped with a magnetic flow meter and controller.

#### 2.3.2.3.4 *Holding Tube*

To prevent air entrapment and ensure that nothing moves more quickly at air pocket limits, the slope must be upwards of 1/4 inches per feet in the direction of flow.

#### 2.3.2.3.5 *Indicating Thermometer*

The indicating thermometer is intended to measure temperatures most precisely. The safety thermal limit recorder (STLR) is set to this official temperature. The probe should be placed as close to the STLR probe as practicable, and it shouldn't be more than 18 inches upstream of the flow diverter.

#### 2.3.2.3.6 *Recorder controller (STLR)*

The milk's temperature and the time of day are both recorded by the STLR. It provides electricity to the FDD during forward flow and monitors, regulates, and records the FDD's position. There are controls that are electronic and pneumatic. The operator must record the following information: date, shift, equipment, ID, product, and amount; thermometer temperature; cleaning cycles; cut-in and cut-out temperatures; any connections for unexpected circumstances; and his or her signature.

#### 2.3.2.3.7 *Flow Diversion Device (FDD)*

This is situated at the downstream end of the upward-sloping holding tube and is also known as the flow diversion valve (FDV). It functions essentially as a three-way valve that opens to forward flow when the temperature reaches 72°C. This step requires power. The valve returns to its usual position and directs milk back to the balance tank at temperatures lower than 72°C. It's vital to remember that the FDD operates at the end of the holding period based on the recorded temperature, not time. Two different FDD types exist:

**Single stem:** An older valve system with a single stem has the drawback that it cannot be cleaned in place.

**Dual stem:** Two valves connected in sequence for more fail-safe mechanisms. This FDD is better suited for automation and can be cleaned on the spot.

##### *2.3.2.3.8 Vacuum breaker*

There is a vacuum breaker that releases ambient pressure at the pasteurized product discharge. It needs to be placed more than 12 inches above the raw product's highest point in the system. It ensures nothing farther downstream will result in a vacuum on the pasteurized side.

#### 2.3.2.4 Auxiliary Equipment

##### *2.3.2.4.1 Booster Pump*

The raw regenerator for the balance tank receives raw milk using a centrifugal "stuffing" pump. It needs to be utilized with a pressure differential controlling device and can only work when the timing pump is running, the regenerator is getting the right pressures, and the system is flowing forward.

##### *2.3.2.4.2 Homogenizer*

One option is to use the homogenizer as a timing pump. If not, it cannot increase flow because it is not a positive pressure pump. The homogenizer's speed must be higher than the timing pump's flow rate to ensure free circulation from the outlet to the intake.

##### *2.3.2.4.3 Magnetic Flow Meter and Centrifugal Pump Arrangements*

The flow rate can be determined using magnetic flow meters. These consist mainly of a small, 25 cm long tube that is encased in a housing, inside of which are coils that produce a magnetic field. Milk induces a voltage as it moves through the magnetic field, and the signal that is produced is inversely proportional to the speed. In order to use the magnetic flow meter in HTST pasteurizing systems, it has primarily been applied to the dairy industry's need to replace positive displacement timing pumps as the metering device, where with certain products, the timing pump rotors reportedly wear out in a relatively short period. When in use, the magnetic flow meter sends an electrical signal to the flow controller, which compares the actual flow to the flow rate set by the operator to determine how much flow is there. The magnetic flow meter continuously measures the flow rate, so if the real flow for any reason exceeds the predetermined flow rate, it will alert the electronic controller. The flow diversion device is inserted into the diverted flow if the flow rate is exceeded for any reason. At this point, a key distinction from the typical HTST system (with timing pump) becomes apparent. This system is capable of being run at a flow rate higher than (or a residence time lower than) the permitted maximum. It will never be in forward flow, only in diverted flow.

It is also feasible to use a centrifugal pump instead of a positive displacement metering pump with an AC variable frequency motor control drive in an HTST pasteurizer. Instead of using a control valve in this system, the magnetic flow meter's signal is sent to the AC variable frequency control, which changes the centrifugal pump's speed. The product's flow rate through the system and how long it stays in the holding tube are then controlled by the pump.

### 2.3.3 UHT Processing

The basic steps of UHT milk processing are illustrated in **Figure 2.15**.

The two main UHT treatments are as follows:

i. Direct heating
ii. Indirect heating

#### 2.3.3.1 Direct Heating Systems

By coming into direct touch with potable or culinary-grade steam, the product gets heated. Direct heating has the main benefit of holding the product at an elevated temperature for a shorter amount of time (**Figure 2.16**). As a result, less harm will be done to a heat-sensitive product like milk (Deeth, 2021; Deeth & Lewis, 2017).

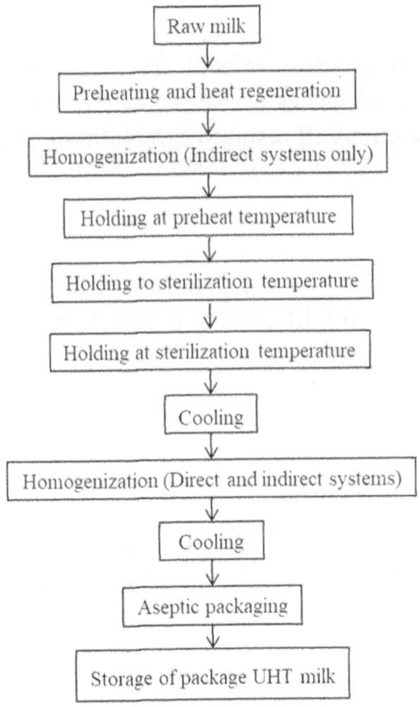


**FIGURE 2.15 Flow diagram of UHT milk processing.** This technique heats milk to at least 135°C for a few seconds and then promptly cools it to ambient temperature.

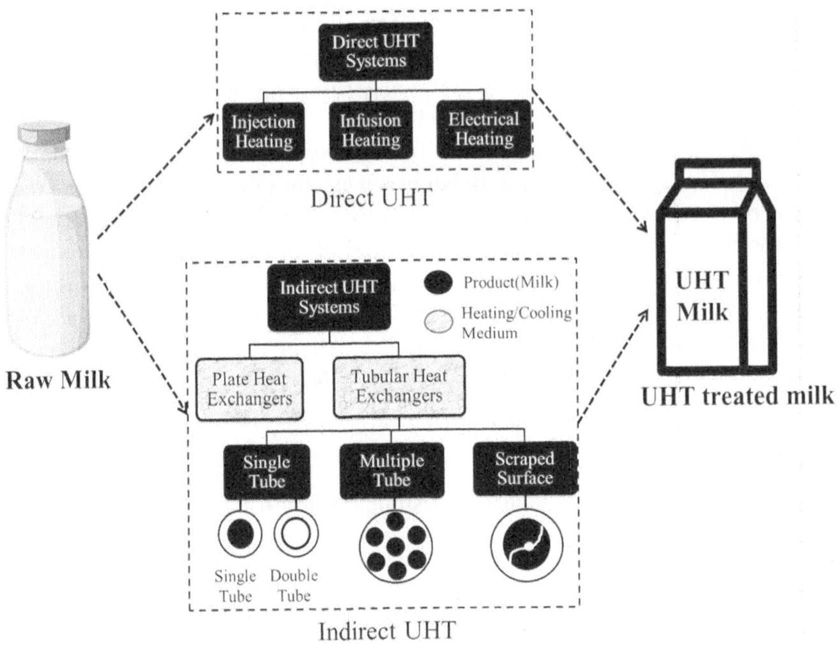


**FIGURE 2.16 Illustration of UHT milk processing.** UHT of milk includes heating for 1–8 seconds at 135–150°C. In the case of a direct heating system, the products are heated by direct contact with steam of potable or culinary quality, which can be obtained from potable water. In the case of indirect heating systems, the heating medium and product are not in direct contact but are separated by the equipment contact surface.

There are two ways of direct heating (please see schematic diagrams of the equipment):

- Injection
- Infusion

### 2.3.3.2 Injection

A steam injector quickly raises the temperature of a liquid by injecting high-pressure steam into it (**Figure 2.17**). To eliminate water equal to the volume of condensed steam used after holding, the product is flash-cooled in a vacuum. This technique only works with certain compounds; however, it allows for quick heating, cooling, and volatile removal. It consumes a lot of energy, and when the product comes into contact with heated machinery, flavor harm is a possibility.

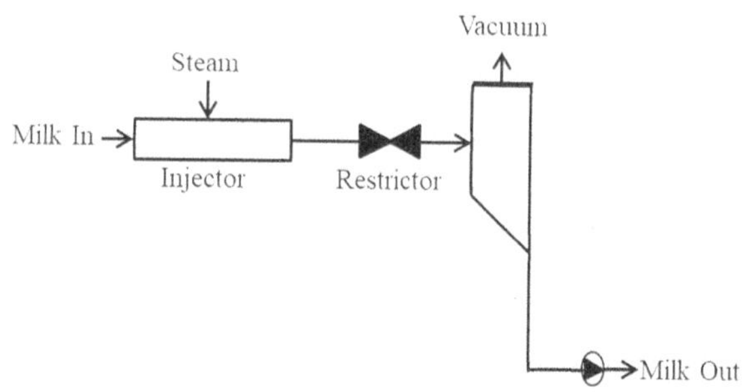


FIGURE 2.17 **Schematic diagram of an injection direct heating system.**

### 2.3.3.3 Infusion

A distributing nozzle pumps the liquid product stream into a steam chamber at high pressure. This system is distinguished by a big steam volume and a small product volume that are dispersed over a sizable amount of product surface area (**Figure 2.18**). Pressure is used to precisely regulate the product's temperature.

Using plate or tube heat exchangers in combination with flash cooling in a vacuum chamber can extend the holding time.

This approach provides the following benefits:

- Instantaneous heating and rapid cooling
- No localized overheating or burn-on
- Suitable for low- and high-viscosity products

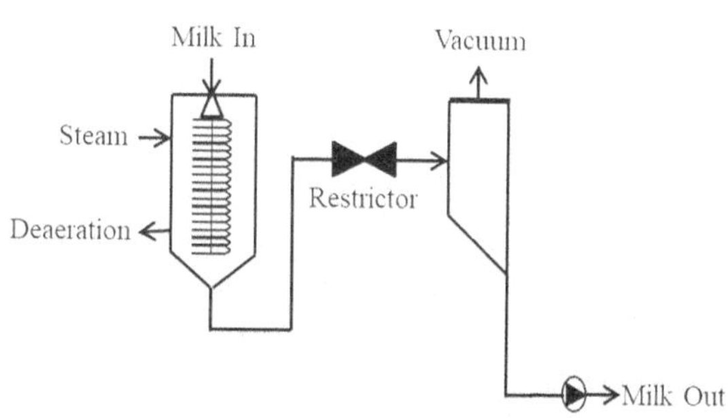


FIGURE 2.18 **Schematic diagram of an infusion direct heating system.**

#### 2.3.3.4 Indirect Heating Systems

Equipment contact surfaces stand between the product and the heating medium to prevent direct contact. Different types of heat exchangers can be used:

- Plate
- Tubular
- Scraped surface

#### 2.3.3.5 Plate Heat Exchangers

Similar to those used in HTST, gaskets limit operating pressures. Low liquid velocities may result in burn-on and uneven heating. This approach uses less floor space, is simple to check, and permits possible regeneration.

#### 2.3.3.6 Tubular Heat Exchangers

There are several types:

- Shell and tube
- Shell and coil
- Double tube
- Triple tube

These tubular heat exchangers all involve fewer seals than plates do. Increased pressures, higher flow rates, and higher temperatures are all made possible by this. The heating is more even, but inspection is challenging.

#### 2.3.3.7 Scraped-Surface Heat Exchangers

A spinning knife scrapes the product's sidewalls as it passes through a jacketed tube that houses the heating medium. This technique can be customized for various goods by altering the rotor's shape. It is suitable for viscous fluids with particles (1 cm), such as fruit sauces. Larger particles pose a problem since their prolonged processing periods would call for longer, useless holding sections. This could lead to damaged solids and excessive sauce processing (Deeth, 2021; Deeth & Lewis, 2017).

### 2.3.4 Homogenization

The process of milk's fat globules being broken down to a small enough size to prevent the creation of a cream layer is known as homogenization. A homogenizer is an instrument that breaks up milk fat globules. The choice of homogenization pressure is a crucial stage in the manufacturing of pasteurized milk to preserve and enhance the sensory quality and stability of the milk. In homogenization, milk is pumped at high pressure through a valve to reduce the size of milk fat globules. An increase in surface area results from the process that reduces fat globules to tiny particles (between 3.5 and 1 μm). Then, casein, a milk protein, coats the freshly formed surface of the fat globules. The homogenization pressure reduces the size of the fat globules, which decreases the phenomenon of fat floating and increases milk stability (D'Incecco et al., 2018). Additionally, dairy products' physicochemical characteristics are impacted by homogenization (**Figure 2.19**), which also changes the texture and flavor of the products (Sfakianakis & Tzia, 2014). The fundamental goal of homogenizing pasteurized milk is to evenly distribute its components, hence raising milk's quality and stability. Through homogenization, milk quality, and stability can be improved through two mechanisms: the reduction of fat globule size and the interaction of the fat with the protein matrix (**Figure 2.19**) (Sodini et al., 2004).

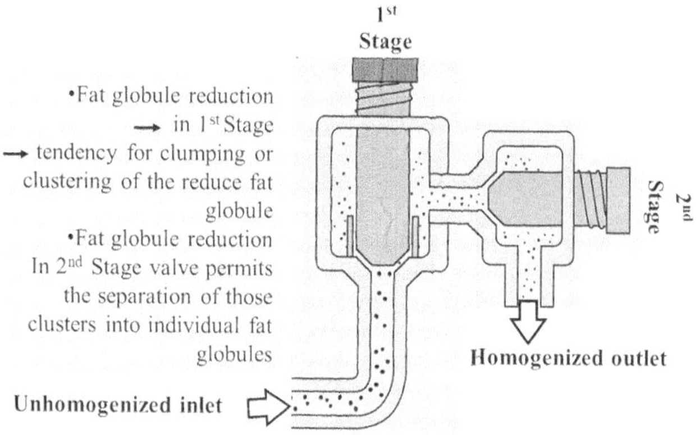


**FIGURE 2.19 Diagram of a homogenizer (breakdown of milk fat globules).** The overall homogenization pressure is measured before the first stage, P1, and the homogenization pressure in the second stage is measured before the second stage, P2. The two-stage approach is often used to get the best homogenization/efficiency. When P2/P1 = 0.2, the best results are obtained. The pressure in the first stage is roughly 2000–2500 psi, while the pressure in the second stage is 500–1000 psi. The temperature is 120°F. In the first stage, small fat particles come together to form groups, which is called post clumping.

#### 2.3.4.1 Types of Homogenization

The mechanical procedure known as homogenization minimizes the size of the fat globules by applying pressure and lessening the separation of the product's creamy portion. Because milk lipase and many microbial lipases are rendered inactive at 45°C (113°F), the homogenization temperature must be higher than this (Olorunnisomo et al., 2014). However, at 50°C, pressure begins to affect the size and distribution of fat globules. Due to the durability of the fat particle membrane, no modifications take place below this temperature.

During the high-pressure pumping of milk, fat globules begin to separate. The homogenizer is single-stage if the pressure drop occurs through a single valve and is suited for low-fat or high-viscosity products like milk and sour cream. Dual-stage homogenizers, on the other hand, are homogenizers that reduce fat particle size in two steps. The second step is intended to break apart the clusters of fat globules created in the first stage to prevent creaming in milk. The first-stage pressure reduces the milk fat globule diameter size to less than 1 m. High fat content, high solids content, or goods where low viscosity is sought might all benefit from dual-stage processing (Thompson et al., 2009). The second stage of dual-stage homogenization increases the free fatty acid concentration and denaturation of whey proteins (**Figure 2.19**) (Thompson et al., 2009).

#### 2.3.4.2 Effects of Homogenization on Milk

##### *2.3.4.2.1 Effects on Fat*

Homogenization enhances the stability of milk fat by lowering the size of milk fat globules (**Figure 2.20 and 2.21**).

##### *2.3.4.2.2 Effect on Microorganisms*

Homogenization is helpful for inactivating harmful bacteriophages and spoilage microorganisms (**Table 2.11**).

The order of microorganism's lethality after high-pressure treatment (>200 Mpa) is: Gram-negative bacteria > Gram-positive bacteria > Yeast >Mold (Massoud et al., 2016).

##### *2.3.4.2.3 Effect on Proteins*

Casein micelles are broken down into tiny pieces during high-pressure homogenization, which also increases calcium phosphate and casein content in the serum phase.

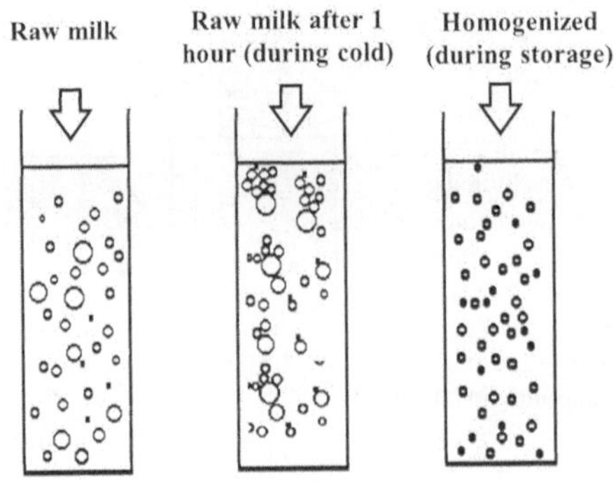


**FIGURE 2.20 Diagram of raw milk, cold raw milk after 1 hour, and homogenized milk during storage.** Appearance of fat globules in raw milk, cold raw milk, and homogenized milk during the storage period.

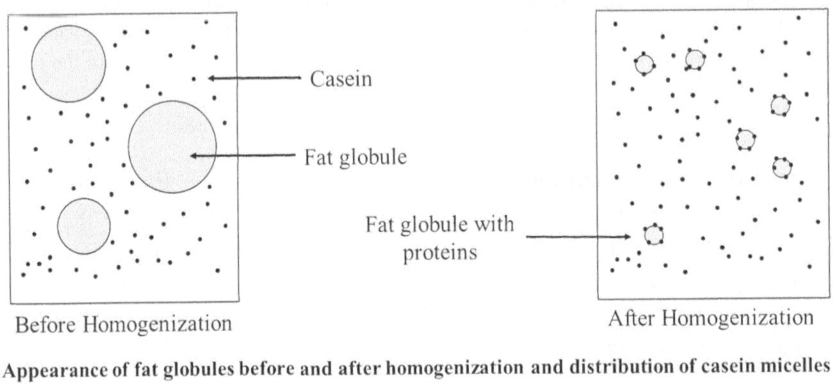


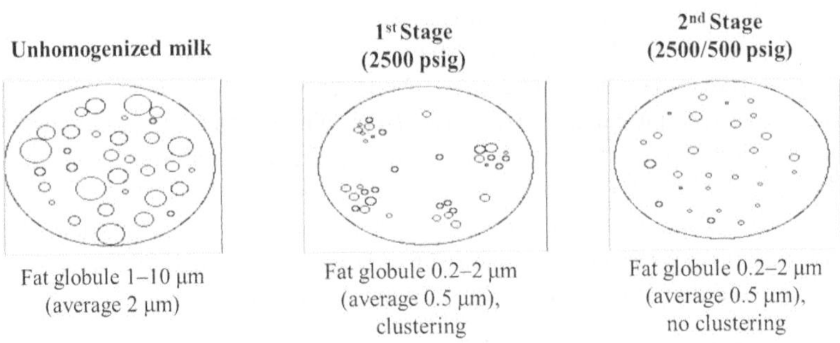


**FIGURE 2.21 Effect of homogenization on milk.** The effects of two-stage homogenization on fat globule size distribution, as observed using a light microscope, are depicted in the diagram.

**TABLE 2.11**
**The Effects of Different Pressures on Microorganisms**

| Pressure (Mpa) | Structural and functional changes in microorganisms |
|---|---|
| 50 | Inhibition of protein synthesis, ribosomes decreasing |
| 100 | Reversible protein denaturation, squeezing of gas vacuoles |
| 200 | Damage of cell membrane, sign of cell contents leakage |
| 300 | Irreversible protein denaturation, leakage of cell contents |

#### *2.3.4.2.4 Effect on Sensory Properties of Dairy Products*

The quality of dairy products like cheese and yogurt is increased by high-pressure homogenized milk's improved sensory features, including its whiter color, superior flavor, viscosity, and stability (Patrignani et al., 2007). Due to the significant changes in the milk, homogenization also enhances the probiotic bacteria's capacity to survive during refrigeration in dairy products, particularly yogurt.

### 2.3.4.3 Theories

The decrease in size of the fat globules during homogenization is most likely explained by a mixture of the two ideas of turbulence and cavitation.

**Turbulence:** The homogenizer valve creates severe turbulent eddies that are the same size as the typical globule diameter as energy is lost in the liquid passing by it. Thus, these eddies currents tear apart globules, reducing their average size.

**Cavitation:** Considerable pressure drop with a charge of the velocity of the fluid. Because its vapor pressure is reached, liquid cavitates. Cavitation generates further eddies that would produce disruption of the fat globules. The liquid has a large kinetic energy due to its high velocity, which is quickly disrupted. Velocity rises as pressure increases. This energy is dissipated, resulting in a high energy density (energy per volume and time). The energy density determines the final diameter.

In simple terms, the homogenization variables include the type of valve pressure (either single or two-stage), the amount of fat, the type of surfactant, and the viscosity temperature. Additionally, we should also think about the size of the droplets (smaller droplets are harder to break apart) and the logarithmic diameter, which decreases in a straight line as the logarithm of pressure decreases and then levels off at higher pressures.

### 2.3.4.4 Advantages of Homogenization

- No formation of cream layer/plug.
- Fat will not churn.
- Thick body, rich appearance, and more full-bodied flavor.
- Produces soft curd, easily digestible.
- Less susceptibility to oxidation.
- Better stability of cultured milk products.

### 2.3.4.5 Disadvantages

- Increased cost of production.
- Fat from returned homogenized milk is difficult to salvage.
- Sediment is greater.
- May produce rancidity if temperature is not kept adequately high.

## 2.4 MICROORGANISMS IN MILK AND DAIRY FOODS

Dairy microbiology is an applied biological science that deals with microorganisms related to the dairy industry. The composition of microorganisms in milk is complex and diverse. These microorganisms can participate in the fermentation or the spoilage of milk and dairy products, which affects their food quality, flavor, nutrition, function, safety, and shelf life.

The families in the suborder Eubacteriineae that are studied by the dairy microbiologist include the following:

i. Lactobacteriaceae
ii. Micrococcaceae

iii. Enterobacteriaceae
iv. Pseudomonadaceae
v. Bacillaceae
vi. Achromobacteriaceae
vii. Bacteriaceae
viii. Corynebacteriaceae
ix. Parvobacteriaceae

### 2.4.1 Family: Lactobacillaceae (Lactic Acid Producing Bacteria)

Lactic acid was discovered in sour milk by the Swedish chemist Scheele in 1782. The microorganisms of this family are divided into two groups:

#### Homofermentative Group

The microorganisms that produce primarily lactic acid from fermentable carbohydrates are known as homofermentative.

#### Heterofermentative Group

The microorganisms that produce acetic acid, glycerol, ethanol, carbon dioxide, and other substances are known as heterofermentative group. They also produce lactic acid.

#### Importance

i. Lactic acid bacteria are very important in the field of applied microbiology. These things are very important to make lactic acid, pickles, and silage.
ii. In the dairy industry, they are essential in the production of fermented milk (buttermilk), cheese, and culture-containing butter.
iii. Under certain circumstances, various species of lactic acid bacteria are considered spoilage agents, for example in the souring of market milk or cream and the production of discoloration in cheddar cheese.

#### 2.4.1.1 Genus: *Streptococcus*

The word "Streptococcus" is derived from the Greek word "*Streptos*" meaning flexible, and "*Kokkos*" meaning seed or grain. All types of *Streptococcus* bacteria are round or oval and have a positive reaction to the Gram stain. They usually form chains or pairs. They are also immobile and do not form spores. Most streptococci can live in environments with or without oxygen, but there are certain strains that need carbon dioxide to grow. In simple terms, they get energy from chemical processes and break down carbohydrates to make lactic and other acids. They need a variety of nutrients, and they are catalase-negative (Tagg et al., 2011). They prefer mild temperatures (thermophilic) and can tolerate only limited quantities of salt (less than 2% NaCl). *S. salivarius* subsp. *Thermophilus* grows at 45°C but not at 10°C and grows in the presence of 2.5% NaCl but not at 4%.

Certain types of microorganisms can be found on the skin, while others can be detected in foods like milk and dairy products (Hardie, 1996).

Some strains of streptococci are pathogenic to humans, such as *S. pneumoniae*, *S. pyogenes*, and *S. agalactiae*. *S. salivarius* subsp. *Thermophilus* has differentiated itself from other streptococci and occupies a well-defined place in the ecological niche of milk (Bintsis, 2018). This species is often used as a starter culture for making fermented foods because it has several helpful abilities. These abilities include breaking down sugars and proteins, making a substance called exopolysaccharide, and creating flavors (Bintsis, 2018).

Generally, the streptococci are divided into four groups (**Figure 2.22**).

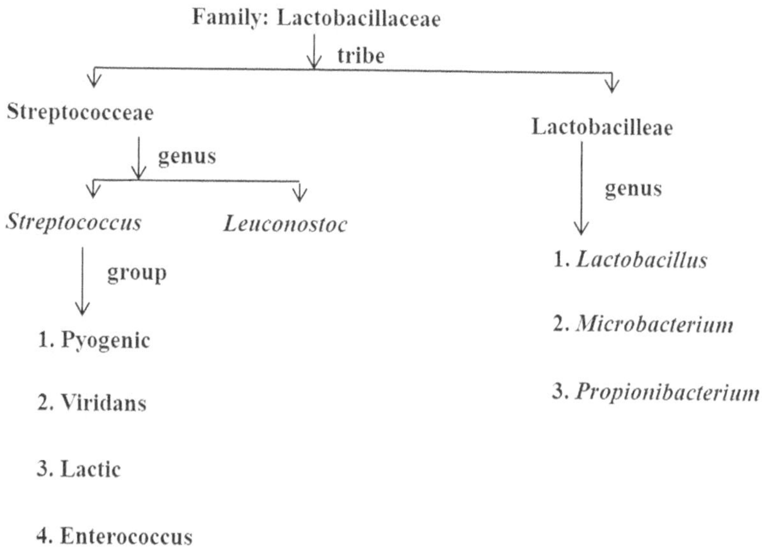


FIGURE 2.22 **Overview of the Lactobacteriaceae family.**

## GROUP 1: PYOGENIC STREPTOCOCCI

The representative organisms of the pyogenic group are:

i. *Streptococcus pyogenes*
ii. *Streptococcus agalactiae*

## SIGNIFICANCE

***Streptococcus agalactiae*:** Can be isolated from the milk and udders of animals affected with mastitis. This species is not known to be pathogenic to humans.

## GROUP 2: VIRIDAN STREPTOCOCCI

The representative organisms of this group are:

i. *Streptococcus thermophilus*
ii. *Streptococcus bovis*

## SIGNIFICANCE

*Streptococcus thermophilus* is a type of bacteria that plays a significant role in making cheese and fermented milk like yogurt and dahi.

## GROUP 3: LACTIC STREPTOCOCCI

Some of the most widely known dairy bacteria are found in this group.

i. *Streptococcus lactis*
ii. *Streptococcus cremoris*

## SIGNIFICANCE

### *Streptococcus lactis*

- It may be considered either useful or harmful in the dairy industry. It is essential in the manufacture of cheese and fermented milk. It is the master organism in the dairy industry.

### *Streptococcus cremoris*

- It is used in "starter cultures" (media containing desirable bacteria in good growing condition for the manufacture of milk products and it is a portion of milk or skim milk)
- *Streptococcus cremoris* will not grow in synthetic medium and citrate, but *Streptococcus lactis* grows under this condition.
- Sometimes this organism may cause ropiness in milk, although the ability to do so is easily lost.
- *Streptococcus cremoris* has many properties in common with *Streptococcus lactis.*

### 2.4.1.2 Genus: *Enterococcus*

Enterococci are Gram-positive, round bacteria that can be found singles, in pairs, or in groups. They can survive with or without oxygen (facultative anaerobes) (Devriese & Pot, 1995). They do not form spores, are mobile, and have a homofermentative metabolism, in which the end product of glucose fermentation via the glycolytic pathway is L-lactic acid. They are catalase-negative, but some strains produce a pseudocatalase and need a lot of nutrients (Devriese & Pot, 1995).

After pasteurization, enterococci can still be present in numerous cheeses, unlike lactococci. Most people think that enterococci are present because the processing is not done in a clean and hygienic way. Some strains have properties that make them useful for technology, but people are not aware of using them because they are also used to check if food is contaminated with feces. Some species, such as *E. faecalis*, are promiscuous and can easily acquire resistance to antibiotics such as vancomycin from plasmids or transposons.

***Streptococcus fecalis*:** It is found in the intestinal tract of humans and animals, as well as raw milk, pasteurized milk, and cheese. It is used as a starter culture by manufacturers of cheddar cheese.

***Streptococcus liquefaciens*:** It is also found in milk and milk products. It coagulates milk and peptonizes the casein at relatively low acidity (sweet curdling) without the presence of lactic acid. It has been found to produce a bitter flavor in milk and soft cheese.

***Streptococcus durans*:** It have been isolated from cow feces, udders, soil, and water. The species are not regarded as pathogenic for humans.

### 2.4.1.3 Genus: *Lactococcus*

Bacteria of the genus *Lactococcus* are characterized by being Gram-positive cocci that occur singly, in pairs, or in a chain; are non-spore-forming, non-motile, facultatively anaerobic, non-β-hemolytic, and catalase negative; and grow at 10°C and at 40°C, but not at 45°C. They produce L-lactic acid when they break down glucose using a metabolic process called fermentation (Carr et al., 2002).

This genus consists of 17 different types of species, including *Lc. Lactis* (subspecies *cremoris, lactis, hordniae*, and *tructae), Lc. Garvieae, Lc. Plantarum, Lc. Raffinolactis, Lc. Piscium, Lc. Chungangensis, Lc. Fujiensis, Lc. Taiwanensis, Lc. Hircilactis, Lc. Nasutitermitis, Lc. urnetii, Lc. Formosensis, Lc. Reticulitismitis, Lc. Laudensis, Lc. Termiticola*, and *Lc. Allomyrinae* (Vinderola et al., 2019). *Lactococcus lactis* is the type of organism usually found in unpasteurized milk and dairy foods (Vinderola et al., 2019). When manufacturing dairy products, it is typical to use lactococci, known for their beneficial urnetiies, to initiate the fermentation procedure (Carr et al., 2002). For example, *Lc. Lactis* subsp. *Lactis* and *Lc. Lactis* subsp. *Cremoris* are the main lactococci used as starter cultures for different cheeses (Lahtinen et al., 2011). The reason these lactococci are selected is due to their capacity to maintain stability during food processing, withstand harmful bacteria, and produce specific substances derived from amino acid degradation (Lahtinen et al., 2011).

#### 2.4.1.4 Genus: *Leuconostoc*

*Leuconostoc* are characterized as Gram-positive cocci with irregular morphology that may be elongated or elliptical. Most types of bacteria appear in liquid as either single round cells, pairs of cells, or groups of cells in a short line (Bintsis, 2018). However, cell morphology can vary depending on growth conditions: when bacteria grow in a glucose medium or in a solid medium, they are elongated, whereas most strains form ovoid cells when they grow in milk (Bintsis, 2018).

They are heterofermentative and produce D-lactate, ethanol, $CO_2$, and small amounts of acetate from glucose metabolism via the phosphoketolase pathway (Bintsis, 2018). Additional methods of breaking down food and generating substances involve converting citrate into diacetyl and acetoin, as well as producing dextrans using sucrose (Bintsis, 2018).

*Leuconostoc* are a type of microorganism that need a lot of different nutrients to survive. They can be found in plants, dairy products, and foods that have been fermented (Dellaglio et al., 1995). *Leuconostoc* are a type of microorganism that need a lot of different nutrients to survive. They can be found in plants, dairy products, and foods that have been fermented. *Leuconostoc mesenteroides* subsp. *Cremoris* and *Ln. paramesenteroides* are less frequently detected in milk, probably due to their slow growth under psychrotrophic conditions (Dellaglio et al., 1995).

*Leuconostoc* are bacteria that have a significant effect on altering the flavor, consistency, and overall quality of food items such as milk, butter, and cheese. (Dellaglio et al., 1995). The texture of certain cheeses can sometimes be altered, and air holes may form due to the production of carbon dioxide by bacteria present in them. However, this can also result in the formation of "eyes" within the cheese. (Dellaglio et al., 1995). Furthermore, *Leuconostoc* are utilized to enhance flavor in combinations of other starter cultures such as *Ln. mesenteroides* subsp. *Dextranicum* and *Ln. mesenteroides* subsp. *Cremoris* (Carr et al., 2002). Some strains also convert citrate to diacetyl and acetoin, adding to dairy products' familiar flavor and smell. (Dellaglio et al., 1995).

## USES

These two bacteria are commonly used in the manufacture of sour cream, buttermilk, and butter. In this regard, the formation of desirable flavor substances from citric acid fermentation is their important function. For this reason, these organisms are sometimes called "aroma bacteria." Biacetyl is the most important of the aroma substances formed.

#### 2.4.1.5 Genus: *Lactobacillus*

The genus *Lactobacillus* comprises a large number of different species (261 species in March 2020) (Zheng et al., 2020) with a relatively high degree of diversity (Samedi & Charles, 2019). Technologically and commercially, *L. acidophilus*, *L. casei*, *L. delbrueckii*, *L. plantarum*, *L. rhamnosus*, and *L. salivarius* are the most important species (Samedi & Charles, 2019). The genus *Lactobacillus* has recently been reclassified into 25 distinct groups according to genomic phylogeny and ecological and metabolic characteristics (Zheng et al., 2020). Zheng et al. (2020) actually proposed 23 new genera, named *Holzapfelia*, *Amylolactobacillus*, *Bombilactobacillus*, *Companilactobacillus*, *Lapidilactobacillus*, *Agrilactobacillus*, *Schleiferilactobacillus*, *Loigolactobacilus*, *Lacticaseibacillus*, *Latilactobacillus*, *Dellaglioa*, *Liquorilactobacillus*, *Ligilactobacillus*, *Lactiplantibacillus*, *Paucilactobacillus*, *Limosilactobacillus*, *Fructilactobacillus*, *Acetilactobacillus*, *Apilactobacillus*, *Levilactobacillus*, *Secundilactobacillus*, and *Lentilactobacillus*. The generic term "lactobacilli" is used to describe all organisms that are classified as Lactobacillaceae.

Lactobacilli are the most common bacteria found in foods like yogurt and cheese that have been fermented. These foods, when consumed, collaborate with the bacteria present in the GIT. Research on traditional raw milk cheeses has found that lactobacilli are the main type of bacteria that grow and develop as the cheese ripens.

Lactobacilli are characterized by being Gram-positive, non-spore-forming, catalase-negative bacilli or coccobacilli (Coelho et al., 2022). They are strictly fermentative, aerotolerant, or anaerobic, and have complex nutrient requirements (e.g., for carbohydrates, amino acids, peptides, fatty acid esters, salts, nucleic acid derivatives, and vitamins). With glucose as a carbon source, lactobacilli can be homofermentative and produce more than 85% lactic acid or heterofermentative and produce lactic acid, $CO_2$, ethanol, and/or acetic acid in equimolar amounts (Hammes & Vogel, 1995). Lactobacilli are therefore classified into three groups based on their fermentation characteristics (Hammes & Vogel, 1995).

**Group I:** Obligate homofermentative lactobacilli. Hexoses are almost exclusively (>85%) fermented to lactic acid via the Embden–Meyerhof–Parnas pathway (EMP). The organisms have fructose 1,6-bisphosphate aldolase but no phosphoketolase, and thus pentoses and gluconate are not fermented. This group includes the species *L. acidophilus*, *L. delbrueckii*, and *L. salivarius*.

**Group II:** Facultative heterofermentative lactobacilli. Hexoses are mostly turned into lactic acid through the EMP pathway. The organisms have two enzymes, aldolase and phosphoketolase, which allow them to break down both hexoses and pentoses through fermentation. The presence of glucose inhibits the functioning of enzymes in the phosphogluconate pathway. This group has several types of lactobacilli (e.g., *L. casei*, *L. paracasei*, *L. plantarum*, and *L. curvatus*) in matured cheese.

**Group III:** Obligate heterofermentative lactobacilli. They have phosphoketolase but not aldolase and therefore ferment sugars in a heterofermentative manner. Hexoses are fermented via the phosphogluconate pathway, producing lactate, ethanol (acetic acid), and $CO_2$ in equimolar amounts. Pentoses enter this pathway and can also be fermented.

The inclusion of numerous lactobacilli in food preparation and preservation enhances its sourness, taste, texture, and nutritional value, ensuring lasting freshness. Their natural habitat is very diverse, as these bacteria are found in virtually all environments where carbohydrates are available. This includes things like food, plants, and wastewater. In addition, they can be located in both humans and animals, including areas like the mouth, genitals, and digestive system (Claesson et al., 2007). Numerous organisms can be found inhabiting the intestines of humans and animals without posing any threat to their well-being. Some types of lactobacilli are considered probiotics because they have a positive impact on the health of the host (Claesson et al., 2007).

## SIGNIFICANCE

They produce a considerable amount of lactic acid from fermentable carbohydrates, and since these organisms are not easily killed by the acid, they are known as "aceduric."

***Lactobacillus casei*:** It is a common organism in raw milk and is important in the ripening of cheese and the natural souring of milk and cream.

***Lactobacillus acidophilus*:** Certain strains of lactobacillus acidophilus have been used in the preparation of fermented milk. It can be implanted in the intestinal tract of man and has been used in the treatment of certain intestinal disorders.

## MISCELLANEOUS LACTOBACILLI

***Lactobacillus thermophilus*:** It may cause difficulty in obtaining a satisfactory reduction of bacterial numbers during pasteurization of milk by the holding method.

***Lactobacillus helveticus*:** It is used in starter cultures in the manufacture of Swiss cheese.
***Lactobacillus bulgaricus*:** It is used in the manufacture of Swiss cheese, fermented milk, and buttermilk.

#### 2.4.1.6 Genus: *Microbacterium*

Microbacteria are small, Gram-positive, non-motile, asporogenic, rod-shaped organisms. They thrive on the media's surface since they are aerobic. This organism produces acid in milk, but coagulation is variable. The optimum growth temperature is 30°C and has a range of 15 to 35°C. Some strains of microbacterium survive 80 to 85°C for 10 minutes. The microbacteriae is very resistant to heat and may be the cause of high bacterial counts in pasteurized milk and milk powder.

#### 2.4.1.7 Genus: *Propionibacterium*

**Species:** *Propionibacterium shermanii, Propionibacterium petersonii.*

They are Gram (+), non-motile, asporogenic, coccobacillary organisms that ferment the lactic acid in cheese to propionic and acetic acids and carbon dioxide. Propionibacteria are essentially anaerobic organisms and require supplements of yeast extract and fermentable carbon compounds for optimum growth. They have an optimum temperature of 30°C with a range of 15–45°C. *Propionibacteria shermanii* and *Propionibacteriua petersonii* are used in starter cultures for the manufacture of Swiss cheese.

### 2.4.2 Family: Micrococcaceae

Bacteria included in this family are spherical or elliptical cells that divide into two or three planes and occur singly or in pairs, packets, or tetrads. They are non-motile, asporogenic, and Gram-positive. They grow at 22°C, and many of them grow best at 30–31°C.

#### 2.4.2.1 Genus: *Micrococcus*

The name is derived from the Greek word "*Micros*" meaning small and "*Kokkos*" which means seed or grain; hence, *Micrococcus* means small seeds. They are spherical cells arranged in irregular masses but never in long chains. Some types of these organisms are found in the lactiferous ducts of the cow's mammary glands and are present in milk obtained from the udder under sterile conditions. Contaminated equipment may be the main source of micrococci in milk. Many species of micrococci are heat resistant and survive at 63°C for 30 minutes.

- There are two clearly defined groups: one produces an acid curd in litmus milk, ferments lactose, grows at 37°C fails to survive at 65°C for 30 minutes, and may be considered *Micrococcus luteus.*
- The other acidifies litmus milk slowly and fails to grow at 37°C and survive at 65°C for 30 minutes and may be considered *Micrococcus varians.*
- Micrococci are found to cause the thickening of sweetened condensed milk and they may be important organisms due to their outbreaks in pasteurizing plants.
- *Micrococcus pyogenes* var. *aureus* often produces a heat-stable toxin. Although ingestion of this toxin is rarely fatal, the symptoms produced are vomiting, distressing diarrhea, and abdominal pains, with a duration generally not more than 1 day.
- *Micrococcus pyogenes* var. *aureus* and *Micrococcus pyogenes* var. *albus* are important organisms for mastitis in cows.

### 2.4.3 Family: Enterobacteriaceae

These are Gram-negative, short, straight rods motile by peritrichous flagella or non-motile and may be capsulated. They are aerobic/facultatively anaerobic chemoorganotrophs that ferment glucose,

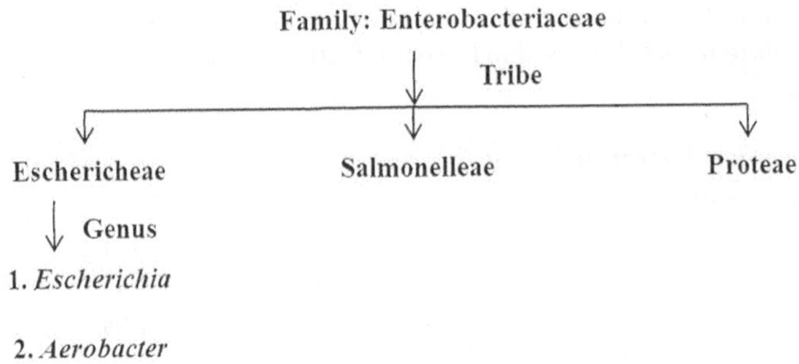


**FIGURE 2.23 Overview of the Enterobacteriaceae family.**

producing acid or acid and gas, and are mainly catalase positive, oxidase negative. They are inhabitants of the intestines of humans and animals, and some may act as pathogens or saprophytes.

### 2.4.3.1 Coliforms

Coliforms may be defined as Gram-negative, oxidase-negative, non-spore-forming rods that can grow aerobically or facultatively anaerobically in the presence of bile salts or surface-active agents with similar growth inhibitory properties and that ferment lactose with the production of acid and gas within 48 h at 37°C. Coliform bacteria have been used as indicators of sanitation in the dairy industry. When bacteria are found in heat-treated dairy products, it typically suggests that either the pasteurization process was not carried out properly or contamination occurred afterwards.

The family is divided into several tribes, of which Eschericheae is of principal interest, although the other two tribes, Proteae and Salmonelleae, are also encountered.

The tribe Eschericheae includes two genera (**Figure 2.23**):

i. *Escherichia*
ii. *Aerobacter*

These two genera are collectively known as coliforms or colon-aerogenes. The name is derived from the Latin word "*colon*" meaning large intestine.

- Coliform bacteria occur singly, in pairs, and in short chains, but many strains are cocco-bacillary.
- They have been defined as aerobic, facultatively anaerobic, Gram-negative, asporogenic, rod-shaped organisms capable of producing gas and acid from lactose.
- The coliform group is completely undesirable in milk and milk products.

#### *2.4.3.1.1 Escherichia coli*

It is generally motile; its optimum growth temperature is 37°C, and the range is 2.5 to 45°C. It can resist 63°C for 30 minutes, which is not always common.

*Escherichia coli* are sometimes known as "pseudolactic acid bacteria" because they produce lactic acid, which makes up around 35% of their acid. The type of acid produced by *E. coli* depends on the sugar fermented and the nature of $N_2$ source.

## SIGNIFICANCE

They are a sign of fecal contamination when they are present in the foods. They are significant food deterioration microbes. They produce gas in dairy products. Dairy products acquire an unpleasant

**TABLE 2.12**
**Characteristics of *Escherichia coli* and *Aerobacter aerogenes***

| Characteristics | *Escherichia coli* | *Aerobacter aerogenes* |
|---|---|---|
| Motility | Motile | Non-motile |
| $CO_2$:$H_2$ | 1:1 | 2:1 |
| Origin | Fecal | Non-fecal |
| IMViC tests | | |
| Indole | Positive | Negative |
| Methyl red | Positive | Negative |
| Voges–Proskauer | Negative | Positive |
| Citrate | Negative | Positive |

taste and ropiness due to their presence. The presence of these in pasteurized dairy food suggests that the production site did not uphold cleanliness standards. Some types of strains make harmful substances called enterotoxins, and some are entero-pathogenic in nature.

#### 2.4.3.1.2 *Aerobacter aerogenes*

This is one of the most important members of the coliform group. Characteristics are similar to those of *E. coli* with some minor differences (**Table 2.12**). This organism grows in milk and ferments the lactose. Gas is not formed unless coagulation occurs. The organisms are mainly proteolytic and produce indole chemicals.

## GENUS

***Escherichia***: *E. coli*, *E. ferousonii*
***Klebsiella***: *K. planticola*
***Proteus***: *P. vulgaris*, *P. mirabilis*
***Salmonella***: *S. typhosa*, *S. paratyphi*
***Aerobacter***: *A. aerogenes*
***Shigella***: *S. boydii*, *S. sonnei*

## TRIBE: PROTEAE

**Genus:** *Proteus* (only one genus)
**Species:** *Proteus vulgaris*

## CHARACTERISTICS

They are rod-shaped. Sometimes they occur as singles, pairs, and short chains. They can be easily killed by pasteurization. They cannot ferment lactose but decompose urea rapidly. Market milk usually is free from this type of organism.

## TRIBE: SALMONELLEAE

**Genus:** *Salmonella*
**Species:** *S. typhosa*, *S. paratyphi*, *S. schottmuelleri*

## CHARACTERISTICS

These types of organisms are usually destroyed by proper pasteurization. These organisms are transmitted in food that has been contaminated directly or indirectly by the fecal materials of infected humans or rodents.

### 2.4.4 Family: Pseudomonadaceae

These bacteria are the important spoilage bacteria originating in refrigerated raw milk. They fit the definition of psychrotrophs because they can thrive at normal refrigerator temperatures (0–15°C). Certain enzymes synthesized by *Pseudomonas flourescens* have the potential to influence milk due to their bacterial characteristics. Milk can be affected by these enzymes, leading to drawbacks like a distasteful flavor, an unpleasant smell, and cardboardy flavors. They can also break down proteins in the milk and make it slimy.

*Pseudomonas aeruginosa* also causes outbreaks of intra-mammary infections. The main sources of *Pseudomonas* sp. Are water and soil. Hose nozzles and milking equipment may be colonized by pseudomonads. *Pseudomonas* sp. Contamination of hoses and water can be very difficult to eliminate (Erskine et al., 1987), but the elimination of *Pseudomonas aeruginosa* has been demonstrated.

### 2.4.5 Other Families

The other families in the suborder Eubacteriineae that are studied by the dairy microbiologist include the followings:

Family: **Bacillaceae**
The family Bacillaceae is divided into two genera, *Bacillus* and *Clostridium.*
*Bacillus cereus, Bacillus coagulans*
*Clostridium perfringens, Clostridium putrefacines*
Family: **Achromobacteriaceae**
*Alcaligenesviscosus* (ropiness), *Alcaligenes metalcaligenes* (gelatinous film on cottage cheese)
Family: **Bacteriaceae**
*Bacterium linens* (proteolysis), *Bacterium erythrogenes* (soft cheeses)
Family: **Corynebacteriaceae**
*Corynebacterium diphtheriae, Corynebacterium pyogenes*
Family: **Parvobacteriaceae**
*Brucella abortu, Mycobacterium tuberculosis*

## 2.5 MILK-BORNE DISEASES/ILLNESSES

Milk can act as a potential means of disease transmission under some circumstances. It provides a suitable culture for numerous types of microbes, both beneficial and harmful, and offers them protection. A variety of pathogens may gain access into milk from different sources and cause different types of milk-borne illness. Milk and dairy foods may carry microbes or their toxins to the consumers. Based on the type of illness produced these are categorized as food infection, food intoxication, and food toxi-infection (**Table 2.13**). The production of toxic chemicals by pathogens poses a significant threat to public health.

### 2.5.1 Outbreaks

A food-borne disease outbreak occurs when two or more people suffer from the same sickness, typically gastrointestinal, after consuming a common food.

**TABLE 2.13**
**Milk-Borne Diseases/Illnesses**

| Disease type | Examples |
|---|---|
| **Food intoxication** | Staphylococcal food poisoning, Botulism, *E. coli* diarrhea, Cholera |
| **Food infection** | Typhoid, Shigellosis, Septic sore throat, Scarlet fever |
| **Food toxi-infection** | *Bacillus cereus* food poisoning, *Clostridium perfringens* gangrene |

### 2.5.2 Food Intoxication

Consumers experience poisoning syndrome when they consume toxins that have already been generated by bacteria in food (pre-formed). Enterotoxins are toxins that affect the GI tract.

### 2.5.3 Food Infection

Viable pathogenic bacteria that are consumed with food become lodged and establish in the organs of the consumers. This is termed a food infection.

### 2.5.4 Food Toxi-Infection

Some organisms can produce toxins "in situ" after getting ingested with food and infecting the intestine.

### 2.5.5 Other Milk-Borne Diseases

**Bacterial:** Tuberculosis, brucellosis, diphtheria, and anthrax
**Rickettsial:** Q fever
**Viral:** Enterovirus, infectious hepatitis, FMD, and tick-borne encephalitis

### 2.5.6 How to Prevent Milk-Borne Infectious Diseases

Avoid drinking raw milk. Keep dairy products chilled until they reach their expiration date, which is indicated on the package. One should be careful when they travel to any place, not consume raw dairy products, and observe the country's sanitary precautions as directed.

### 2.5.7 Control of Milk-Borne Diseases

i. **Techniques:** For the specialized control of milk-borne illnesses, four approaches are used. These techniques serve to lengthen the lag phase of the growth curve of microorganisms.

a. The inspection of cattle and elimination of sick and infected animals.
b. All dairy workers and those who handle milk should get regular medical examination.
c. Proper pasteurization of milk should be done to destroy pathogens.
d. Proper chilling of milk during storage.

ii. **Pasteurization:** Milk is heated during pasteurization in order to kill pathogenic bacteria. This is followed by rapid cooling. Louis Pasteur first developed the procedure to eliminate the microbes that might contaminate wine, not milk. Now that it eliminates all pathogens, it is crucial primarily for assuring safe milk. One of the most difficult disease agents to destroy in milk is the rickettsial agent *Coxiella burnetii* which causes Q fever. Some of these organisms will be able to survive if the pasteurization temperature is reduced by even 4°F (2.2°C). Pasteurization significantly reduces the number of non-pathogens such as *Streptococcus lactis* and different *Lactobacillus* species while also eradicating the pathogens in milk. This enhances the keeping quality of the milk because the lactic acid produced by non-pathogens is what causes milk to sour. As a result, less lactic acid is produced and the milk takes longer to turn sour when there are fewer microbes present.

### 2.5.8 Control of Microorganisms in Milk and Dairy Food Processing

In the 1960s, a technique for ensuring pathogen-free food for the space program was developed by the US Army and NASA. This system, called hazard analysis and critical control points (HACCP), focuses on critical food safety areas as part of total quality programs (**Figure 2.24**). It includes a thorough analysis of every step of the food production process to identify any instances when the food may become physically, chemically, or microbiologically contaminated, making it dangerous or unsuitable for human consumption. The use of the HACCP system is not new to the dairy food industry. Now, the HACCP application is a must for the food industry, including the dairy sector. It's high time to establish consistent regulations for food safety across all stages of food production, including agricultural farms. HACCP is a logical, simple, effective, but highly structured system of food safety control (Sayler, 2009).

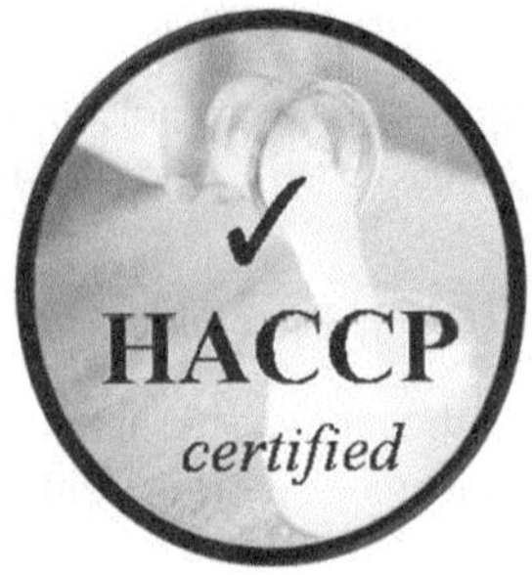


**FIGURE 2.24** HACCP logo illustrations.

#### 2.5.8.1 Principles of HACCP

Suherman et al. (2021) and Jan et al. (2016) define HACCP principles (**Figure 2.25**) as follows:

i. Perform a risk analysis of the planting, harvesting, processing, manufacturing, distribution, and marketing of raw materials and ingredients, preparation, and consumption of dairy food.
ii. Determine the critical control points (CCPs) needed to manage the identified hazards in the process.
iii. Establish critical limits for preventive measures associated with each identified CCP.
iv. Establish CCP monitoring requirements. Establish mechanisms for modifying the process and maintaining control based on monitoring outcomes.
v. Establish corrective actions to be taken when monitoring indicates there is a deviation from an established critical limit.
vi. Develop efficient systems for keeping records that reflect the HACCP strategy.
vii. Establish methods for confirming the HACCP system's effectiveness.

#### 2.5.8.2 Prerequisite Program

The HACCP prerequisite program is defined as follows by Zecchini et al., 2003:

##### *2.5.8.2.1 Premise Control*

Buildings and surroundings must be designed, constructed, and maintained to prevent conditions that may result in the contamination of dairy products. Premises include all elements of the building and building surroundings: outside property, roadways, drainage, building design and construction, product flow, sanitary facilities, and water quality.

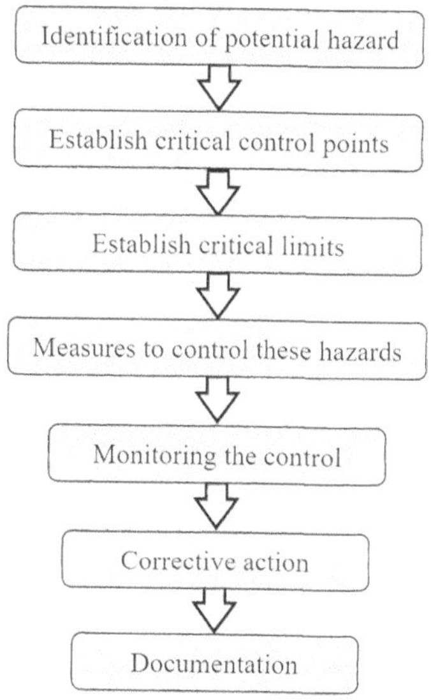


**FIGURE 2.25** **Illustration of a picture diagram showing the seven HACCP principles.**

#### *2.5.8.2.2 Receiving and Storage Control*

Plants must receive, inspect, and store ingredients, packaging material, and incoming materials in ways to prevent conditions that may result in the contamination of dairy foods. All elements in this area must be monitored and controlled by plants, and they must keep the necessary records.

#### *2.5.8.2.3 Equipment Performance and Maintenance Control*

Dairy facilities must install and maintain equipment in such a way as to prevent situations that might lead to food contamination. Dairy facilities must utilize equipment that is suited for the production of dairy foods. All elements in this area must be monitored and controlled by plants, and they must also keep the necessary records.

#### *2.5.8.2.4 Personnel Training*

Dairy facilities must have a sufficient program in place to oversee and manage training initiatives and keep accurate records. Making sure that safe food handling procedures are followed must be the goal of the personnel training program. The appropriate training for production staff must be continuously provided by the personnel training program. A procedure must be developed to verify the effectiveness of the training program.

#### *2.5.8.2.5 Sanitation*

The equipment and facilities need to be cleaned and sanitized according to a planned schedule. Regular inspections should be conducted to verify the cleanliness of the equipment. Before usage, all residue and extraneous matter must be removed from the equipment.

#### *2.5.8.2.6 Recall Procedure*

The aim of the recall process is to promptly and efficiently remove a dairy product from the market by implementing a flexible plan that can be employed as necessary. To confirm the program's effectiveness, tests must be conducted.

### 2.5.8.3 Preliminary Setup (HACCP implementation)

Lievaart et al., 2005; Jan et al., 2016 define HACCP preliminary setup (HACCP implementation) (**Figure 2.26**) as follows:

*Step 1: Gain Management Commitment and Assemble the HACCP Team*

The team is responsible for developing each step of the HACCP plan. As they are most acquainted with the operation, the team should be multidisciplinary and comprise all employees who are directly involved in the daily process operations.

*Step 2: Describe Dairy Food and Methods of Distribution*

The dairy product should be defined in terms of composition, structure, processing, packaging system, storage, necessary shelf life, and usage directions. Whether the dairy food is to be distributed frozen, refrigerated, or shelf-stable should be included along with the distribution method.

*Step 3: Identify Intended Use and Potential Consumers*

The general public, a particular segment of the population, another food (dairy or non-dairy), or a non-food product may all be considered intended customers or uses.

*Step 4: Develop and Verify a Flow Diagram*

The goal of the flow diagram is to give a concise, clear explanation of the procedures involved in making dairy products. The flow diagram should be adjusted as necessary.

*Step 5: Conduct a Hazard Analysis (Principle 1)*

Any microbiological, chemical, or physical characteristic that could render a dairy product dangerous for human ingestion is referred to as a hazard. The team must decide if any preventive measures can be used for each hazard.

*Step 6: Critical Control Points (Principle 2)*

Examples of CCPs include the temperature of incoming raw milk, animal drug residue monitoring in raw milk, the storage temperature of raw milk or cream, pasteurization temperature and time, and the use of metal detectors.

*Step 7: Critical Limits (Principle 3)*

Critical limits may be established for preventive measures such as temperature, time, pH, titratable acidity, drug residues, and microbiological numbers and kinds.

*Step 8: Monitoring/Inspection (Principle 4)*

A scheduled series of observations or measurements is known as monitoring. Its purpose is to determine whether a CCP is under control and to create an accurate record that can be used for verification in the future.

*Step 9: Corrective Actions (Principle 5)*

Corrective activities are the steps that must be taken when a deviation occurs. Each CCP needs a different corrective action plan because of the complexity of potential deviations and variations across dairy products.

*Step 10: Records (Principle 6)*

HACCP team and assigned responsibilities; description of the dairy product and its intended use; and a flow diagram for the entire dairy manufacturing process indicating CCPs, hazards, records for all

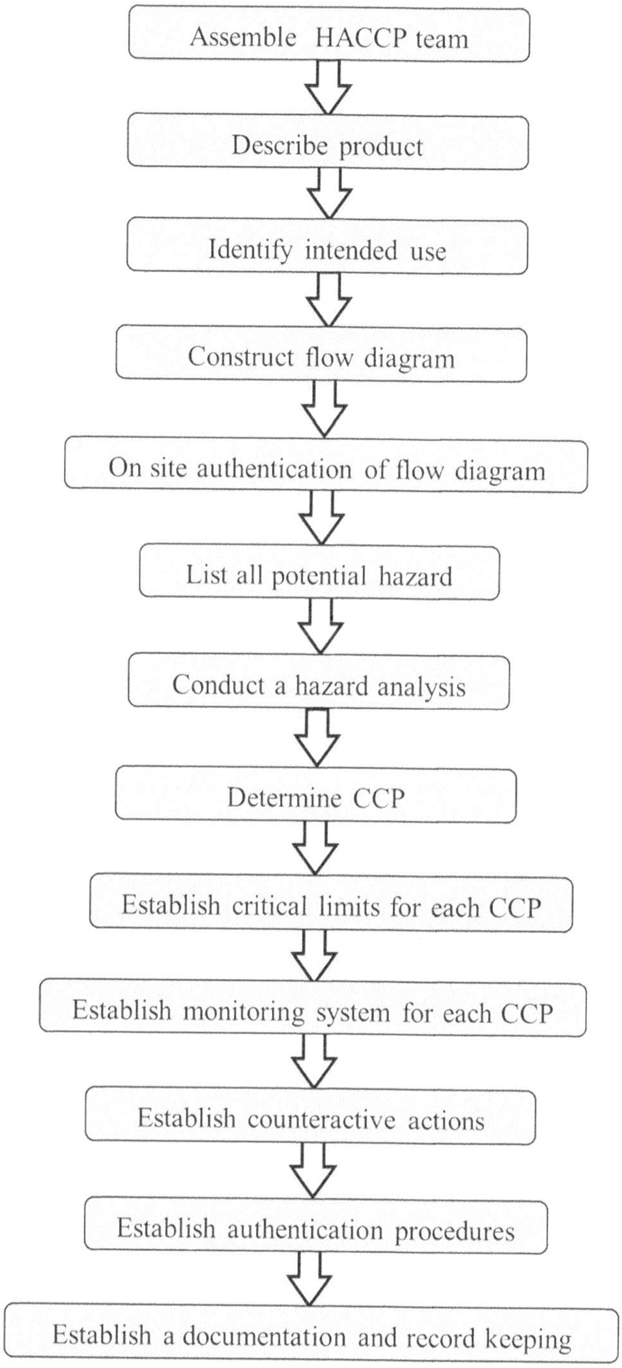


**FIGURE 2.26 A logical sequence for implementing HACCP.**

CCPs, preventive measures, critical limits, monitoring systems, corrective action plans for deviations from critical limits, and processes for HACCP system verification are all included with each CCP.

*Step 11: Verification (Principle 7)*

Verification reports should include (i) information about the existence of a HACCP plan and persons responsible for administering and updating the HACCP plan, (ii) status of records associated with CCP monitoring, (iii) direct monitoring data of the CCP while in operation, (iv) a certification that monitoring equipment is properly calibrated and in working order, (v) deviations and corrective actions, (vi) any samples analyzed to verify that CCPs are under control (analyses may involve microbiological, chemical, physical, or organoleptic methods), (vii) modifications to the HACCP plan, and (viii) training and knowledge of individuals responsible for monitoring CCPs.

*Step 12: Evaluating and Revising HACCP Systems*

The CCP should be validated and evaluated as part of a thorough review that occurs at least once a year.

## 2.6 CONCLUSIONS

Milk has a wide range of physiological functions in addition to the basic nutrients for human growth and development that it provides. The digestion of milk proteins leads to the synthesis of bioactive peptides, which have been found to have human health-promoting benefits. Milk is typically subjected to pasteurization or sterilization to maintain stability and increase shelf life. During the industrial processing and storage of milk products, many chemical changes in milk components occur. These changes majorly affect the sensory characteristics and/or nutritional value of the milk product. It is important to emphasize HACCP regulations from the industry to the whole chain of food production, including farms. New methods of processing need to be commercialized to improve the quality of dairy products for the consumer markets.

## REFERENCES


Bintsis, T. (2018). Lactic acid bacteria as starter cultures: An update in their metabolism and genetics. *AIMS Microbiology*, *4*(4), 665.

Carr, F. J., Chill, D., & Maida, N. (2002). The lactic acid bacteria: A literature survey. *Critical Reviews in Microbiology*, *28*(4), 281–370.

Cashman, K. D., & Kiely, M. (2016). Tackling inadequate vitamin D intakes within the population: Fortification of dairy products with vitamin D may not be enough. *Endocrine*, *51*, 38–46.

Christie, W. W. (2006). Composition and structure of milk lipids. In P. F. Fox (Ed.), *Advanced dairy chemistry* (Vol. 2. Lipids, 2nd ed., pp. 1–36). Chapman & Hall. (Original work published 1995)

Claesson, M. J., Van Sinderen, D., & O'Toole, P. W. (2007). The genus Lactobacillus—a genomic basis for understanding its diversity. *FEMS Microbiology Letters*, *269*(1), 22–28.

Coelho, M. C., Malcata, F. X., & Silva, C. C. (2022). Lactic acid bacteria in raw-milk cheeses: From starter cultures to probiotic functions. *Foods*, *11*(15), 2276.

Cui, L., Fan, X., Wang, P., Wang, Q., & Fu, G. (2011). Casein and transglutaminase-mediated modification of wool surface. *Engineering in Life Sciences*, *11*(2), 201–206.

D'Incecco, P., Rosi, V., Cabassi, G., Hogenboom, J. A., & Pellegrino, L. (2018). Microfiltration and ultra-high-pressure homogenization for extending the shelf-storage stability of UHT milk. *Food Research International*, *107*, 477–485.

Deeth, H. C. (2021). Heat treatment of milk: Extended shelf life (ESL) and ultra-high-temperature (UHT) treatments. In J. McNamara & P. McSweeney (Eds.), *Encyclopedia of dairy sciences* (3rd ed., Vol. 4, pp. 618–631). Academic Press.

Deeth, H. C., & Lewis, M. J. (2017). *High temperature processing of milk and milk products*. Wiley Blackwell. ISBN 978-1-118-46050-4.

Dellaglio, F., Dicks, L., & Torriani, S. (1995). The genus leuconostoc. In *The genera of lactic acid bacteria* (pp. 235–278). Springer.

Devriese, L., & Pot, B. (1995). The genus enterococcus. In *The genera of lactic acid bacteria* (pp. 327–367). Springer.

Di Stefano, M. (2022). Il Malassorbimento e L'intolleranza al Lattosio Fisiopatologia, Diagnosi e Approccio Terapeutico.

Erskine, R. J., Unflat, J. G., Eberhart, R. J., Hutchinson, L. J., Hicks, C. R., & Spencer, S. B. (1987). Pseudomonas mastitis: Difficulties in detection and elimination from contaminated wash-water systems. *Journal of the American Veterinary Medical Association*, *191*(7), 811–815.

Facioni, M. S., Raspini, B., Pivari, F., Dogliotti, E., & Cena, H. (2020). Nutritional management of lactose intolerance: The importance of diet and food labelling. *Journal of Translational Medicine*, *18*, 1–9.

Fantuz, F., Todini, L., Ferraro, S., Fatica, A., Marcantoni, F., Zannotti, M., & Salimei, E. (2022). Macro minerals and trace elements in milk of dairy buffaloes and cows reared in mediterranean areas. *Beverages*, *8*(3), 51.

Fassio, F., Facioni, M. S., & Guagnini, F. (2018). Lactose maldigestion, malabsorption, and intolerance: A comprehensive review with a focus on current management and future perspectives. *Nutrients*, *10*(11), 1599.

Fox, P. F., & Kelly, A. L. (2006a). Indigenous enzymes in milk: Overview and historical aspects-Part 1. *International Dairy Journal*, *16*(6), 500–516.

Fox, P. F., & Kelly, A. L. (2006b). Indigenous enzymes in milk: Overview and historical aspects-Part 2. *International Dairy Journal*, *16*(6), 517–532.

Hammes, W. P., & Vogel, R. F. (1995). The genus lactobacillus. In *The genera of lactic acid bacteria* (pp. 19–54). Springer.

Hardie, J., & Whiley, R. (1996). The genus streptococcus. In *The genera of lactic acid bacteria*. Springer.

Huot, P. S., Sarkar, B., & Ma, D. W. (2010). Conjugated linoleic acid alters caveolae phospholipid fatty acid composition and decreases caveolin-1 expression in MCF-7 breast cancer cells. *Nutrition Research*, *30*(3), 179–185.

Jan, T., Yadav, K. C., & Borude, S. (2016). Study of HACCP implementation in milk processing plant at Khyber Agro Pvt. Ltd in Jammu & Kashmir. *Journal of Food Processing and Technology*, *7*(610), 2.

Jayaratne, N., Hughes, M. C. B., Ibiebele, T. I., van den Akker, S., & van der Pols, J. C. (2013). Vitamin D intake in Australian adults and the modeled effects of milk and breakfast cereal fortification. *Nutrition*, *29*(7–8), 1048–1053.

Jensen, R. G. (2002). The composition of bovine milk lipids: January 1995 to December 2000. *Journal of Dairy Science*, *85*(2), 295–350.

Kaur, N., Sharma, P., Jaimni, S., Kehinde, B. A., & Kaur, S. (2020). Recent developments in purification techniques and industrial applications for whey valorization: A review. *Chemical Engineering Communications*, *207*(1), 123–138.

Lahtinen, S., Ouwehand, A. C., Salminen, S., & von Wright, A. (2011). *Lactic acid bacteria: Microbiological and functional aspects*. CRC Press.

Lievaart, J. J., Noordhuizen, J. P. T. M., Van Beek, E., Van der Beek, C., Van Risp, A., Schenkel, J., & Van Veersen, J. (2005). The hazard analysis critical control point's (HACCP) concept as applied to some chemical, physical and microbiological contaminants of milk on dairy farms. A prototype. *Veterinary Quarterly*, *27*(1), 21–29.

Mahony, J. A., Fox, P. F., & Kelly, A. L. (2013). Indigenous enzymes of milk. In P. McSweeney & P. Fox (Eds.), *Advanced dairy chemistry*. Springer.

Massoud, R., Belgheisi, S., & Massoud, A. (2016). Effect of high pressure homogenization on improving the quality of milk and sensory properties of yogurt: A review. *International Journal of Chemical Engineering and Applications*, *7*(1), 66–70.

Medhammar, E., Wijesinha-Bettoni, R., Stadlmayr, B., Nilsson, E., Charrondiere, U. R., & Burlingame, B. (2012). Composition of milk from minor dairy animals and buffalo breeds: A biodiversity perspective. *Journal of the Science of Food and Agriculture*, *92*(3), 445–474.

Misselwitz, B., Butter, M., Verbeke, K., & Fox, M. R. (2019). Update on lactose malabsorption and intolerance: Pathogenesis, diagnosis and clinical management. *Gut*, *68*(11), 2080–2091.

Olorunnisomo, O. A., Ososanya, T. O., & Adedeji, O. Y. (2014). Homogenization of milk and its effect on sensory and physico-chemical properties of yoghurt. *African Journal of Food Science*, *8*(9), 465–470.

Patrignani, F., Iucci, L., Lanciotti, R., Vallicelli, M., Mathara, J. M., Holzapfel, W. H., & Guerzoni, M. E. (2007). Effect of high-pressure homogenization, nonfat milk solids, and milkfat on the technological performance of a functional strain for the production of probiotic fermented milks. *Journal of Dairy Science*, *90*(10), 4513–4523.

Potočnik, K., Gantner, V., Kuterovac, K., & Cividini, A. (2011). Mare's milk: Composition and protein fraction in comparison with different milk species. *Mljekarstvo: Časopis Za Unaprjeđenje Proizvodnje I Prerade Mlijeka*, *61*(2), 107–113.

Samedi, L., & Charles, A. L. (2019). Isolation and characterization of potential probiotic Lactobacilli from leaves of food plants for possible additives in pellet feeding. *Annals of Agricultural Sciences*, *64*(1), 55–62.

Sayler, A. (2009). Hazard analysis (appraisal) critical control point (HACCP) in milk processing—a practical overview. In A. Y. Tamime (Ed.), *Milk processing and quality management.* Blackwell Publishing Ltd.

Ségurel, L., & Bon, C. (2017). On the evolution of lactase persistence in humans. *Annual Review of Genomics and Human Genetics, 18*, 297–319.

Sfakianakis, P., & Tzia, C. (2014). Conventional and innovative processing of milk for yogurt manufacture: Development of texture and flavor: A review. *Foods, 3*(1), 176–193.

Shahani, K. M., Chandan, R. C., Kelly, P. L., & Macquiddy E. L. (1962). Determination of lysozyme in milk and factors affecting its concentration and properties. *Proceeding of Internation Dairy Congress* 16th vol C, 285–294.

Sodini, I., Remeuf, F., Haddad, S., & Corrieu, G. (2004). The relative effect of milk base, starter, and process on yogurt texture: A review. *Critical Reviews in Food Science and Nutrition, 44*(2), 113–137.

Sola-Larrañaga, C., & Navarro-Blasco, I. (2009). Chemometric analysis of minerals and trace elements in raw cow milk from the community of Navarra, Spain. *Food Chemistry, 112*(1), 189–196.

Spitsberg, V. L. (2005). Invited review: Bovine milk fat globule membrane as a potential nutraceutical. *Journal of Dairy Science, 88*(7), 2289–2294.

Stabel, J. R., & Lambertz, A. (2004). Efficacy of pasteurization conditions for the inactivation of Mycobacterium avium subsp. paratuberculosis in milk. *Journal of Food Protection, 67*(12), 2719–2726.

Storhaug, C. L., Fosse, S. K., & Fadnes, L. T. (2017). Country, regional, and global estimates for lactose malabsorption in adults: A systematic review and meta-analysis. *The Lancet Gastroenterology & Hepatology, 2*(10), 738–746.

Suherman, S., Janitra, A. A., Budhiary, K. N. S., Pratiwi, W. Z., & Idris, F. A. (2021, February). Review on hazard analysis and critical control point (HACCP) in the dairy product: Cheese. *IOP Conference Series: Materials Science and Engineering, 1053*(1).

Tagg, J. R., Wescombe, P. A., Burton, J. P., & Wescombe, P. (2011). Streptococcus: A brief update on the current taxonomic status of the genus. In *Lactic acid bacteria: Microbiological and functional aspects* (pp. 123–146). CRC Press, Taylor & Francis Group.

Tay, T., & Chua, Y. (2015). High temperature short time (HTST) camel milk pasteurization pilot plant. *ARPN Journal of Engineering and Applied Sciences, 10*, 6241–6245.

Thompson, A., Boland, M., & Harjinder, S. (2009). *Milk proteins: From expression to food* (1st ed., pp. 205–227). Elsevier, ch. 7.

Udenigwe, C. C., & Aluko, R. E. (2012). Food protein-derived bioactive peptides: Production, processing, and potential health benefits. *Journal of Food Science, 77*(1), R11–R24.

Vandevelde, A. J. J. (1908). A lactose-destroying enzyme in milk. *Biochemische Zeitschrift, 11*, 61.

Vinderola, G., Ouwehand, A., Salminen, S., & von Wright, A. (2019). *Lactic acid bacteria: Microbiological and functional aspects.* CRC Press.

Zecchini, G. I., Schiavi, A. M., Guidi, E., Schatzle, A., Albonetti, S., & Rosmini, R. (2003). Food safety and HACCP system in the milk and milk products chain: Significance of the farm. *Industrie Alimentari, 42*, 1–4.

Zheng, J., Wittouck, S., Salvetti, E., Franz, C. M., Harris, H. M., Mattarelli, P., O'Toole, P. W., Pot, B., Vandamme, P., Walter, J., Watanabe, K., Wuyts, S., Felis, G. E., Gänzle, M. G., & Lebeer, S. (2020). A taxonomic note on the genus Lactobacillus: Description of 23 novel genera, emended description of the genus Lactobacillus Beijerinck 1901, and union of lactobacillaceae and leuconostocaceae. *International Journal of Systematic and Evolutionary Microbiology, 70*(4), 2782–2858.

# 3 Fermented (Cultured) Dairy Food—Yogurt

## 3.1 LEARNING OBJECTIVES

By the end of the chapter, the reader will be able to:

- Understand the classification and composition of yogurt
- Gain recent knowledge on the production, processing, and nutritional attributes of yogurt
- Learn about yogurt chemistry
- Understand how microorganisms of starter cultures can help speed up the process and make yogurt taste better
- Make yogurt enterprises profitable
- Learn how to judge and improve the quality of the yogurt
- Inquire about the key potential health benefits of yogurt
- Discover yogurt innovations from production to nutritional and health attributes

Yogurt gets its natural sweetness from new lactic acid bacteria (LAB). Researchers have developed a new and natural way of cleaving milk sugar that relies on safe LAB to fulfil consumer demand. By producing natural sweetness in the yogurt, the new LAB minimizes the need for additional sugar.

## 3.2 INTRODUCTION

Fermented foods, including yogurt, have been staples of the human diet for thousands of years (**Figure 3.1**). Foods that have been fermented typically have better nutritional and health-promoting qualities. Yogurt, for example, contains live, functional bacteria that can improve human health by supporting the maintenance of a balanced intestinal flora. Additionally, research has revealed that yogurt has additional health advantages over merely providing nourishment because of the distinctive bioactive chemicals produced during fermentation. In fact, new research documents yogurt's positive benefits on metabolic health and related risk factors in both healthy and

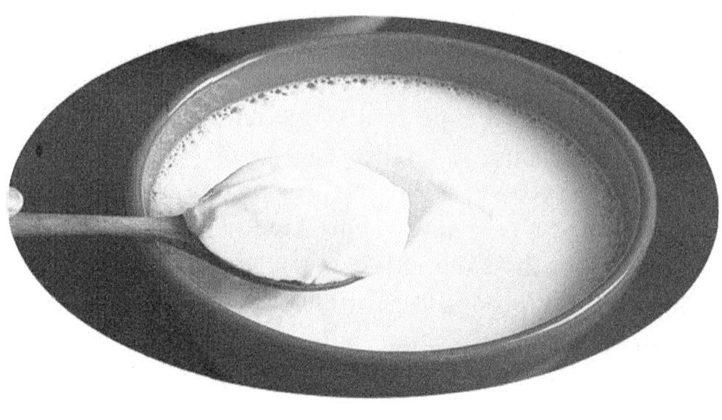

FIGURE 3.1 **Image of yogurt.** Yogurt has been a mainstay of the human diet for thousands of years.

DOI: 10.1201/9781003397786-3

unhealthy people (e.g., individuals with obesity or type 2 diabetes). On the other hand, dahi is a popular fermented traditional dairy product in the Indian subcontinent, having a similar appearance to that of yogurt (Bari et al., 2017; Kober et al., 2007; Amin et al., 2022). Yogurt is a cultured milk product. It is formed by heating milk and mixing it with *Lactobacillus bulgaricus* and *Streptococcus thermophilus*, two living cultures (**Figure 3.5a** and **3.5b**). The warm milk provides the ideal atmosphere for the bacteria to expand and thicken the milk to make yogurt. Yogurt or dahi contains beneficial bacteria that promote good health. Probiotics are found in both yogurt and dahi. Other lactic acid bacteria such as *Streptococcus thermophilus*, *Lactobacillus bulgaricus*, *Lb. acidophilus*, *Lb. casei*, *Lb. GG*, *Lb. plantarum*, *Lb. reuteri*, *B. bifidum*, *B. longum*, and *Bifidobacterium* spp. are used to make probiotic yogurt. By regulating the microorganisms within our bodies, probiotics contribute to our overall health and well-being. They can also help with weight management and fighting obesity (Kobyliak et al., 2016).

### 3.2.1 Definition

Yogurt is a form of fermented milk with a characteristic flavor. It is an acidic food product due to the production of lactic acid through lactic acid fermentation. It is produced by adding a "starter" of active yogurt containing a culture of *Lactobacillus bulgaricus* and *Streptococcus thermophilus*. Yogurt, often similar to dahi, is believed to have therapeutic properties that can aid in the prevention and treatment of different illnesses, including gastrointestinal disorders, heart diseases, and tumor development. This is true for both people and animals (Rao et al., 2016). Dahi is a fermented dairy product popular in the Indian subcontinent that resembles yogurt in appearance. The product made from pasteurized or boiled milk by souring, whether naturally or artificially, by a safe lactic acid culture is known as dahi or curd. In addition to lactic acid bacteria cultures, other harmless bacterial cultures can also be utilized for souring. It is a popular fermented milk product throughout South Asian countries such as Bangladesh, India, Nepal, Pakistan, Sri Lanka, etc. (Bari et al., 2017; Kober et al., 2007; Akter et al., 2019)

## 3.3 HISTORY OF YOGURT AND DAHI

### 3.3.1 Yogurt History

It is believed that the word "yogurt" comes from the Turkish word "*yoğurmak*" which means to thicken, coagulate, or curdle. It is an ancient food that has gone by many names over the millennia: *katyk* (Armenia), *dahi* (India), *zabadi* (Egypt), *mast* (Iran), *lebenraib* (Saudi Arabia), *matsoni* (Georgia, Russia, and Japan), *cuajada* (Spain), *roba* (Sudan), *coalhada* (Portugal), *dovga* (Azerbaijan), *laban* (Iraq and Lebanon), and *iogurte* (Brazil). Yogurt's origins are uncertain; however, it is assumed to have originated in Mesopotamia around 5000 BC. The combination of yogurt and honey is known as "the food of the gods" in ancient Indian chronicles. Ancient Greek cuisine includes *oxygala*, a dairy product thought to be a kind of yogurt. It is quite likely that it did not originate in a single nation. Nations all across the world create it; they simply don't always name it yogurt. The word originated from Turkish, though it has already been used by everyone else for ages. According to Fisberg and Machado (2015), the medieval Turks were the first to evaluate yogurt's medicinal use for a variety of illnesses and symptoms. At the beginning of the twentieth century, yogurt was sold in pharmacies as a medicine. Yogurt was commercially produced in France, starting in 1932. In the United States, yogurt production began in 1941.

### 3.3.2 Dahi History

In accordance with popular legend, as some Turks journeyed across the desert, they kept milk within a sack made from the skin of a goat and slung it onto the back of their camel. When they opened the bag some hours later, they found that it had turned into a thick, tangy custard. The hot sun in the desert and the microorganisms in the bag helped to make this curd, which is known as dahi. Dahi has been an extremely popular fermented food in India, Pakistan, Bangladesh, Nepal, Sri Lanka, etc., mainly originating from the Indian subcontinent. The ancient Hindu documents make significant mention of this product. The product's therapeutic value is well established. It is primarily a traditional yogurt or fermented milk product from the Indian subcontinent that is typically made from cow's milk; however, occasionally it can also be made from buffalo or goat milk. It is called dahi and is widely consumed across the Indian subcontinent (Fisberg & Machado, 2015).

## 3.4 TYPES OF YOGURT AND DAHI

### 3.4.1 Types of Yogurt

i. Types based on the chemical composition:
   Yogurt can be classed according to its fat content:
   a. Full-fat yogurt (above 3.0%).
   b. Medium-fat yogurt (0.5–3.0%).
   c. Low-fat yogurt (0.5% or below).
ii. Types based on the method of production or physical structure of the coagulum:
   a. **Set yogurt:** It is the product that is incubated and cooled in the final package. It has a firm, jelly-like texture.
   b. **Stirred yogurt:** It is the type of yogurt produced after the fermentation has been carried out in bulk and the coagulum is broken before cooling and packaging by stirring.
   c. **Fluid yogurt:** It can be considered stirred yogurt with low viscosity, e.g., 11% total solids or less.
iii. Types based on the flavor:
   i. **Natural or plain yogurt:** This is the traditional type with a sharp, acidic taste.
   ii. **Fruit yogurt:** This can be made by the addition of fruits and sweetening agents to the natural yogurt.
   iii. **Flavored yogurt:** It is another type in which fruit ingredients are replaced with synthetic flavoring and coloring compounds.
iv. Types based on post-incubation processing:
   a. **Pasteurized yogurt:** This type of yogurt can be processed by conventional methods, but after fermentation, yogurt is heat treated to extend its shelf life.
   b. **Frozen yogurt:** Blend of sugars, stabilizers, emulsifiers, and flavors in naturally stirred yogurt.
   c. **Dietetic yogurt:** These are low-calorie, low-lactose, or vitamin/protein-fortified yogurts.
   d. **Concentrated yogurt:** It has total solids of around 24%.
   e. **Dried yogurt:** It has total solids between 90–94%.
v. Others:
   a. **Greek and Greek-style yogurt:** Delicious thick and creamy texture.
   b. **Drinking yogurt:** Stirred, diluted, and mixed with flavors of fruit juices.

c. **Labneh (yogurt cheese balls):** Drained of whey to form a fresh yogurt cheese. It is flavored and rolled into balls.
d. **Made with active cultures:** It is not heat-treated and retains live and active cultures.
e. **Sundae or fruit on the bottom:** Fruit on the bottom, so that turned upside down.

### 3.4.2 Types of Dahi

i. Dahi can be classified into two types:
   a. For churning into desi butter (Makhan)
   b. For direct consumption:
      1. Whole milk dahi
      2. Skim milk dahi
      3. Sweet dahi (with 0.7% acidity)
      4. Sour dahi (with 1% acidity)
      5. Sweetened dahi
ii. Others:
   a. Plain dahi
   b. Probiotic dahi
      1. Additional beneficial bacteria
      2. Added advantage to consumers

## 3.5 DIFFERENCES BETWEEN DAHI AND YOGURT

Dahi typically has a milder flavor, as its fermentation process is less controlled. Yogurt, on the other hand, undergoes a more controlled fermentation, resulting in a thicker, custard-like consistency (smooth and firm coagulation), and a distinct tangy taste. According to Mudgal and Prajapati (2017), the existing differences between dahi and yogurt are shown in **Table 3.1**.

**TABLE 3.1**
**The Differences between Dahi and Yogurt**

| Dahi | Yogurt |
|---|---|
| More acidity. | Relatively less acidity. |
| Starter includes *Lactobacillus bulgaricus* and *Streptococcus thermophilus*. | Starter includes *Lactococcus lactis*, *Streptococcus thermophilus*, *lactobacillus bulgaricus*, and lactose-fermenting yeasts. |
| Dahi is produced from the milk of cows, water buffalo, sheep/ewes, yaks, reindeer, llamas, camels, and goats. | Yogurt is produced from the milk of cows, water buffalo, goats, ewes, mares, camels, and yaks. |
| Dahi slightly tastes more tangy or sour than yogurt. It may squeak against teeth while eating. | The bacteria in yogurt cultures may produce lactic acid, giving yogurt a tart, acidic flavor. |
| Dahi is nutritious and high in probiotics. Four ounces of curd contains 111 calories, 13 g protein, 5 g fat, and 3 g carbohydrates. It contains saturated fat and oleic acid. It also contains certain amounts of vitamin A, E, K, $B_1$, $B_2$, $B_3$, $B_5$, $B_9$, and $B_{12}$. Minerals include Ca, Fe, Mg, P, K, Na, Zn, Cu, Mn, F, and Se. | Yogurt is a good source of vitamin $B_2$, $B_5$, and $B_{12}$ and a good source of Ca, P, Zn, K, and Mn minerals. Yogurt is also high in probiotics. |
| Dahi can be eaten just like that or it can be salted or sweetened. It is usually served with sandwiches, salads, and desserts. | Yogurt can be eaten just like that or it can be salted or sweetened. Yogurt can also be flavored with other ingredients. In several recipes, yogurt is often used in place of heavy cream. Indian lassi and chaas are two more beverages that can be made using it. |

## 3.6 NUTRITIONAL FACTS

Yogurt provides a significant percentage of the daily reference nutrient intake of key nutrients to humans. Panjagari et al. (2013) demonstrated the chemical (**Table 3.2**) and nutritional composition (**Table 3.3, 3.4**) of yogurt in the following amounts.

**TABLE 3.2**
**Nutritional Composition of Whole-Milk and Skim-Milk Yogurt**

| Components | Whole-milk yogurt (%) | Skim-milk yogurt (%) |
|---|---|---|
| Water | 85–88 | 90–91 |
| Fat | 5–8 | 0.05–0.1 |
| Protein | 3.2–3.4 | 3.3–3.5 |
| Lactose | 4.6–5.2 | 4.7–5.3 |
| Lactic Acid | 0.5–1.1 | 0.5–1.1 |
| Ash | 0.7–0.75 | 0.7–0.75 |

**TABLE 3.3**
**Nutritional Composition of Yogurt**

| Components | Value (per 100 g) |
|---|---|
| Energy | 179 kcal |
| Fat | 6 g |
| Carbohydrates | 27 g |
| Sugars | 23 g |
| Proteins | 4 g |
| Dietary fiber | 5 g |
| Calcium | 85 mg |

**TABLE 3.4**
**Nutritional Composition of Low-Fat Plain Yogurt***

| Components | Value (per 100 g) |
|---|---|
| Energy | 56 kcal |
| Protein | 5.1 g |
| Carbohydrate | 7.3 g |
| Fat | 0.8 g |
| Saturated fat | 0.5 g |
| Monounsaturated fat | 0.2 g |
| Polyunsaturated fat | Trace |
| Sodium | 83 mg |
| Dietary fiber | Nil |
| Vitamin A | 9 µg |
| Vitamin $B_{12}$ | 0.2 µg |
| Pantothenic acid | 0.45 mg |
| Biotin | 2.9 µg |

*(Continued)*

**TABLE 3.4** ***(Continued)***
**Nutritional Composition of Low-Fat Plain Yogurt***

| Components | Value (per 100 g) |
|---|---|
| Vitamin C | 1.0 mg |
| Vitamin D | 0.01 μg |
| Vitamin E | 0.01 mg |
| Vitamin K | NA |
| Calcium | 190 mg |
| Chlorine | 150 mg |
| Copper | Trace |
| Iodine | 63 μg |
| Iron | 0.1 mg |
| Magnesium | 19 mg |
| Phosphorus | 160 mg |
| Potassium | 250 mg |
| Selenium | 1 μg |
| Zinc | 0.6 mg |

* Chemical/nutritional composition can vary depending on the milk and types of yogurt/dahi

## 3.7 WORLDWIDE YOGURT PRODUCTION AND CONSUMPTION TRENDS

Global yogurt production is projected to reach more than 329,000 metric tons by 2026, up from 278,000 in 2021. **Table 3.5** illustrates yogurt production in various countries of the world in 2020. France is Europe's largest yogurt user, followed by Ireland, with an annual consumption of 21.3 and 13.2 kg per person, respectively (Production of Yoghurt, 2020). China is one of the major yogurt markets in the Asia–Pacific region. In 2020, the average per capita consumption was 6.8 kg. The average per capita intake in the United States (6.7 kg/year) was still less than half of what many individuals in Europe eat.

## 3.8 MICROFLORA OF YOGURT AND DAHI

### 3.8.1 Microflora of Yogurt

The microbiological standard of yogurt is shown in **Table 3.6.** The microflora of yogurt can be divided into three groups:

i. **Essential microflora:** These consists of *S. thermophilus* and *L. delbrueckii* subsp. *bulgaricus.*
ii. **Non-essential microflora:** These are represented by homofermentative lactic acid strains and heterofermentative lactic acid bacteria. Some of them might be utilized beneficially to supplement the natural flora, e.g., *L. acidophilus, Bifidobacterium bifidum, Propionibacterium shermanii,* and *L. lactis* subsp. *diacetylactis.*
iii. **Contaminants:** Yeasts (*Candida mycoderma, C. tropicalis, C. krusei*), molds, coliforms, and other undesirable microorganisms may be present as contaminants.

**TABLE 3.5**
**Yogurt Production in Various Countries of the World in 2020**

| Country | Production in 2020 (metric tons) |
|---|---|
| Germany | 886,440 |
| Russian Federation | 530,000 |
| France | 460,020 |
| Belarus | 336,048 |
| Poland | 265,890 |
| Spain | 255,860 |
| Saudi Arabia | 205,191 |
| Greece | 195,510 |
| Jordan | 192,158 |
| Austria | 151,590 |

**TABLE 3.6**
**Microbiological Standard of Yogurt**

| Parameters | Value (per g) |
|---|---|
| Total viable count | $\geq 10^6$ CFU |
| Coliform | 10 (maximum) |
| Yeast and mold count | 100 (maximum) |

### 3.8.2 Microflora of Dahi

The starter of khatta (jaman) used for the preparation of dahi is a mixture of lactococci and lactobacilli. The organisms commonly found in the inoculums are *L. lactis* subsp. *cremoris*, *L. lactis* subsp. *lactis*, S. *thermophilus*, *L. acidophilus*, *L. delbrueckii* subsp. *Bulgaricus*, and *L. helveticus*.

The recommended level of inoculum is 2.0–2.5% with 1–2% acidity to obtain good-quality dahi. The National Culture Collection Centre at Karnal recommends the use of LF-40 (a mixed culture) as dahi culture for the preparation of dahi of superior quality (Ghosh & Rajorhia, 1990).

### 3.8.3 Lactic Acid Bacteria

Lactic acid bacteria (LAB) are Gram-positive, non-spore-forming coccobacilli. Generally, they are non-respiratory and lack catalase. They mainly ferment glucose into lactic acid or lactic acid, $CO_2$, and ethanol. Both LAB types grow anaerobically, but they emerge as "aerotolerant anaerobes" in the presence of $O_2$, unlike most anaerobes. Although lactic acid is a primary or secondary end product of fermentation produced by a number of bacterial genera, traditionally, genera of the order Lactobacillales are the only ones that use the term "lactic acid bacteria" and include *Lactobacillus*, *Leuconostoc*, *Pediococcus*, *Lactococcus*, *Streptococcus*, *Carnobacterium*, *Enterococcus*, *Oenococcus*, *Tetragenococcus*, *Vagococcus*, and *Weisella*.

There are three categories of lactic acid bacteria:

i. Homolactic (*Streptococcus*, *Pediococcus*)
ii. Heterolactic (*Leuconostoc*)
iii. Facultative (*Lactobacillus*)

Most LAB generate bacteriocins that minimize the use of chemical preservatives, such as nisin (bacteriocin) produced by *Lactobacillus lactis*, which inhibits the growth of *Clostridium botulinum* and *Listeria monocytogenes* (Juodeikiene et al., 2012). Some LAB have properties of stabilization and viscosity formation. This allows the use of synthetic stabilizers and emulsifiers to be avoided.

## 3.9 INGREDIENTS OF YOGURT

The main ingredient in yogurt is milk. The type of yogurt depends on the type of milk used.

i. Full-fat yogurt (whole milk)
ii. Low-fat yogurt (low-fat milk)
iii. Non-fat yogurt (skimmed milk)

Different flavors, sweeteners, and fruit preparations are utilized in yogurt to satisfy a variety of consumers.

For dahi, it is best to use full-fat milk or whole milk only. Diluted milk or low-fat milk will not set dahi well and make it watery with more whey.

## 3.10 MANUFACTURING PROCESS

Dahi and yogurt are produced by the inoculation of certain species of lactic acid bacteria to milk in the form of a starter culture. According to Kanawjia (2006), the dahi and yogurt preparation method is classified as follows:

*i. Traditional Method:* Dahi is prepared on a small scale in this approach, either in the household of the consumer or in the confectionery shop (*Halwais*). The milk is boiled in the household, cooled to room temperature, inoculated with 0.5 to 1.0% starter (dahi or buttermilk from the previous day), and then incubated overnight. The dahi setting vessel is generally bundled up with woolen cloth in cold weather to maintain a comfortable temperature. The process used for the preparation of dahi is more or less the same in the confectionery shops, except that the milk is condensed before inoculation in an open pan and typically dahi is set in earthenware.

*ii. Standardized method:* The existing method was built on the basis of scientific lines for dahi development in the organized sector. Fresh, sweet, high-quality milk is collected, preheated, filtered, and clarified. Milk is standardized to 2.5 to 3.0% fat and 10% non-fat solids, preheated to 60°C, and homogenized using single-stage pressure of 176 kg/sq cm. For 15–30 minutes, the milk is heated to 85–90°C, cooled to 22–25°C, and inoculated with 1–2% of the particular dahi starter culture. It is then filled into appropriate containers of the required size and incubated for 16–18 hours at 22–25°C. The acidity of dahi reaches 0.6 to 0.7% after the proper setting of the dahi, and a stable curd is formed. The curd is cooled around the containers by circulating chilled water or air and then moved to a cold room sustained at about 4–5°C. The flow diagram for the development of dahi and yogurt is given in **Figure 3.2** and **Figure 3.3**, respectively.

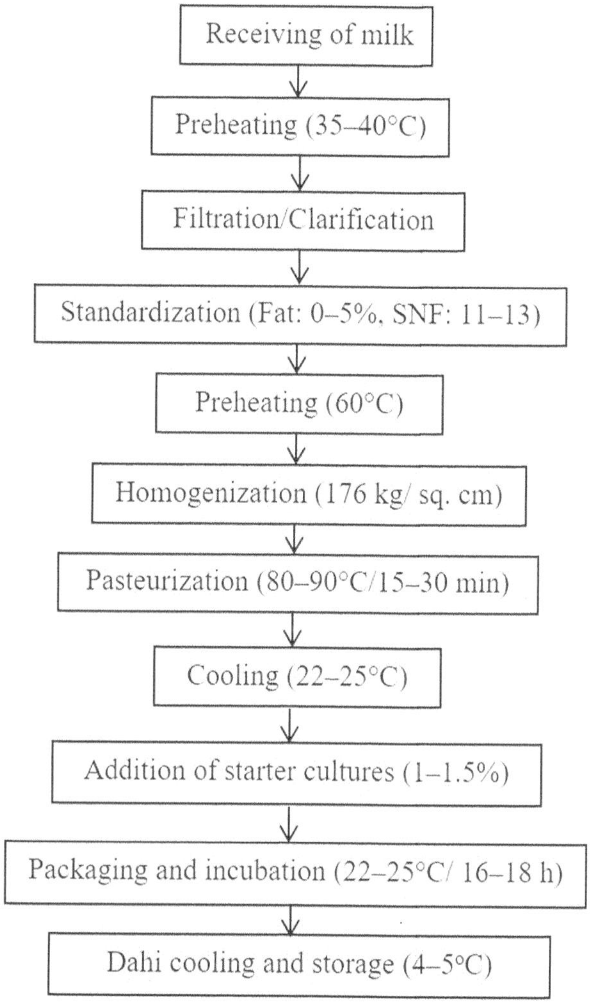


**FIGURE 3.2 Flow diagram for the manufacturing process of dahi.**

## 3.11 YOGURT AND DAHI CHEMISTRY

When bacteria ferment the sugar lactose into lactic acid, the lactic acid causes the proteins in the milk to coagulate. While the increase in lactic acid decreases pH and causes the milk to clot or form a soft gel, lactose is responsible for flavor.

- Starter cultures in yogurt.
- Lactic acid produced by fermenting lactose.
- Lactic acid:
  a. Delivers the sour yogurt flavor.
  b. Induces the development of a gel structure.
  c. Reduces pH.
- This results in the milk clotting.
- Milk gel:
  a. A solid structure composed of a protein matrix with other components.
  b. Can immobilize the liquid phase of milk.
- Proteolytic enzymes, lactic acid, heat, and other factors can cause curdling.

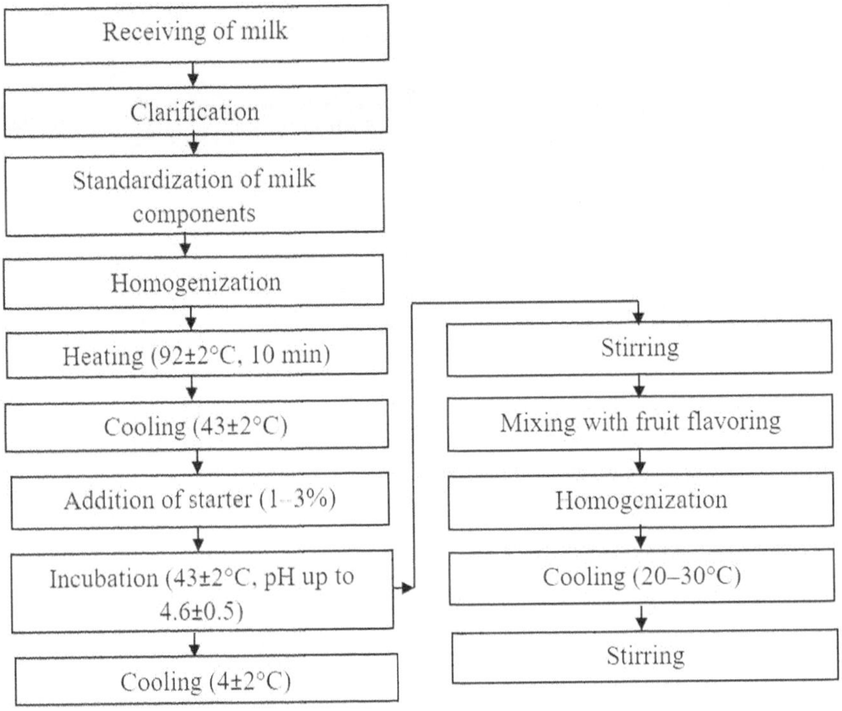


FIGURE 3.3 **Flow diagram for the manufacturing process of yogurt.**

## 3.12 BIOCHEMICAL CHANGES IN FERMENTATION

### 3.12.1 Change-Inducing Bacteria

Mostly lactic acid bacteria (LAB) are used in dahi preparation, and they are greatly responsible for the occurring changes in yogurt or dahi.

i. **Heterolactic bacteria/starter cultures:**
*Lactobacillus lactis, Lactobacillus brevis, Lactobacillus fermentum* and *Leuconostoc* sp., contribute to flavor compounds including acetic acid, butanone, diacetyl, acetaldehyde, ethanol, and some other volatile compounds.

ii. **Homolactic bacteria/starter cultures:**
Homolactic starter cultures bacteria in yogurt include *Lactobacillus* and *Lactococcus* bacteria. They produce 95% of the lactic acid (acts as a preservative and provide sharp acidic taste).

### 3.12.2 Biochemical Changes during Yogurt/Dahi Preparation

Biochemical changes which occur during the preparation of yogurt/dahi are as follows:

i. **Carbohydrates:** Lactose, a major carbohydrate in milk is converted to lactic acid via LAB. Small quantities of flavor compounds are also produced through carbohydrate catabolism.

$$\text{Lactose} \xrightarrow{\text{LAB}} \text{Lactic acid}$$

Lactic acid has two main roles:

a. Gives sharp acidic taste.
b. Destabilization of casein micelles.

ii. **Proteins:** LAB convert casein into free amino acids and peptides by a complex proteolytic system.

$$\text{Casein} \xrightarrow{\text{LAB}} \text{Free amino acid}$$

Free amino acids are required for the growth of microbes.

iii. **Lipids:** Lipase activity of microbial contaminants of milk results in the generation of minor amounts of free fatty acids and volatile fatty acids.

$$\text{Lipid} \xrightarrow{\text{Lipase activity}} \text{Free fatty acid + volatile fatty acid}$$

iv. **Flavor compounds:** Due to carbohydrate metabolism, fat metabolism, and proteolytic activity, lactic acid, acetaldehyde, acetone, ketone, diacetyl, etc. are produced.

v. **Cell mass:** During fermentation, LAB starters multiply to a minimum number of $10^6$ to $10^7$ colony forming units (CFUs)/gm of viable cells in the products. LAB cells contain cell walls, nucleic acid, enzymes, cellular proteins, lipids, and carbohydrates that occupy about 1% volume of yogurt products.

### 3.12.3 Enzymatic Reactions in Yogurt Production

#### 3.12.3.1

Reagents | End Products

$$\text{Lactose} \xrightarrow{\text{Lactase}} \text{Glucose + Galactose} \xrightarrow{\text{Glycolysis + Fermentation}} \text{Lactic acid + Acetaldehyde}$$

## 3.13 FUNCTIONAL PROPERTIES OF PROBIOTIC YOGURT

Yogurt is abundant in probiotics (Hoseinifar et al., 2018). Its functional properties are as follows:

i. After eating yogurt, *Lactobacillus delbrueckii* sbsp. *bulgaricus* was found in 73% of fecal samples from people who eat yogurt, but only in 28% of samples from people who don't eat yogurt (Wang et al., 2013).

ii. According to randomized controlled research, healthy adults who consumed yogurt with *Bifidobacterium animalis* subsp. *lactis* BB-12 while taking antibiotics had slightly greater fecal *B. lactis* levels, and it was safe and well tolerated (Merenstein et al., 2015).

iii. Having probiotic yogurt containing *Lactobacillus acidophilus* La5 and *Bifidobacterium lactis* Bb12 by Non-alcoholic fatty liver disease (NAFLD) patients resulted in lowering of 4.67, 5.42, 4.10 and 6.92% in serum levels of alanine aminotransferase, aspartate aminotransferase, total cholesterol, and low-density lipoprotein cholesterol, respectively, in contrast to the control group (Zaharuddin et al., 2019).

iv. Administration of probiotics such as *B. infantis*, *S. thermophilus*, and *B. lactis* (Jacobs et al., 2013) or *Lactobacillus reuteri* may be safe and is reducing the incidence of Necrotizing enterocolitis (NEC) in very-low-birth-weight premature infants.

v. In comparison to yogurt containing *Lactobacillus rhamnosus* PRA331, yogurt supplemented with *Lactobacillus casei* PRA205 had higher levels of antihypertensive and antioxidant peptides, and this culture could be used as an adjunct in the production of bi-functional yogurt that is enriched in bioactive peptides (Rutella et al., 2016).

## 3.14 NEW YOGURTS USING FUNCTIONAL PROBIOTICS

### 3.14.1 Functional Probiotics

Functional probiotics can be defined as live microbial food supplements that have a beneficial effect on the host by improving intestinal microbial balance (Kober et al., 2022). Probiotics that beneficially regulate the immune system of the host are called immunobiotics (Clancy, 2003). Lately, as nutritional supplements and in several food products, commercial probiotics have become available, exclusively in dairy products such as yogurt (**Table 3.7**).

Undoubtedly, since dairy products are excellent sources of calcium, they are functional foods. Nonetheless, research has specifically concentrated on other elements of dairy products. Fermented milk and yogurt are considered healthy sources of vitamins and minerals that supply lactic acid bacteria (LAB) at the same time, which may have additional health benefits. However, traditional cultures of yogurt with enhanced nutritional quality and digestibility show limited survival after ingestion. Adequate numbers of more than $10^6$ CFU/ml viable cells need to be eaten daily to exert probiotic advantages to consumers. An important concern is probiotic cell survival over the shelf life of the product. The survival of probiotic cells in fermented dairy products may be impaired by many factors, such as conditions of culture, strain selection, the extent of inoculation, the composition of medium fermentation, interactions between organisms, final acidity, nutrient availability, growth promoters and inhibitors, sugar concentration, dissolved oxygen, the temperature of incubation and storage, and fermentation period. These criteria and ways of reducing their effect on the viability of LAB are being studied by many researchers. However, to ensure health advantages, probiotic viability during the preparation, distribution, and ingestion of the substance is necessary. In the case of probiotic yogurts, there is a range of regulatory criteria, especially the number of viable bacteria found and the pH value. First, about the content of the substance, it is important that the probiotics are alive at the time of use, and the viable CFU count must be shown to impart a health advantage on humans or animals at a certain level.

Plessas et al. (2012) in their studies showed that probiotic microorganisms usually make a weak contribution to the product's organoleptic properties and steadily grow in milk. *Lactobacillus plantarum* and *Lactobacillus paracasei* subsp. *tolerans* have potential use in the manufacture of conventional Greek set-type yogurt as adjuncts. Studies have shown that the survival and viability of yogurt probiotics are lower than those required for the prescribed daily intake. Commercial yogurts have been found to have low numbers of *Lactobacillus acidophilus* and, in particular, bifidobacteria. Several practices have been suggested to encourage probiotic growth and viability during storage and to enhance the sensory characteristics of the finished product, such as milk supplementation.

**TABLE 3.7**
**Functional Probiotic Organisms Used in Yogurt Production**

| Microorganism | Strain |
|---|---|
| Lactic acid bacteria | *Lactobacillus rhamnous GG*<br>*Lactobacillus casei*<br>*Lactobacillus cascishirota*<br>*Lactobacillus acidophillus*<br>*Lactobacillus johnsonii* |
| Bifidobacteria | *Bifidobacterium breve*<br>*Bifidobacterium bifidum*<br>*Bifidobacterium infantis*<br>*Bifidobacterium animalis* |
| Yeasts | *Saccharomyces cerevisiae boulardi* |

## 3.15 CRITERIA FOR THE SELECTION OF FUNCTIONAL PROBIOTICS AND LAB

Nowadays, the use of probiotics depends on the following criteria (**Figure 3.4**):

i. They must be of human origin, as it is intended for human consumption.
ii. They should be recognized as safe: GRAS (generally recognized as safe).
iii. They should survive when passing through the GI tract and arrive alive to be able to act.
iv. They should have the ability to attach to the GI tract.
v. They should survive the acidic conditions produced in the human GI tract (several metabolic products appear in the food product, including acetic acid and lactic acid).
vi. Additionally, the functional properties encompass the probiotics' capacity to survive in the gastrointestinal tract, aid in digestion, strengthen immunity, and inhibit mutations. (Culligan et al., 2009).
vii. Furthermore, the probiotic strains should not deconjugate bile salts or have transmissible antibiotic-resistance genes.

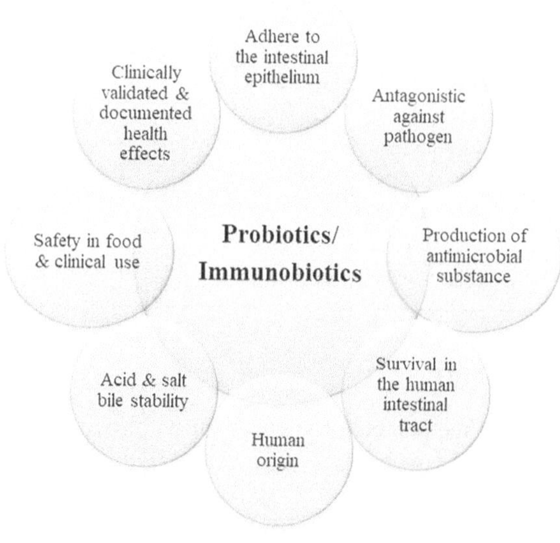


**FIGURE 3.4 Major features of functional probiotics.** Many functional qualities such as resistance to stomach acidity, bile, and salt are used to select probiotics.

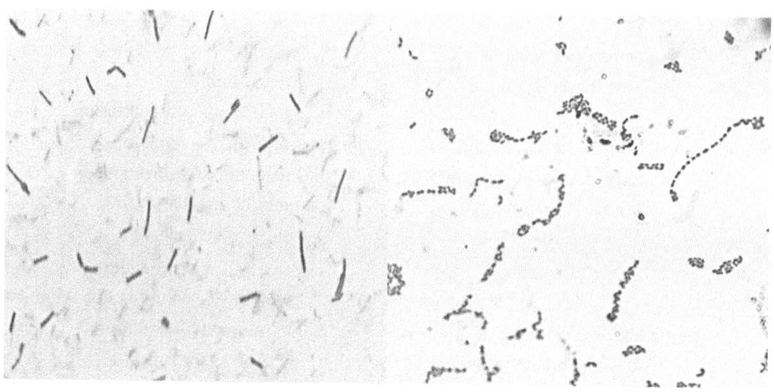

a b

**FIGURE 3.5 Bacteria in yogurt.** (**a**) *Lactobacillus* sp. and (**b**) *Streptococcus thermophilus*.

## 3.16 QUALITY JUDGING OF YOGURT

The Hedonic Type scale is used to assess the sensory qualities of yogurt (Shekhar et al., 2012). The Hedonic Type scale is illustrated in the example below (**Table 3.8**).

**TABLE 3.8**
**Score Card for Sensory/Organoleptic Evaluation of Yogurt**

| Name: | | Sample no: | | | Date: | |
|---|---|---|---|---|---|---|
| Sl. no | Color and appearance | Aroma | Taste | Body and texture | Overall acceptability | Total remarks |
| 1 | | | | | | |
| 2 | | | | | | |
| 3 | | | | | | |
| 4 | | | | | | |
| 5 | | | | | | |

| Rate | Organoleptic score |
|---|---|
| Like extremely | 9 |
| Like very much | 8 |
| Like moderately | 7 |
| Like slightly | 6 |
| Neither like nor dislike | 5 |
| Dislike slightly | 4 |
| Dislike moderately | 3 |
| Dislike very much | 2 |
| Dislike extremely | 1 |

## 3.17 DEFECTS IN YOGURT

Aneja et al. (2002) described the defects of yogurt/dahi with their possible causes and remedies, which are shown in (**Table 3.9**).

**TABLE 3.9**
**Defects, Probable Causes, and Remedies in Yogurt/Dahi**

| Name of the defects | Probable cause | Remedies |
|---|---|---|
| **Flavor defects** | | |
| Insufficient flavor | i. Low citrate level in milk<br>ii. Low diacetyl content | i. Add 0.02–0.05% sodium citrate before mixing the starter culture.<br>ii. Cool rapidly after culturing. |
| Oxidized flavor | i. Copper contamination<br>ii. Exposure to fluorescent light, exposure to sunlight | i. Avoid the usage of copper utensils.<br>ii. Prevent product from being exposed to UV or sunlight directly. |
| Yeast/cheesy flavor | i. Yeast growth | i. Sanitation check |
| Rancid flavor | i. Lipolytic activity | i. Prior to homogenization, raw and pasteurized dairy components should not be combined. |
| High acidity | i. Excessive culture addition<br>ii. Prolonged incubation period<br>iii. Using sour milk | i. Optimum culture addition<br>ii. As soon as the product's pH is at its ideal level, blast-cool it.<br>iii. Use fresh milk. |

**TABLE 3.9 *(Continued)***

| Name of the defects | Probable cause | Remedies |
|---|---|---|
| **Body and textural defects** | | |
| Weak body | i. Insufficient heat treatment<br>ii. Inadequate milk non-fat solids<br>iii. Severe agitation after homogenization | i. Recommended heat treatment temp. is 85°C for 30 min.<br>ii. Homogenization before fermentation<br>iii. By adding skim milk powder, raise the non-fat solids content to 11%. |
| Grainy texture | i. Higher acidity<br>ii. Improper distribution of skim milk powder | i. As soon as the product reaches the ideal acidity, rapidly cool it to 5°C.<br>ii. Apply an inner screen/filter. |
| Syneresis | i. Improper heat treatment<br>ii. Improper standardization and too low milk non-fat solids<br>iii. Agitation/disturbances during fermentation | i. Recommended heat treatment temp. is 85°C for 30 min.<br>ii. By adding skim milk powder, raise the non-fat solids content to 11%.<br>iii. The cups during fermentation should not be disturbed. |
| Ropiness | i. Psychotropic microorganisms<br>ii. Culture contamination | i. Proper heat treatment of milk; avoid cold storage of milk before pasteurization.<br>ii. Use pure culture. |

## 3.18 FUTURE STRATEGIES TO PROTECT THE HUMAN GUT

Tiwari et al. (2012) demonstrated the strategies to protect the human gut, which are described in the following subsections:

i. Produce genetically modified (GM) probiotics to strengthen the effect of the existing strain. To prevent damage and inflammation in the gut, they are utilized as food additives to regulate the release of human growth factors by modified bacteria. As an example, the genetically altered probiotic bacterium *Bacteroides ovatus* in the human gut may be stimulated by a plant sugar called xylan to create certain proteins that can heal damaged cells that suppress the immune system in the intestine and contribute to sickness and inflammation.
ii. Using microencapsulated probiotic cells in acidic products is becoming popular to help the probiotics survive and remain effective. The process of microencapsulation protects probiotic cells and minimizes their vulnerability to damage in challenging conditions.
iii. Improving the survival of an included probiotic is to formulate the food product in such a way that it assists probiotics.
iv. Probiotics should be non-resistant to low pH and should be safe for humans; they should survive when they pass through the GI tract and arrive alive to be able to act.
v. Low-cost production of probiotics.
vi. Expansion of proven strains to benefit the oral cavity, respiratory tract, stomach, bladder, and skin as well as for cancer, allergies, and recovery from surgery and injury.
vii. Improvement of the viability of probiotics.
viii. Development of probiotics organisms that carry vaccines or other beneficial substances.

## 3.19 BEST TIME TO CONSUME YOGURT

Obviously, the stomach is a challenging environment that exposes any probiotics taken to a low (acidic) pH; however, the exact pH changes constantly, dependent on the time of day and the presence or absence of food. It is recommended that our probiotics are taken with breakfast each day, as stomach acid is naturally at its weakest in the mornings, and this is then buffered (or diluted) still further by the presence of food in the stomach. Taking probiotic supplements at this time of day offers the greatest percentage survival of bacteria and therefore the greatest health benefits from the product.

Looking at yogurt and examining the survival of probiotic bacteria through digestive acids, usually bifidobacteria survive the stomach's gastric acidity at a level of a tenth of a percent to a percent. So, if there include 10 billion CFUs in the initial product, a percent or a tenth of a percent makes it into the gut (Deep Dive, 2016).

A strain might get good results by supplying a certain health or wellness benefit at 10 billion CFUs. About 24% to 78% survival of probiotic bacteria through gastric acid is expected.

- The right dose of probiotics will depend on an individual's purpose for taking probiotics.
- A daily dose of 10–15 billion CFU is advisable for individuals seeking everyday immune and digestive support.

## 3.20 HEALTH BENEFITS OF YOGURT

Yogurt is among the most popular fermented foods in the world, and enjoyed by wide consumer due to its taste and health benefits. The significance of disease prevention grows as the population ages. When ingested, probiotics in yogurt are said to have a number of important health benefits (Isolauri, 2004). The major benefits provided by probiotics in yogurt are as follows:

### 3.20.1 Association of Yogurt Consumption with Metabolic Health

Consumers of yogurt typically have better diets and greater intakes of potassium, calcium, magnesium, and zinc, as well as vitamins $B_2$ and $B_{12}$. Additionally, they have lower levels of insulin resistance, systolic blood pressure, circulating lipids, and glucose (Wang et al., 2013). **Figure 3.6 and 3.8** summarize the metabolic health claims connected with the intake of yogurt, advocating them as potential vehicles for future functional food development (Hadjimbei et al., 2022). Yogurt

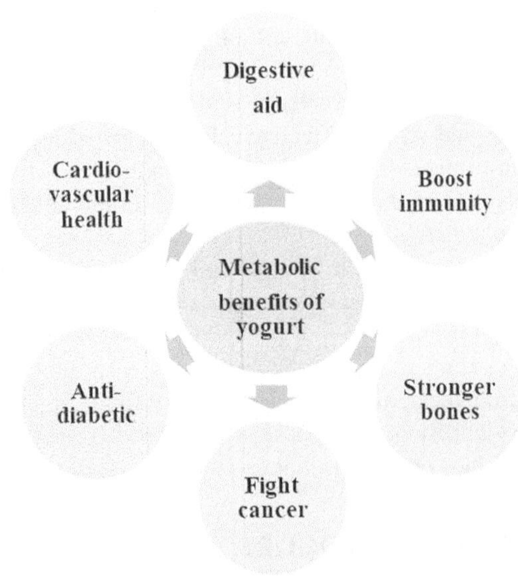


**FIGURE 3.6 Key potential metabolic health benefits of yogurt.** Yogurt contains live bacteria that can benefit human health by promoting a healthy gut microbiome.

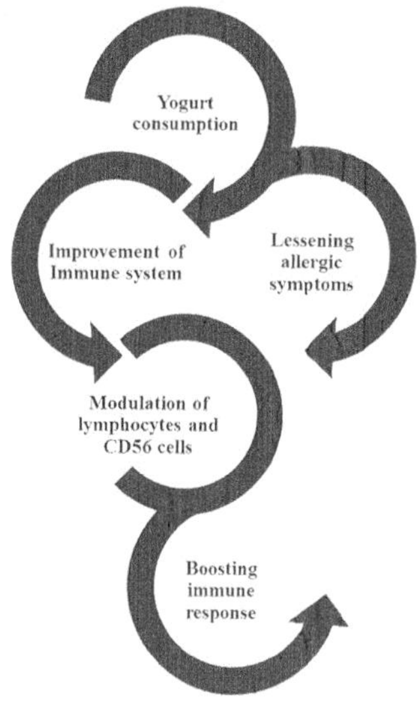


**FIGURE 3.7 Effects of yogurt on the immune system.** Yogurt contains live bacteria that can beneficially regulate the host's immune system. Yogurt possesses a natural "cluster" of nutrients that protect health and enhance the immune system.

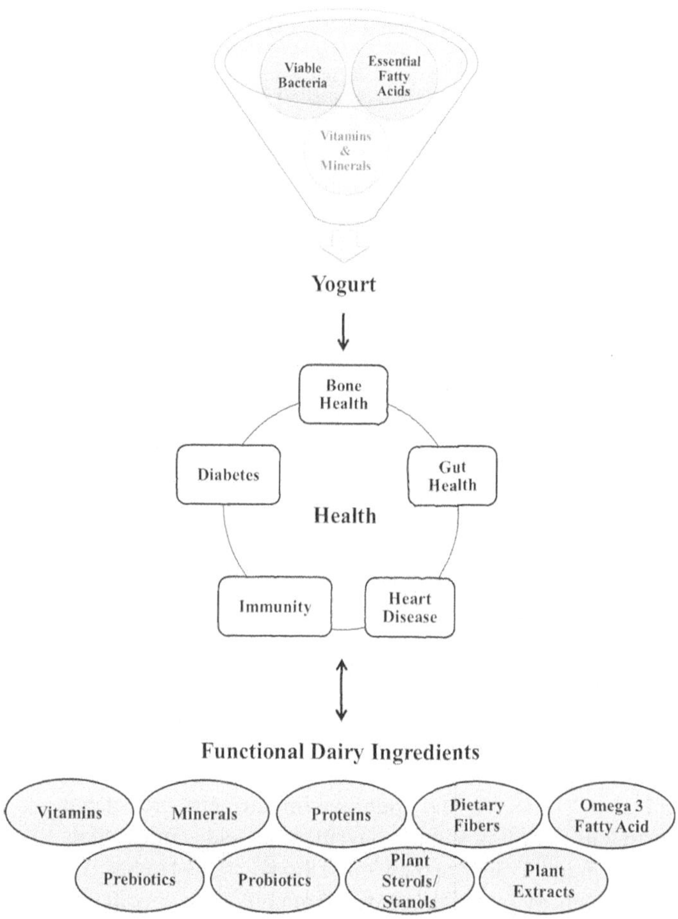


**FIGURE 3.8 Key potential health benefits of yogurt, driving the perfect vehicle for functional dairy food development.** Functional foods offer great potential to improve health and/or help prevent certain diseases when taken as part of a balanced diet and healthy lifestyle. The subject of health claims is becoming increasingly important, and there is broad consensus that there needs to be a regulatory framework that will protect consumers, promote fair trade, and encourage product innovation in the food industry.

includes living microorganisms that can help the host's immune system (Kamada et al., 2013) (**Figure 3.6, 3.7**).

### 3.20.2 Association of Yogurt Consumption with Bone Health

A more recent randomized controlled experiment found that, when consumed regularly, fat-free plain Greek yogurt following 12 weeks of high-impact loading exercise promotes bone growth in university-aged individuals compared to a carbohydrate-based placebo that was lacking in protein and calcium (Bridge et al., 2020). Yogurt's advantages for bone health are outlined in **Figure 3.9** (Hadjimbei et al., 2022).

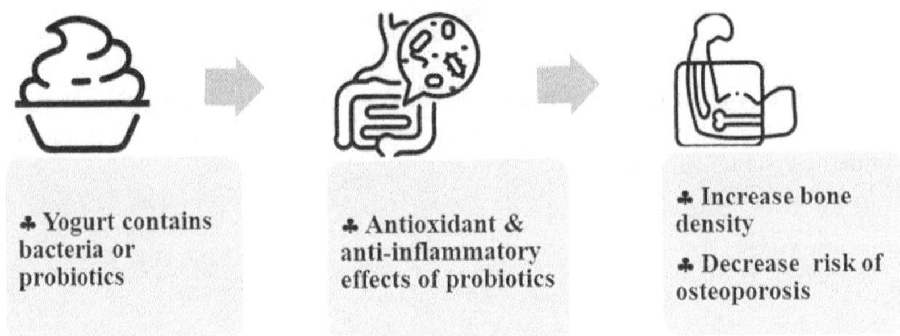


**FIGURE 3.9 Bone health benefits of yogurt.** Yogurt containing live bacteria and those with additional prebiotics may enhance bone health by altering the gut flora and improving calcium absorption.

### 3.20.3 Association of Yogurt Consumption with Gut Health

It is suggested to incorporate dairy products, especially those that include probiotics (probiotic yogurt), in the diet on a daily basis as a dietary supplement because pregnancy-related constipation is a result of a combination of mechanical and hormonal factors (Mirghafourvand et al., 2016). The health benefits of yogurt and fermented milks on gut health, including improvement of gut integrity and cognitive processes, are summarized in **Figure 3.10** (Hadjimbei et al., 2022).

### 3.20.4 Association of Yogurt Consumption with Healthy and Active Aging

Consuming yogurt has been related to health advantages in persons of all ages. Nevertheless, information on the nutritional and health benefits of yogurt for older persons is accessible. Yogurt is an excellent source of protein, rich in calcium, zinc, B vitamins, probiotics, and can be supplemented with vitamin D and more probiotics to improve health benefits. Numerous nutritional deficiencies and health issues linked to under and overnutrition, such as musculoskeletal disability, immunosenescence, cardiometabolic illnesses, and cognitive impairment, are related with aging (El-Abbadi et al., 2014). Yogurt is also accessible and convenient for older individuals to consume, making it a workable strategy to improve older persons' nutritional status (Lebeer et al., 2010). Only a small number of studies, the majority of which are observational, have specifically examined the effect of yogurt on the dietary and health status of older persons. However, the reported results thus far have been encouraging, implying that yogurt has the potential to enhance the nutrition and overall health of older individuals. These studies also encourage additional research on the contribution of yogurt to healthy and active aging (El-Abbadi et al., 2014).

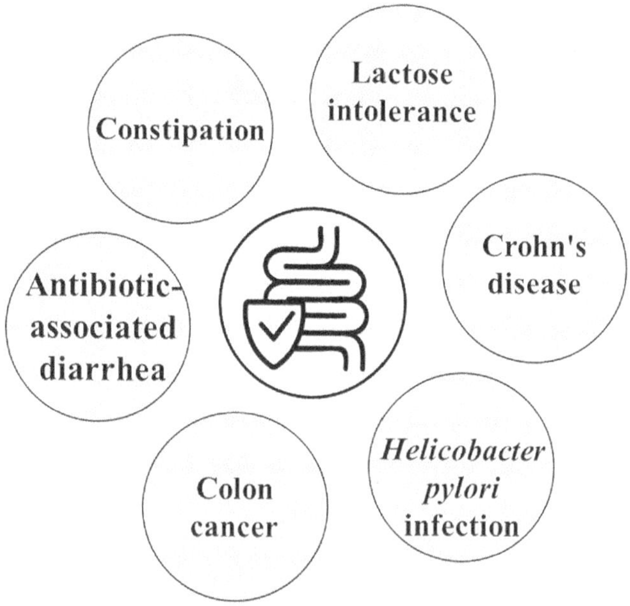


**FIGURE 3.10 Human gut health benefits of yogurt.** Yogurt contains probiotics, which may improve digestive health by alleviating symptoms of common gastrointestinal diseases such bloating, diarrhea, and constipation.

## 3.21 YOGURT INNOVATIONS

Innovations and advancements in yogurt have experienced tremendous change over the period of time and running, especially in sensory and nutritional attributes. These innovations involve the use of new technologies, research findings, or consumer preferences to create a better yogurt experience. Fortification is a major concern in yogurt mainly focused on the consumers' health, done by incorporating fruit extract, cereals, fiber, protein, vitamins, and minerals. High-protein, low-sugar, and plant-based yogurt with added functional ingredients like vitamin D and probiotics is a hot topic in the yogurt industry. On the other way, technological innovations were made in the packaging system to increase the shelf life. This results in an increasing demand for yogurt throughout the world. **Figures 3.11,** and **3.12** illustrate yogurt innovations in nutritional and health attributes.

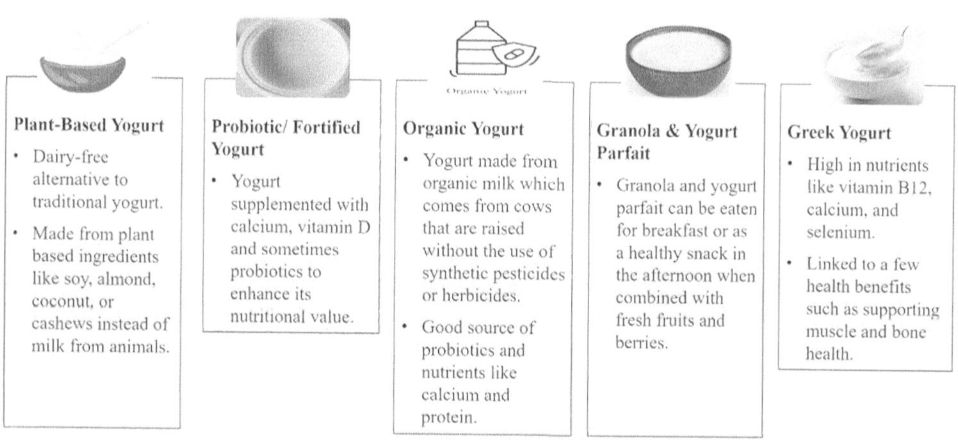


**FIGURE 3.11 Yogurt innovations in nutritional attributes.**

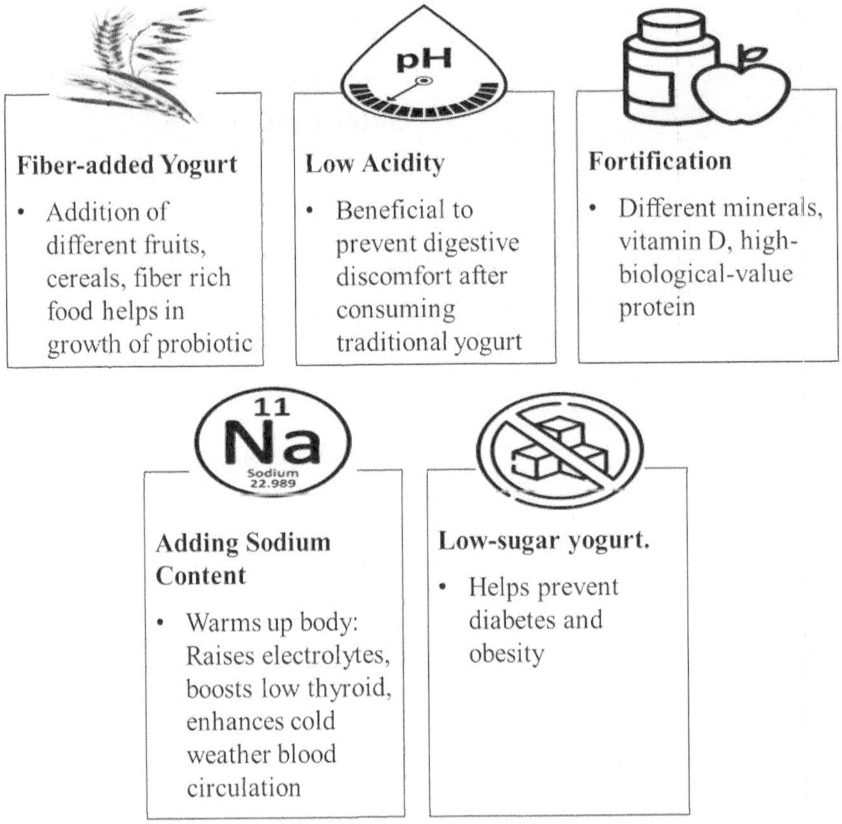


**FIGURE 3.12 Yogurt innovations in health attributes.**

## 3.22 SAFETY, SPOILAGE, AND SHELF LIFE OF YOGURT

Yogurt production has two characteristics that provide barriers to pathogen growth: heat and acidity (low pH) (Matin et al., 2018). Both of these factors are necessary to ensure a safe product. Recent outbreaks of food poisoning by *E. coli*, which is acid-tolerant, bring into question the protective mechanism of acidity alone. However, *E. coli* is easily destroyed by pasteurization.

Yogurt generally has a 10- to 21-day shelf life when made properly and stored in the refrigerator at temperatures below 40°F. To ensure a long shelf life, always use clean and sanitized equipment and containers.

## 3.23 YOGURT YIELD

One liter of milk yields approximately 1 kg of yogurt. It depends on the type of milk and the method used to manufacture the yogurt, but in general, 1 kg of yogurt for 1 liter of milk is to be expected. The amount of yogurt produced will be nearly identical to the amount of milk used to manufacture it. All that is done during manufacture is the inclusion of starter culture. In theory, a small amount of lactose is transformed into lactic acid and carbon dioxide is produced, although these have no practical effect on weight.

## 3.24 CONCLUSIONS

Yogurt consumption exhibits favorable health effects on a number of pathological illnesses, as is abundantly obvious from the accumulating scientific research. Along with gut health promotion and immune system regulation, treated conditions include osteoporosis, cardiovascular conditions, and diabetes. The health benefits of consuming yogurt and fermented milks are becoming more and more evident; therefore, it can be a good idea to promote regular intake of these foods as a complement to meals or as a tasty substitute for other snacks. Additionally, since yogurt products are generally accepted and consumed, they may make a great delivery system for beneficial substances that offer alternative methods for the prevention of disease and the promotion of good health. The stability of functional components and their interactions with the product matrix must be thoroughly investigated in order to ensure the functionality of novel products over the course of their commercial life. Despite these encouraging findings, there are still unsolved issues regarding the mechanisms underlying yogurt's positive effects and its food matrix effects in terms of overall dietary patterns, metabolic health, and its risk factors. An emphasis on the development of novel, functional dairy products that are not yet available on the market, along with the use of next-generation probiotics, should be made possible by the literature's increasingly positive findings, which should serve as leverage for the food industry.

## REFERENCES


Akter, S., Akter, N., & Kober, A. K. M. H. (2019). *Isolation of Escherichia Coli and Salmonella sp from Dahi marketed in Chattogram Metropolitan Area* (p. 116). 4th Young Scientist Congress', Dhaka, Bangladesh (Abstr- PP 10).

Amin, U. S., Kober, A. K. M. H., Akter, N., Hossain, M. A., & Rana, E. A. (2022). Isolation and identification of lactic acid bacteria from traditional fermented milk "Dahi" towards developing probiotic dahi in Bangladesh. *Journal of Modern Agriculture and Biotechnology*, *1*(1), 2.

Aneja, R. P., Mathur, B. N., Chandan, R. C., & Banerjee, A. K. (2002). *Technology of Indian milk products: Handbook on process technology modernization for professionals, entrepreneurs and scientists*. Dairy India Yearbook.

Bari, M. S., Mokbul, S. B., & Kober, A. K. M. H. (2017). Isolation of exopolysaccharide producing *Lactobacillus bulgaricus* organism from yoghurt. *International Journal of Natural Sciences*, *6*(3), 123–127.

Bridge, A. D., Brown, J., Snider, H., Ward, W. E., Roy, B. D., & Josse, A. R. (2020). Consumption of Greek yogurt during 12 weeks of high-impact loading exercise increases bone formation in young, adult males-a secondary analysis from a randomized trial. *Applied Physiology, Nutrition, and Metabolism = Physiologie Appliquee, Nutrition Et Metabolisme*, *45*(1), 91–100.

Clancy, R. (2003). Immunobiotics and the probiotic evolution. *FEMS Immunology and Medical Microbiology*, *38*(1), 9–12.

Culligan, E. P., Hill, C., & Sleator, R. D. (2009). Probiotics and gastrointestinal disease: Successes, problems and future prospects. *Gut Pathogens*, *1*(1), 19.

Deep Dive. (2016). *Probiotics are alive, active and not just in yogurt*. www.fooddive.com/news/probiotics-are-alive-active-and-not-just-in-yogurt/425873/.

El-Abbadi, N. H., Dao, M. C., & Meydani, S. N. (2014). Yogurt: Role in healthy and active aging. *The American Journal of Clinical Nutrition*, *99*(Suppl. 5), 1263S–1270S.

Fisberg, M., & Machado, R. (2015). History of yogurt and current patterns of consumption. *Nutrition Reviews*, *73*(Suppl. 1), 4–7.

Ghosh, J., & Rajorhia, G. S. (1990). Selection of starter culture for production of indigenous fermented milk product (Misti dahi). *Le Lait*, *70*(2), 147–154.

Hadjimbei, E., Botsaris, G., & Chrysostomou, S. (2022). Beneficial effects of yoghurts and probiotic fermented milks and their functional food potential. *Foods (Basel, Switzerland)*, *11*(17), 2691.

Hoseinifar, S. H., Sun, Y. Z., Wang, A., & Zhou, Z. (2018). Probiotics as means of diseases control in aquaculture, a review of current knowledge and future perspectives. *Frontiers in Microbiology*, *9*, 2429.

Isolauri, E. (2004). Dietary modification of atopic disease: Use of probiotics in the prevention of atopic dermatitis. *Current Allergy and Asthma Reports*, *4*(4), 270–275.

Jacobs, S. E., Tobin, J. M., Opie, G. F., Donath, S., Tabrizi, S. N., Pirotta, M., Morley, C. J., Garland, S. M., & ProPrems Study Group. (2013). Probiotic effects on late-onset sepsis in very preterm infants: A randomized controlled trial. *Pediatrics*, *132*(6), 1055–1062.

Juodeikiene, G., Bartkiene, E., Viskelis, P., Urbonaviciene, D., Eidukonyte, D., & Bobinas, C. (2012). Fermentation processes using lactic acid bacteria producing bacteriocins for preservation and improving functional properties of food products. *Advances in Applied Biotechnology*, 63–100.

Kamada, N., Chen, G. Y., Inohara, N., & Núñez, G. (2013). Control of pathogens and pathobionts by the gut microbiota. *Nature Immunology*, *14*(7), 685–690.

Kanawjia, S. K. (2006). *Technological innovations in the manufacture of dahi and misti dahi*. Developments in Traditional Dairy Products.

Kober, A. K. M. H., Mannan, M. A., Debnath, G. K., & Akter, S. (2007). Quality evaluation of dahi/yogurts sold in Chittagong metropolitan area in Bangladesh. *International Journal of Sustainable Agricultural Technology*, *3*, 41–46.

Kober, A. K. M. H., Riaz Rajoka, M. S., Mehwish, H. M., Villena, J., & Kitazawa, H. (2022). Immunomodulation potential of probiotics: A novel strategy for improving livestock health, immunity, and productivity. *Microorganisms*, *10*(2), 388.

Kobyliak, N., Conte, C., Cammarota, G., Haley, A. P., Styriak, I., Gaspar, L., Fusek, J., Rodrigo, L., & Kruzliak, P. (2016). Probiotics in prevention and treatment of obesity: A critical view. *Nutrition & Metabolism*, *13*, 14.

Lebeer, S., Vanderleyden, J., & De Keersmaecker, S. C. (2010). Host interactions of probiotic bacterial surface molecules: Comparison with commensals and pathogens. *Nature Reviews. Microbiology*, *8*(3), 171–184.

Matin, A., Banik, T., Badsha, M. R., Hossain, A., Haque, M. M., & Ahmad, M. (2018). Microbiological quality analysis of yoghurt in some selected areas of Bangladesh. *International Journal of Natural and Social Sciences*, *5*(4), 82–86.

Merenstein, D. J., Tan, T. P., Molokin, A., Smith, K. H., Roberts, R. F., Shara, N. M., Mete, M., Sanders, M. E., & Solano-Aguilar, G. (2015). Safety of *Bifidobacterium animalis* subsp. lactis (B. lactis) strain BB-12-supplemented yogurt in healthy adults on antibiotics: A phase I safety study. *Gut Microbes*, *6*(1), 66–77.

Mirghafourvand, M., Homayouni Rad, A., Mohammad Alizadeh Charandabi, S., Fardiazar, Z., & Shokri, K. (2016). The effect of probiotic yogurt on constipation in pregnant women: A randomized controlled clinical trial. *Iranian Red Crescent Medical Journal*, *18*(11), e39870.

Mudgal, S. P., & Prajapati, J. B. (2017). Dahi-An Indian naturally fermented yogurt. In *Yogurt in health and disease prevention* (pp. 353–369). Academic Press.

Panjagari, N. R., Behare, P., Devraja, M., Khetra, Y., Kharui, K., & Hussain, S. A. (2013). *Dairy products technology*. Central Board of Secondary Education, Delhi.

Plessas, S., Bosnea, L., Alexopoulos, A., & Bezirtzoglou, E. (2012). Potential effects of probiotics in cheese and yogurt production: A review. *Engineering in Life Sciences*, *12*(4), 433–440.

Production of Yoghurt. (2020). *Fact sheet food*. www.teagasc.ie/media/website/rural-economy/rural-development/diversification/1-Production-of-Yoghurt.pdf.

Rao, S. C., Athalye-Jape, G. K., Deshpande, G. C., Simmer, K. N., & Patole, S. K. (2016). Probiotic supplementation and late-onset sepsis in preterm infants: A meta-analysis. *Pediatrics*, *137*(3).

Rutella, G. S., Tagliazucchi, D., & Solieri, L. (2016). Survival and bioactivities of selected probiotic lactobacilli in yogurt fermentation and cold storage: New insights for developing a bi-functional dairy food. *Food Microbiology*, *60*, 54–61.

Shekhar, S., Joe, J., Kumar, R., Jyothis, J., Kumar, K., Priya, Y. A., Rao, K. J., & Pagote, C. N. (2012). Effect of heat treatment of milk on the sensory and rheological quality of dahi prepared from cow milk. *Journal of Food and Dairy Technology*, *1*(1), 8–14.

Tiwari, G., Tiwari, R., Pandey, S., & Pandey, P. (2012). Promising future of probiotics for human health: Current scenario. *Chronicles of Young Scientists*, *3*(1), 17–17.

Wang, Z. H., Gao, Q. Y., & Fang, J. Y. (2013). Meta-analysis of the efficacy and safety of Lactobacillus-containing and Bifidobacterium-containing probiotic compound preparation in Helicobacter pylori eradication therapy. *Journal of Clinical Gastroenterology*, *47*(1), 25–32.

Zaharuddin, L., Mokhtar, N. M., Muhammad Nawawi, K. N., & Raja Ali, R. A. (2019). A randomized double-blind placebo-controlled trial of probiotics in post-surgical colorectal cancer. *BMC Gastroenterology*, *19*(1), 131.

# 4 Protein-Rich Dairy Food—Cheese (Preservation of Milk)

## 4.1 LEARNING OBJECTIVES

By the end of the chapter, the reader will be able to:

- Understand the classification and composition of cheese
- Learn about cheese varieties and their characteristics
- Gain knowledge of cheese production and processing
- Learn about cheese analogue
- Understand how technology can help speed up the process and make cheese taste better
- Make cheese enterprises profitable
- Learn about cheese judging and how to improve the quality of the cheese
- Learn about the key potential health benefits of cheese
- Discover cheese innovations from production to nutritional and health attributes

Recent research demonstrates that the flavoring of various soft cheeses is due in part to the bacteria that colonize them during ripening. Scientists have developed new cheese recently using vegetable rennet instead of traditional rennet. These cheeses have similar taste and texture to regular cheeses. This aims to address the requirements of customers, particularly those who practice a vegetarian lifestyle. On the other hand, wooden vats are often employed in the production of traditional cheeses, as they contain abundant biofilms that transfer considerable amounts of bacteria to the cheese.

## 4.2 INTRODUCTION

Cheese is a type of food that is made from milk (**Figure 4.1**). To make cheese, casein (milk protein) is thickened using substances like rennet or certain enzymes, along with lactic acid produced by bacteria that are intentionally added or naturally present. The cheese is then cut, cooked, pressed, molded, and allowed to ripen at the proper temperature and humidity. Over a few thousand years, the art of manufacturing cheese has almost reached the level of science. Cheese variations have multiplied to accommodate various conditions and needs. More than 1000 types are thought to exist.

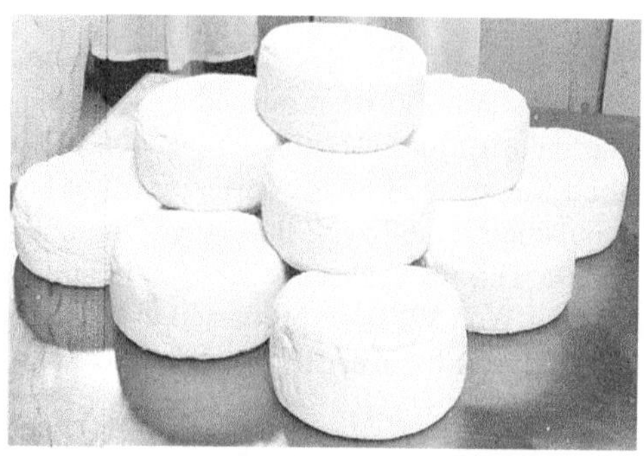

FIGURE 4.1 **Image of cheese (Gouda).** Over time, humans have created many different types of cheese with various flavors, textures, and shapes.

DOI: 10.1201/9781003397786-4

Cheese is the most popular milk product worldwide and is known as the "meat of milk" due to its high amount of protein. Concerning proteins, vitamins, and minerals, it is also just as nutrient dense as milk. Additionally, because of the proteolytic activity during cheese ripening, the digestibility of proteins increases. Cheese is also a healthy dietary choice for those with diabetes or lactose sensitivity due to the low milk-to-sugar ratio it contains.

### 4.2.1 Definition

Cheese is a product prepared from the curd derived from whole, partially skimmed, or skimmed milk from cows or other animals, with or without adding cream, by coagulating the casein with rennet, lactic acid, or another suitable enzyme or acid, with or without further treatment of the separated curd by heat or pressure, or by using ripening ferments, special molds, or seasoning. Cheese is a way to store extra milk. The average composition of cheese consists of water (34–39%), protein (23–27%), fat (30–36%), vitamins (1%), and calcium (4%).

## 4.3 HISTORY OF CHEESE

Around 8000 BC, it is believed that the first cheese was produced around the time when sheep were domesticated. The enzyme rennet, which is required to manufacture cheese, is naturally found in the stomachs of ruminants. Animals' bladder-like organs and leak-proof stomachs were typically used to store and carry milk and other liquids. In the production of the earliest types of cheese, the milk would have naturally curdled due to the intense summer heat and leftover rennet in the stomach lining. The result of straining these milk curds and adding salt for additional preservation is what we now refer to as "cheese." Most cheeses were consumed fresh and prepared every day, even without the addition of salt. Early Roman writings mention how frequently cheese was consumed in ancient Rome. They ate a wide range of cheeses, and manufacturing cheese was already regarded as an art. The Roman legions received hard cheese from them. The Latin word "*caseus*" from which the English term "cheese" derives, has a proto-Indo-European root that means to ferment or turn sour (Moncel, 2019).

### 4.3.1 European Cheeses

In northern Europe, the cheese had a more delectable flavor since it didn't require excessive salt for preservation, leading to a smoother and more tender consistency. In these colder regions, aged, matured, and blue cheeses were also manufactured. Cheddar, Gouda, Parmesan, and Camembert were among the cheeses that were originally produced in Europe throughout the Middle Ages (Moncel, 2019).

### 4.3.2 Modern Cheeses

It wasn't until 1815 that the first cheese manufacturing facility was created in Switzerland when cheese started to be produced in large quantities. Later, when rennet could be mass produced, the industrial cheese production took off just like wildfire. A revolution in American industrial food was sparked by the development of processed cheese. Natural cheese is combined with milk, emulsifiers, stabilizers, flavorings, and colors to manufacture processed cheese (Alavi & Momen, 2020). This inexpensive cheese is popular among Americans, as it melts smoothly and reliably. During World War II, processed cheese was produced in greater quantities. Since then, manufactured cheese has steadily overtaken real cheese in American diets (Moncel, 2019).

## 4.4 TYPES OF CHEESE

There are lots of different kinds of cheese. Cheeses may be classified based on their moisture and fat substance as "hard cheese," "semi-hard cheese," or "soft cheese" (**Figure 4.2**).

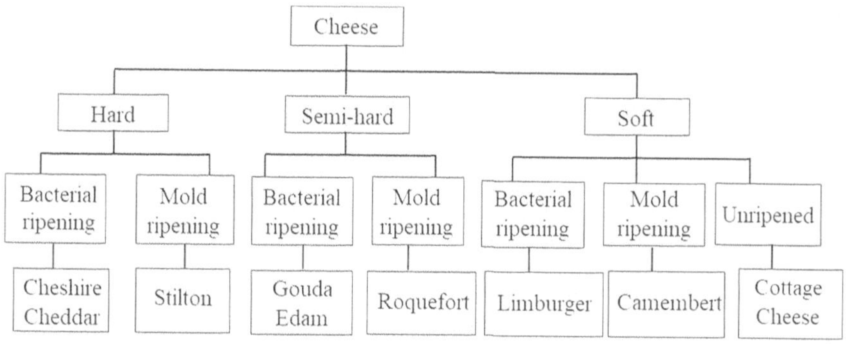


**FIGURE 4.2 Classification of cheese.** Cheese is often classified according to hardness, which varies with moisture content. Firm cheeses can have moisture content as low as about 30%, whereas soft or fresh cheeses can have moisture content as high as 80%.

### 4.4.1 Hard Cheese (49–56% Moisture)

Hard cheese is produced when a significant amount of moisture from the curd is removed during production, leaving the final product hard and dry. The starter culture used to produce close-textured hard cheese releases very little carbon dioxide, and all the lactose is fermented before the cheese is finally formed. Parmigiano, Grana Padano, Pecorino, Cheddar, Gruyere, Emmental, and Mimolette are all highly popular examples of hard cheeses.

### 4.4.2 Semi-Hard Cheese (54–69% Moisture)

i. Ripened by bacteria
ii. Ripened by molds
iii. Ripened by whey

Semi-hard cheese is consumed by a large group of people around the globe. These cheeses need at least 4 weeks to ripen, and the longer the period, the better and more flavorful the cheese will be. This means that cheeses that are ripened for a short time, like Gouda, have a relatively mild flavor, whereas cheeses that are ripened for a longer time, like Appenzeller, have a flavor that is considerably more potent and intense. Gouda, Edam, and Maasdam are types of well-liked semi-hard cheese.

### 4.4.3 Soft Cheese (69–80% Moisture)

i. Unripened
ii. Ripened by bacteria
iii. Ripened by molds

White soft cheese (Gibnabeida) is a type of pickled cheese that is soft or semi-soft. Although fresh consumption of the cheese was an option, it was more frequently consumed after ripening in sealed containers of salt brine or salt-cured whey. The cheese's flavor is enhanced and it is preserved by the brine solution and salted whey. The pickling process is what sets this group apart from other conventional soft cheeses found in temperate regions.

Cheese quickly turns sour in warm weather before it ripens; therefore, salting is crucial for its preservation. Gibnabeidal and Domiati cheeses are essentially salt-cured in the first stage of production when salt is added to milk before renneting, distinguishing them from other soft pickled cheeses.

**Casein** is the main component of cheese. Different cheese varieties are distinguished by their:

- Flavor
- Texture
- Type of milk
- Added salt and seasonings
- Type of bacteria and mold species used in ripening
- Manufacturing method

## 4.5 NUTRITIONAL FACTS

The different types of cheese can be classified based on the kind of milk that is used (cow, sheep, goat, buffalo), their manufacture (rennet, sour milk cheese, ultrafiltration), consistency (extra-hard, hard, semi-hard, semi-soft, soft cheese), fat content (double cream, cream, full fat, three-quarters fat, half fat, quarter fat cheese), fermentation type (lactic acid, lactic and propionic acid, butyric acid), surface (hard, soft, with smear, molds), and interior (eyes, molds). The flavors and bioactive compounds are primarily produced during the various ripening stages when the primary ingredients lactose, protein, and fat are broken down by fermentation, proteolysis, and lipolysis. Thus, the variety of cheese on the market is enormous, which is also reflected in the variability within the composition of the different kinds of cheese (**Table 4.1**). In most countries, cheese is majorly produced from cow's milk, which consists of fat, protein, water, vitamins, minerals, and lactose (rarely present).

**TABLE 4.1**
**Nutritional Composition of Fresh, Soft, Semi-Hard, Hard, and Extra-Hard Cheeses (g/kg)**

| Cheese | Water | Protein | Fat | Lactose |
|---|---|---|---|---|
| Fresh cheese | 700 | 110 | 80 | 30 |
| Soft cheese | 520 | 200 | 220 | 0 |
| Semi-hard cheese | 400 | 250 | 270 | 0 |
| Hard cheese | 350 | 270 | 310 | 0 |
| Extra-hard cheese | 300 | 290 | 330 | 0 |

*Source:* Fox et al., 2015

## 4.6 WORLDWIDE CHEESE PRODUCTION AND CONSUMPTION TRENDS

The USA is the world's largest cheese manufacturer with 6,220,001 tonnes of production per year. Germany comes in second with 3,170,500 tonnes of production annually. France is the third-largest cheese manufacturer in the world, producing 2,233,225 tonnes annually. According to the International Dairy Federation (IDF), France is believed to be the country where people eat the most cheese per person each year. However, Finland is not far behind and comes in second place. **Figure 4.3** illustrates cheese consumption per capita information from various countries of the world.

## 4.7 PRINCIPLE OF CHEESE MAKING

Cheese comprises a concentration of milk's ingredients, mainly milk casein, milk fat, and salts (insoluble), as well as water, within which small amounts of soluble salts, albumin, and lactose are found. Milk is coagulated either by adding rennet, lactic acid produced by bacteria, or both to keep

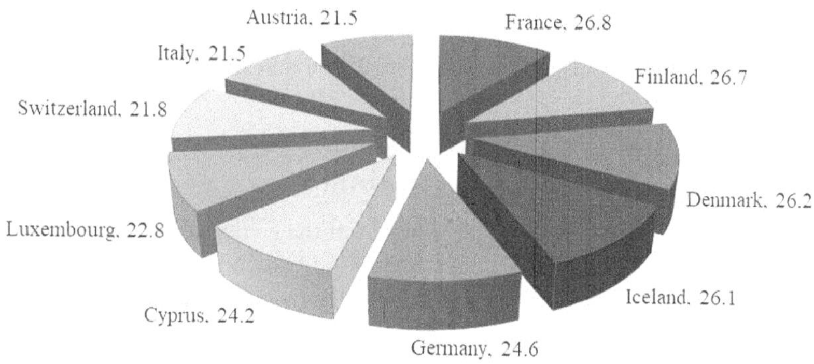


**FIGURE 4.3 Consumption of cheese in various countries (kg per capita).** France is the top country for cheese consumption, with 26.8 kg of cheese per person each year (OECD-FAO, 2016).

these components in concentrated quantities (Kanawjia & Khetra, 2016). It is crucial to remember that the conditions under which cheese is produced have a big impact on its productivity, nutritional content, safety, and sensory quality (Sevenich et al., 2016).

The thousands of varieties vary significantly in shape, size, hardness, color, odor, texture, and style. Regardless of its place of origin or manufacturing method, all cheeses include the following traits:

i. They are manufactured from the milk or milk derivatives of specific mammals
ii. Sourness
iii. Clotting with rennet or the same enzyme preparations
iv. Cutting or breaking up of the coagulum to liberate the whey
v. Consolidation or matting of curd
vi. Maturation

These traits are common to all or any cheeses; however, the conditions vary significantly. Factors responsible for variations in the final cheeses are:

i. Type of milk used
ii. Degree and kind of souring organisms added
iii. Temperature of renneting and subsequent cooking or blistering of the curd in the whey
iv. Milling and salting the curd before putting it in the hoop or mold
v. Pressing of the green cheese
vi. Ripening period, temperature, and relative humidity
vii. Special treatments like stabbing the cheese, bathing within the brine, and surface treatment to provide a definite variety of coats

### 4.7.1 Pasteurization

To eradicate pathogenic bacteria like *Salmonella* and *Campylobacter*, pasteurization is crucial to ensure the safety of cheese (Rankin et al., 2017). The milk should be pasteurized at a temperature of 72°C for 15 seconds. A curd that has been over-pasteurized becomes overly soft; this can or cannot be fixed by adding soluble $CaCl_2$ salt earlier. The ripening period for cheese manufactured from raw milk must be prolonged, and only pasteurized milk may be used to make fresh cheese varieties.

### 4.7.2 Standardization

The qualities of cheese are greatly affected by the milk it's made from. The fat-to-protein ratio is standardized at 1:0.7.

## 4.8 MILK QUALITY USED FOR CHEESE MAKING

Cheese is produced by partially draining the whey after the coagulation of milk by rennet or other coagulating agents. Fresh cheeses like Cottage cheese or Quark are produced when the cheese curd is not ripened; nevertheless, when the cheese curd is pressed and salted, ripened soft, semi-hard, and extremely hard cheese kinds are produced. Novel techniques such as ultrafiltration may be used for cheese making, but the cheese obtained should have similar physical, chemical, and organoleptic characteristics to cheese made by traditional means. Cheese's whey protein-to-casein ratio shouldn't be higher than that of milk's. Milk of good quality for cheese making should have a low content of microorganisms (preferably $<10^4$ CFU/ml milk) and somatic cells (<100,000/ml). To achieve this, the milk must be produced by healthy animals, be as fresh as possible, and have the shortest possible storage period in the bulk tank (El-Salam & El-Shibiny, 2011). Cold storage may cause the growth of psychotropic microorganisms and the leakage of calcium phosphate from the micelles. If storage of the milk is required, the milk should be thermized before storage to avoid the growth of microorganisms. The milk should have a high protein content, which has good cheese-making properties. The variants of lactoglobulin and casein should ideally be present in milk protein. The flavor of the milk must be of good quality, with no off-flavors. The milk should be free of pathogens and clostridium; however, it might include healthy lactic acid bacteria. The milk should contain no antimicrobial agents (Skeie, 2010).

## 4.9 MANUFACTURING PROCESS

The process of making different types of cheese is similar, but small changes can make a difference in the taste of the final cheese. **Figures 4.4 and 4.5** provide flowcharts/pictorials to emphasize the importance of each stage. It will help clarify the procedure better and will supplement the following specific stages.

## 4.10 CHEMICAL CHANGES DURING CHEESE MAKING

All forms of cheese go through the fundamental process of coagulation, which changes milk from liquid to gel. Gel formation happens when proteins become unstable. Rennet, containing acid proteinases like chymosin, can cause this by reducing the pH to the isoelectric point of proteins or through a combination of acidification and heating (Jacob et al., 2011).

### 4.10.1 Action of Rennet

Rennet is an enzyme (**Figure 4.6**) in the stomach lining of young animals that helps in milk digestion. It can made from plant enzymes as well. Milk separates into curds and whey when rennet is added.

The content of the milk, specifically the amount and types of caseins, fat, pH, and calcium, all have an impact on the curd development phases (enzymatic coagulation, curd firming, and syneresis) (Fox et al., 2017). In the initial phase of rennet coagulation, the hydrolysis of κ-casein results in para-κ-casein micelles, which destabilize the casein micelle.

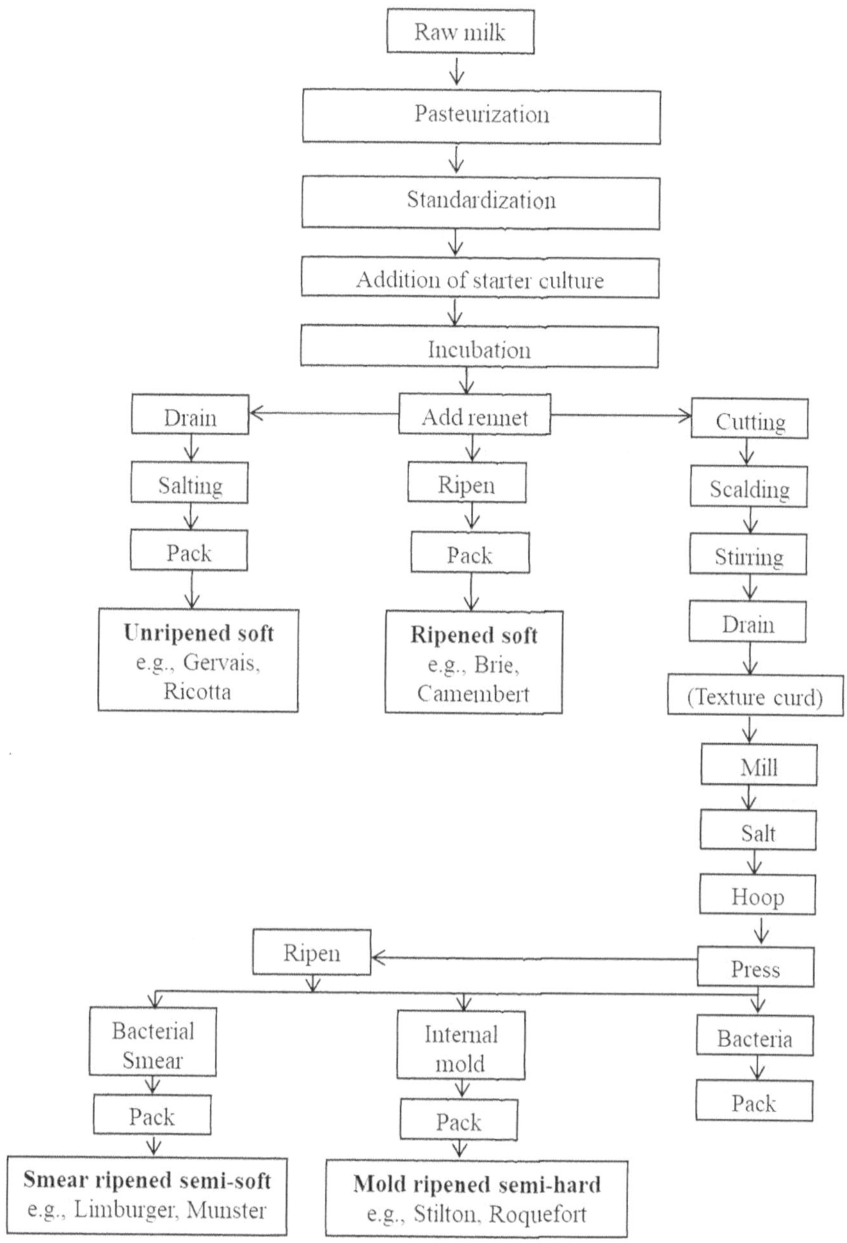


**FIGURE 4.4 Flow chart for the cheese manufacturing process.** It is observed that the cheese-making process comprises multiple phases.

The paracasein micelles then undergo limited aggregation in the secondary calcium-mediated step. A temperature of at least 20°C and quiescent conditions are necessary for the secondary stage. The hydrolysis of κ-casein primarily involves cleavage of the peptide bond. A para-κ-casein, common to all caseins, and a macropeptide specific to each component are produced by this cleavage. The curd is solid enough to cut after the inclusion of rennet, which typically occurs 30 minutes later for most cheese kinds. Depending on the type of cheese, the curd is given various procedures after being cut.

$$\text{Casein} \xrightarrow[\text{Rennet}]{\text{Water}} \text{paracasein} + \text{glycomacropeptide}$$

$$\kappa\text{-casein} \xrightarrow[\text{Rennet}]{\text{Water}} \underset{\text{(insoluble)}}{\text{para-}\kappa\text{-casein}} + \underset{\text{(soluble)}}{\text{glycomacropeptide}}$$

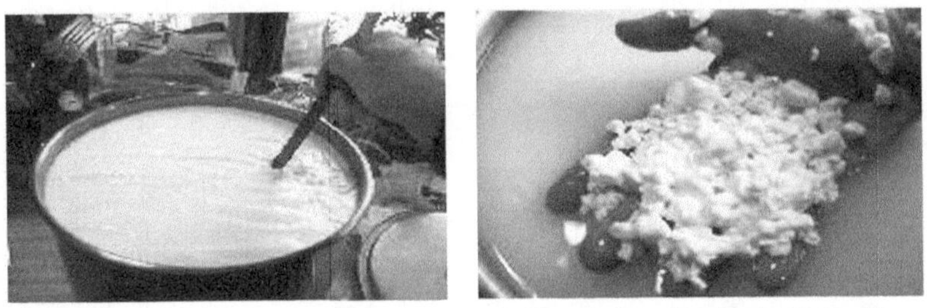

❶ As milk separates into two parts, we call it "curdling" or "clabbering". Curdling happens naturally as the milk sours, but it is done intentionally as the first step in making cheese. Young calves' stomachs are used to extract the enzyme rennin. It makes the milk protein casein clabber when added to raw, whole milk in liquid or tablet form.

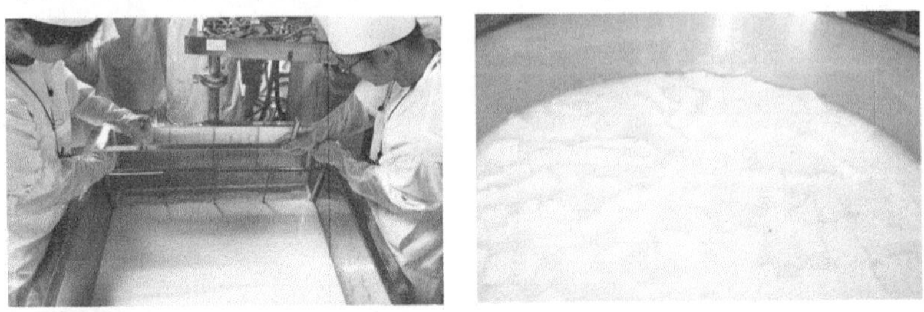

❷A knife is used to cut the clumped milk into cubes.

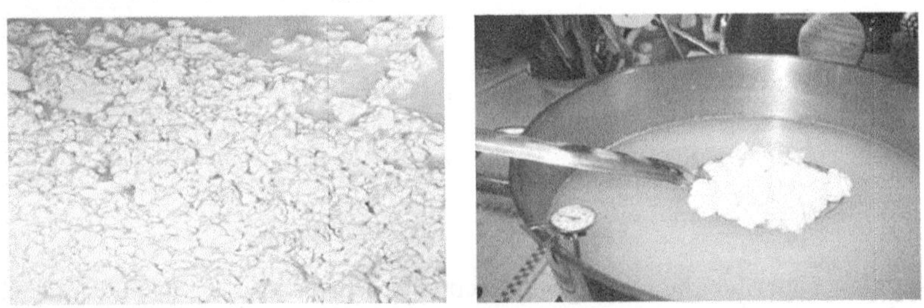

❸ The curds are broken up after the liquid whey has been removed from them. During cheese making at home, a 'cheese cloth' need to be used to drain the curds.

**FIGURE 4.5 Pictorial representation of the various stages of Gouda cheese manufacturing.** The earlier stages are involved in the manufacturing of cheese.

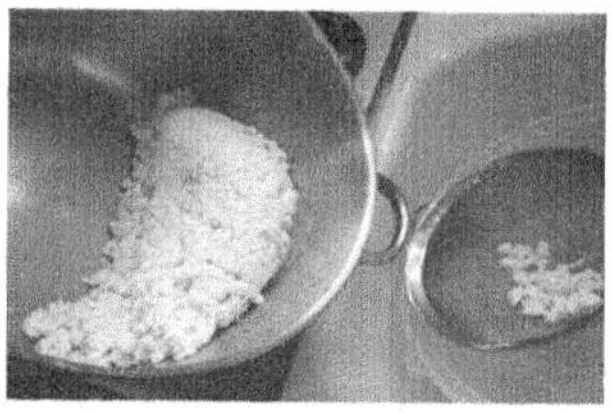

❹ The soft, moist curds are ready for the finishing steps. Some of the curds are crushed into smaller ones, while others are left as large curds.

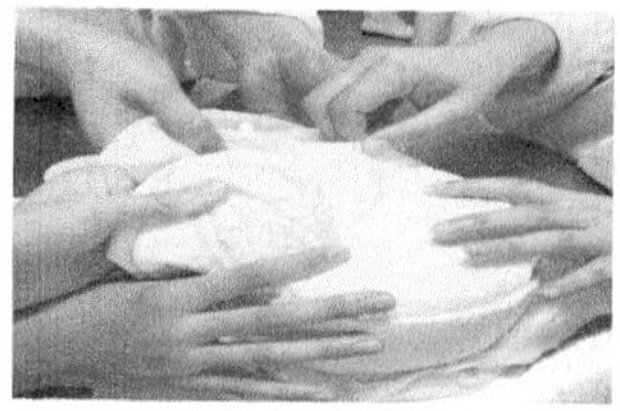

❺ It is Gouda cheese! After the curd is drained and crumbled, the whey is replaced with cream or milk.

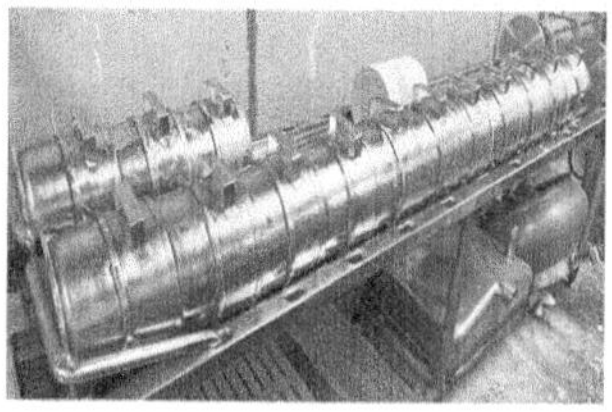

❻ The majority of the soft curds are salted (as a preservative) and compressed under weights, while some of the curds are reconstituted with milk and processed into cottage cheese. The cheese takes on a variety of shapes as a result of this pressure.

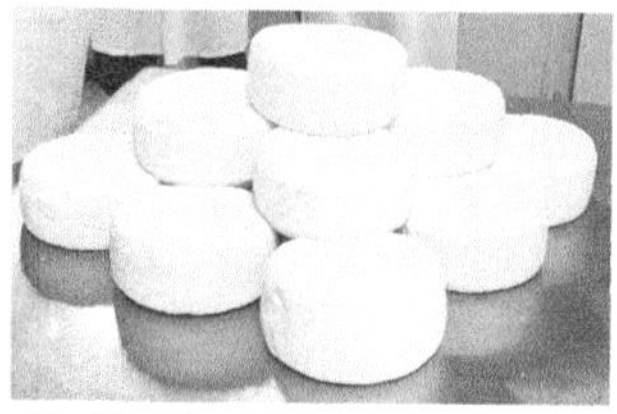

❼ The cheese pieces are currently covered in clear or colored wax or wrapped in fabric to block air and keep the cheese from drying out. The well-known gouda cheese is usually covered in a bright red wax.

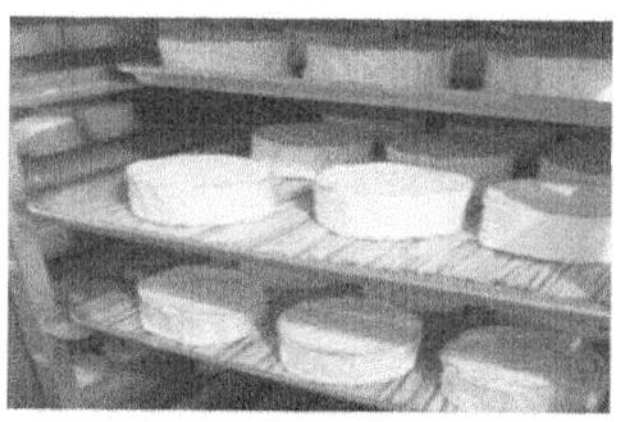

❽ The cheese must mature for 60 days to many years before being sold and consumed. "Green" cheese undergoes a change in texture during the curing process, eventually transforming into a soft and smooth consistency as it ripens. The cheese forms an edible "rind" as it ages. Cheese aged for a short period has a 'mild' flavor. The flavor becomes more potent or "sharp" when the aging process is extended (**TABLE 4.2**). Sharp cheeses are more dry and crumbly than mild cheeses.

**FIGURE 4.5** (Continued)

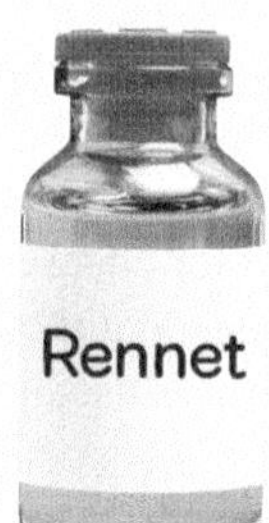


**FIGURE 4.6 Rennet.** Rennet, as a coagulant, assists in the curdling or coagulation of milk.

## 4.11 STARTER CULTURES

Starter cultures are now sold dry or frozen with liquid nitrogen at –196°C after being lyophilized with milk components, nutrients, and energizers (**Table 4.2**).

**TABLE 4.2**
**Bacterial Cultures Used to Make Different Types of Cheese**

| Culture | Major functions | Cheese types |
|---|---|---|
| *Lactobacillus bulgaricus*<br>*Lactobacillus lactis*<br>*Lactobacillus helveticus* | Acid and flavor | Swiss, Emmental, and Italian cheese |
| *Streptococcus thermophiles* | Acid | Emmental, Cheddar, and Italian cheese |
| *Propionibacterium shermanii* | Flavor and eye formation | Emmental and Swiss cheese |
| *Lactobacillus acidophilus* | Acid | |
| *Leuconostoc citrovorum*<br>*Leuconostoc dextranicum* | Flavor | Cottage cheese |
| *Lactococcusdia etilactis* | Acid and flavor | Cheese |
| *Lactococcus lactis*<br>*Lactococcus cremoris* | Acid | Cottage cheese |
| *Enterococcus durans*<br>*Enterococcus faecalis* | Acid and flavor | Soft Italian, Cheddar, and some Swiss cheese |

*Source:* Surono & Hosono, 2011

### 4.11.1 Classification of Starter Cultures

The best growth temperature for mesophilic starters, which include *Lactococcus* and *Leuconostoc*, is 30°C. The optimal growth temperature for thermophilic starters, which include the more prevalent *Lactobacillus* species and *Str. salivarius* ssp. *thermophilus*, is 40–45°C (**Table 4.3**). The top participants in the dairy starter culture market are shown in **Table 4.4.** Probiotics are typically found in aged but not cooked cheeses (**Table 4.5**). Products of lactic acid bacteria with their target organisms are illustrated in **Table 4.6.**

## 4.12 ROLE OF STARTER MICROORGANISMS IN MAKING CHEESE

Besides pathogens, microorganisms that are helpful in cheese ripening are also eliminated during pasteurization. Therefore, technical advancement is required to add a starter culture to compensate for this loss. In current practice, starter cultures of the lactic acid bacteria (LAB) group are added to milk with the primary goal of producing lactic acid through the fermentation of lactose. The fresh acidic flavor of unripened cheese is due to lactic acid, which is also crucial for the production and texturizing of the curd. Additionally, starters perform other critical functions such as the production of lipolytic and proteolytic enzymes needed for cheese ripening as well as the formation of volatile flavor compounds like diacetyl and aldehydes and the inhibition of pathogenic and some spoilage microorganisms. As a result, the starter cultures used to make cheese are crucial in determining its quality (Abou-Soliman et al., 2020).

Both milk acid production and flavor development are influenced by the starter's proteolytic activity. Producing amino acids for their own development is the goal of LAB's proteolytic activity. Compared to *Bacillus*, *Pseudomonas*, and *Enterococcus*, LAB have less proteolytic activity,

**TABLE 4.3**
**Characteristics of Starter Culture Bacteria**

| ***L. lactis* and *L. cremoris*** | ***E. faecalis* and *E. durans*** |
|---|---|
| Gram-positive cocci | Gram-positive oval-shaped cocci |
| Growth at 10°C | Growth at 10°C |
| No growth at 45°C | Growth at 45°C |
| Reduce litmus strongly | Reduce litmus strongly |
| Non-salt tolerant <6.5% | Salt tolerant >6.5% |
| No spores | No spores |
| Non-thermoduric | Thermoduric |
| | Growth at pH 9.6 |
| ***S. thermophilus*** | ***Leuconostoc citrovorum*** |
| | ***Leuconostoc dextranicum*** |
| Gram-positive cocci | Gram-positive cocci |
| No growth at 10°C | Growth at 10°C |
| Growth at 45°C | No growth at 45°C |
| Reduce litmus milk | Reduce litmus milk weakly |
| Non-salt tolerant <6.5% | Non-salt tolerant <6.5% |
| No spores | No spores |
| Thermoduric | Non-thermoduric |
| No growth at pH 9.6 | |
| ***L. bulgaricus*** | ***L. acidophilus*** |
| Gram-positive rods, medium or long | Gram-positive rods, long |
| No growth at 10°C or 20°C | No growth at 10°C |
| Growth at 45°C | Growth at 45°C |
| Reduce litmus strongly | Does not reduce litmus milk |
| Non-salt tolerant <6.5% | Non-salt tolerant <6.5% |
| No spores | No spores |
| Thermoduric | Non-thermoduric |

*Source:* Surono & Hosono, 2011

**TABLE 4.4**
**Commercial Suppliers of Dairy Starter Cultures**

| Company | Country |
|---|---|
| Chr. Hansen | Denmark |
| Danisco | Denmark |
| ASCRC | Australia |
| CSK | Netherlands |
| DSM | Netherlands |
| Centro Sperimentale del Latte | Italy |

*(Continued)*

**TABLE 4.4 *(Continued)***
**Commercial Suppliers of Dairy Starter Cultures**

| Company | Country |
|---|---|
| Alce | Italy |
| Degussa | Germany |
| Gewürzmüller | Germany |
| Lallemand | Canada |
| NZDRI | NewZealand |
| Quest International Nederlands | Netherlands |
| Rhodia | France |

**TABLE 4.5**
**Most Common Beneficial Bacteria (Probiotics) Used to Make Cheese**

| Types | Probiotics |
|---|---|
| *Lactobacillus* species | *Lactobacillus bulgaricus, Lactobacillus cellebiosus, Lactobacillus dellbrueckii, Lactobacillus acidophilus, Lactobacillus reuteri, Lactobacillus brevis, Lactobacillus casei, Lactobacillus plantarum, Lactobacillus rhamnosus, Lactobacillus helveticus, Lactobacillus salivarus* |
| *Streptococcus* species | *Streptococcus thermophilus, Streptococcus intermedius* |
| *Propionibacterium* species | *Propionibacterium shermanii, Propionibacterium freudenreichii* |
| *Bacillus* species | *Bacillus subtilis, Bacillus pumilus, Bacillus lentus, Bacillus licheniformis, Bacillus coagulans* |
| *Pediococcus* species | *Pediococcus cerevisiae, Pediococcus acidilactici, Pediococcus pentosaceus* |
| *Bifidobacterium* species | *Bifidobacterium adolescentis, Bifidobacterium bifidum,* *Bifidobacterium breve, Bifidobacterium infantis, Bifidobacterium thermophilum* |
| *Leuconostoc* species | *Leuconostoc mesenteroides* |
| *Bacteriodes* species | *Bacteriodes capillus, Bacteriodes suis, Bacteriodes ruminicola, Bacteriodes amylophilus* |
| Yeast | *Saccharomyces cerevisiae, Candida torulopsis* |
| Mold | *Aspergillus niger, Aspergillus oryzae* |

*Source:* Surono & Hosono, 2011

**TABLE 4.6**
**Products of Lactic Acid Bacteria with their Target Organisms**

| Product | Main target organisms |
|---|---|
| Acetic acid | Putrefactive bacteria, clostridia, some fungi and yeasts |
| Hydrogen peroxide | Pathogens and spoilage organisms, especially in protein-rich foods |
| Lactic acid | Gram-negative and putrefactive bacteria, some fungi |
| Low-molecular-weight metabolites | |
| Bacteriocin | Gram-positive bacteria and some LAB, notably endospore formers |
| Niacin | |
| Fatty acids | Different bacteria |
| Reuterin (3-OH-propionaldehyde) | Wide spectrum of bacteria, yeasts, and molds |
| Diacetyl | Gram-negative bacteria |

*Source:* Wang et al., 2021

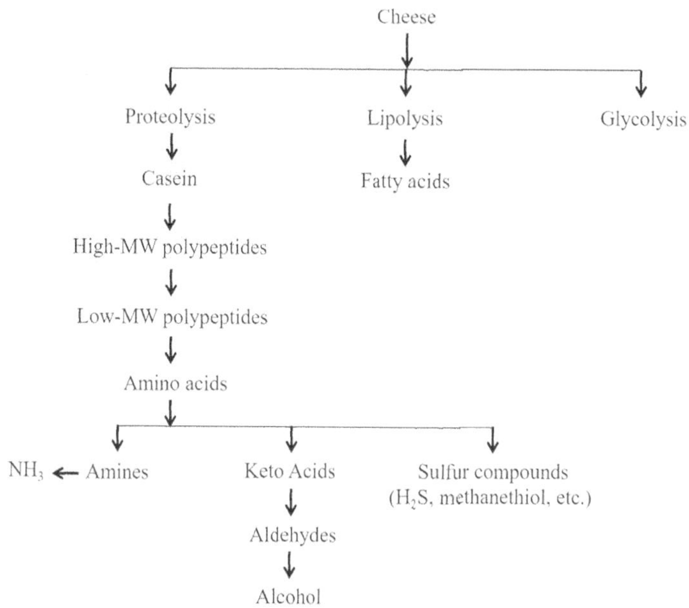


**FIGURE 4.7 Biochemical aspects of cheese ripening.**

although this activity is crucial for the ripening of cheese (**Figure 4.7**). LAB may hydrolyze large protein molecules into tiny peptides because proteases are attached to their cell walls. These peptides are converted into oligopeptides with the aid of peptidases that are found outside of the cell wall. The cell absorbs oligopeptides that are no longer than six amino acids and hydrolyzes them into amino acids. In ripened cheeses, peptidases are still in function. Particularly after the lysis of LAB, they become active. While starter cultures with significant proteolytic activity are utilized for ripened hard cheeses, unripened proteolytic strains are not used for cheeses consumed fresh. Low proteolytic activity is necessary for semi-hard Salted White cheese as well, which is aged for 2–3 months. If the ratio of proteases to peptidases in cheese is higher than normal, this might lead to bitterness and texture issues. Bitterness is caused by a variety of factors, not just proteases. In addition to this, the casein coagulation process parameters and enzymes (rennet, etc.) added to milk can also result in bitterness. The most popular starters are species from the genera *Lactobacillus*, *Lactococcus*, *Leuconostoc*, and *Streptococcus*. More recently, the use of *Pediococcus*, a fifth genus, has been suggested.

### 4.12.1 Ripening: Flavor and Texture Development

i. Primary proteolysis.
   a. 60 days; residual chymosin.
   b. Caseins are broken down into medium-molecular-weight peptides.
ii. Secondary proteolysis.
   a. Starter cultures break down peptides to lower-molecular-weight peptides.
   b. Temperature: 5–7°C.
   c. pH: 4.7– 5.0.
   d. Inhibits the growth of spoilage organisms.
   e. Inhibits enzyme activity.

## 4.13 CHEESE FLAVOR

Cheese flavor is primarily an outcome of enzymatic activity. The flavor of the cheese is concentrated in the water-soluble fraction (peptides, amino acids, organic acids, amines, and NaCl), while the aroma of cheese is mostly in the volatile fraction. Initially, it was thought that only one or a limited number of compounds were responsible for the flavor of cheese, but it was soon discovered that each cheese actually included the same flavoring ingredients. This was acknowledged, which gave rise to the component balance theory, according to which the concentration and harmony of a variety of chemicals give the cheese its distinctive flavor (**Figure 4.8**). Though significant info on the flavor compounds in several cheese varieties has been accumulated, it's not possible to explain fully the flavor of any variety, with the potential exception of Blue cheeses, the flavor of which is dominated by alkan-2-ones (Fox et al., 2015).

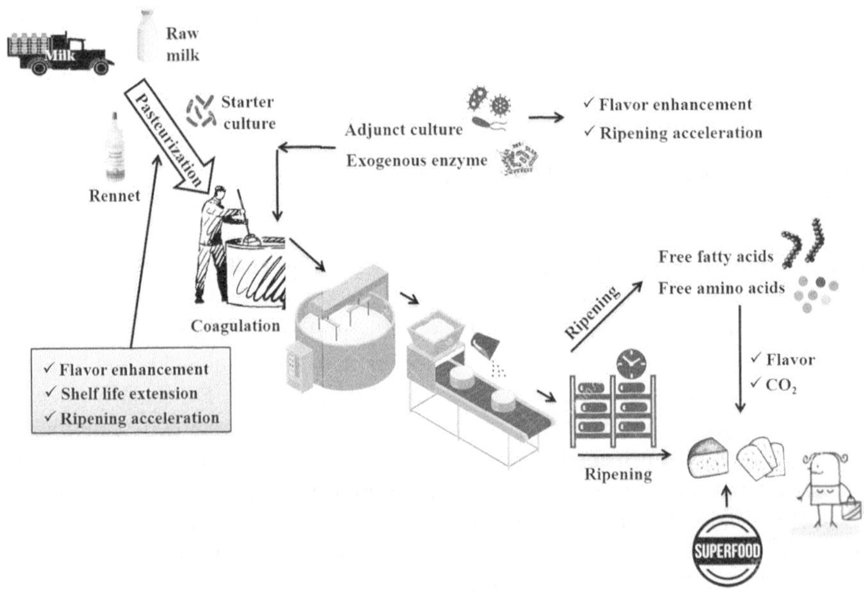


**FIGURE 4.8 An illustration of the cheese ripening process and intervention of technology for accelerating the process and improving cheese flavor.** Accelerated ripening can be utilized to change flavor and produce new varieties. Extended ripening periods result in greater costs owing to cool storage, space, manpower, weight loss, and higher capital costs.

## 4.14 CHEESE COLOR

The color of cheese is controlled by different factors, and the final color of cheese can be influenced by a mixture of one or all of these. The yellowish color of dairy foods produced from cow's milk may make them less acceptable than products produced from sheep, goat, or buffalo milk in regions where the latter are traditional. The supplementation of milk for English-type cheeses, like Cheddar and Gloucester, with carotenoid pigments is common (some people think that that the flavor of red cheddar is superior to that of white cheddar); however, for other kinds, the practice is either uncommon or nonexistent. Soft cheeses have a more orange/red color with some white spots due to the proliferation of *G. candidum*.

## 4.15 POPULAR TYPES OF CHEESE

### 4.15.1 White Cheese

White cheese is a product category that includes both conventional and ultra-filtered varieties. The cheese is often made from cow's milk. Feta, or white cheese, is creamy and heavy in fat, making it ideal for adding a creamy feel to recipes. Instead of heavy cream, use a lump of white cheese in soups and sauces. Combi White is a vegetable-fat-based cheese alternative to ultra-filtrated white cheese. Traditional white cheese, created in the same way as feta, made with cow's milk all over the world. Outside the European Union (EU), feta is a type of cheese manufactured partially or entirely of cow's milk; inside the EU, this is known as white cheese or salad cheese.

#### 4.15.1.1 Manufacture of White Cheese

The schematic of the white cheese manufacturing steps is shown in **Figure 4.9**.

Milk
↓
Pasteurization (72°C, 5 min)
↓
Cooling (32°C)
↓
Starter addition (1%)
↓
Incubation (30 min)
↓
Rennet (0.05%) and $CaCl_2$ (0.1%) addition
↓
Coagulation (90 min)
↓
Cutting
↓
Draining → Whey
↓
Pressing
↓
Salting (15%)
↓
Storage

FIGURE 4.9 **Flow chart of the white cheese manufacturing process.**

#### 4.15.1.2 Qualities of Starter Cultures Used in Making White Cheese

The starter needs include the followings: (i) capacity to produce a lot of acids, (ii) excellent creation of taste and flavor in the appropriate dose and combination, (iii) low proteolytic activity to avoid rapid ripening and bitterness, (iv) high antagonistic activity essential to stop pathogens, (v) resistance to phages, (vi) resistance to antibiotics, (vii) growth at cheese production temperature, and (viii) resistance to certain salt concentrations.

### 4.15.2 Dhaka Cheese

Dhaka cheese is a type of traditional dairy product that comes from a small village called Austagram in Bangladesh. It has been in existence for approximately a century. The unique style of making a basket using bamboo is used to prepare Dhaka cheese (**Figure 4.10**). The Dhaka cheese fermentation method is made in a similar way to other traditional fermented dairy products. It relies on the natural bacteria found in the milk and the surrounding area. Backstopping is a method where a small amount of old fermented milk or sour cream is used to start fermentation in a new batch. This helps speed up the fermentation process.

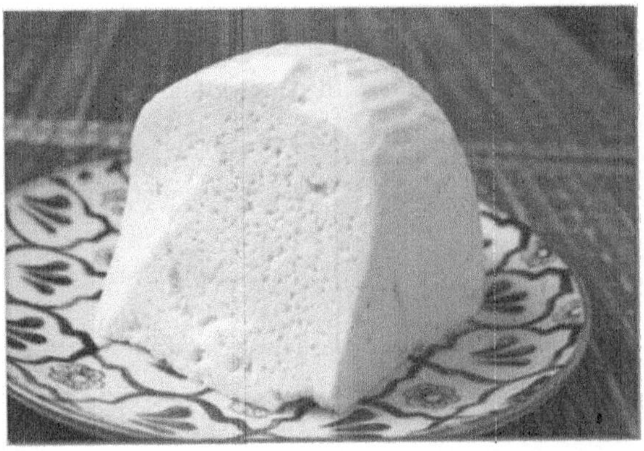

FIGURE 4.10 **Image of Dhaka cheese.** Over time, humans have created many different types of cheese with various flavors, textures, and shapes.

#### 4.15.2.1 Manufacture of Dhaka Cheese

The diagram for how Dhaka cheese is made is shown in **Figure 4.11**.

### 4.15.3 Cottage Cheese

Cottage cheese, also known as Pot cheese, is a type of fresh cheese that is made by curdling cream with acid. It has a low level of acidity and is repeatedly washed during the making process. Cottage cheese has a slightly sour and salty taste, with delicate diacetyl or creamy flavor and smell (**Figure 4.12**). The ideal texture of cottage cheese is smooth and meaty, with individual curd pieces that are not soft and pasty. Cottage cheese makes up about 5% of all the cheese produced in the world (Lucey, 2011).

A key part of making cottage cheese different from fresh cheese is adding a dressing to the curd grains, usually cream. This dressing is mostly responsible for the taste of the cottage cheese.

Cottage cheese has fewer calories than other types of cheese, so it's popular among people who are trying to lose weight or be healthy. People often use it with many different foods like yogurt, fruit, toast, and granola. It can also be used in salads as a dressing and as a substitute for mayonnaise.

To make cottage cheese, it's best to use fresh, tasty, and clean skim milk with very few bacteria. After being separated, skim milk is quickly heated/pasteurized to kill any harmful bacteria. A very good lactic starter is used. Skim milk is used to make a large amount of starter culture. (Kanawjia & Khetra, 2016).

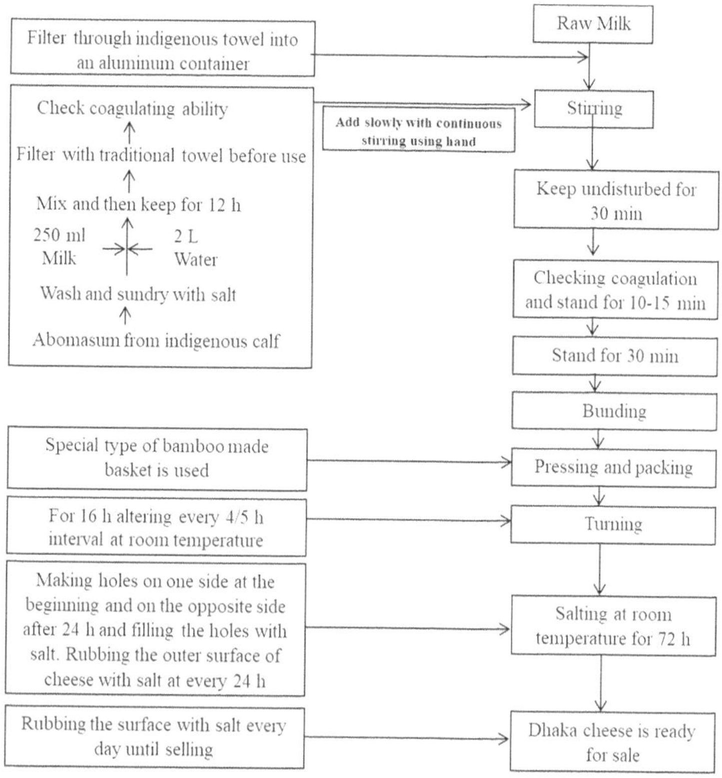


**FIGURE 4.11 Flow chart of the Dhaka cheese manufacturing process.**

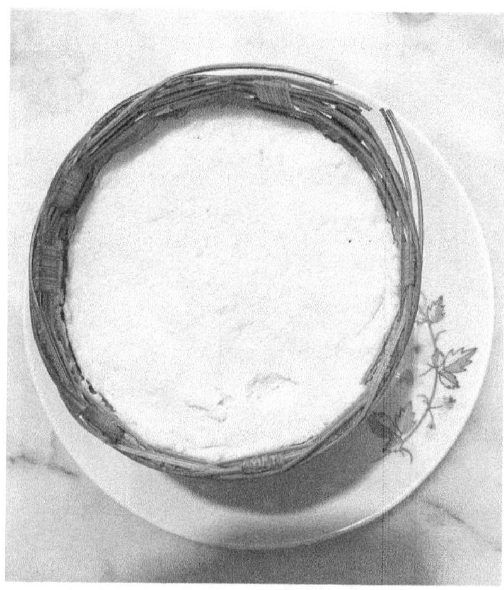

**FIGURE 4.12 Image of Cottage cheese.** The term "Cottage cheese" is thought to have come from the fact that the cheese was traditionally prepared in cottages using surplus milk. Cottage cheese can be eaten on its own, with fruits and toast, or in salads.

#### 4.15.3.1 Manufacture of Cottage Cheese

**Figure 4.13** illustrates a schematic of the Cottage cheese production procedure.

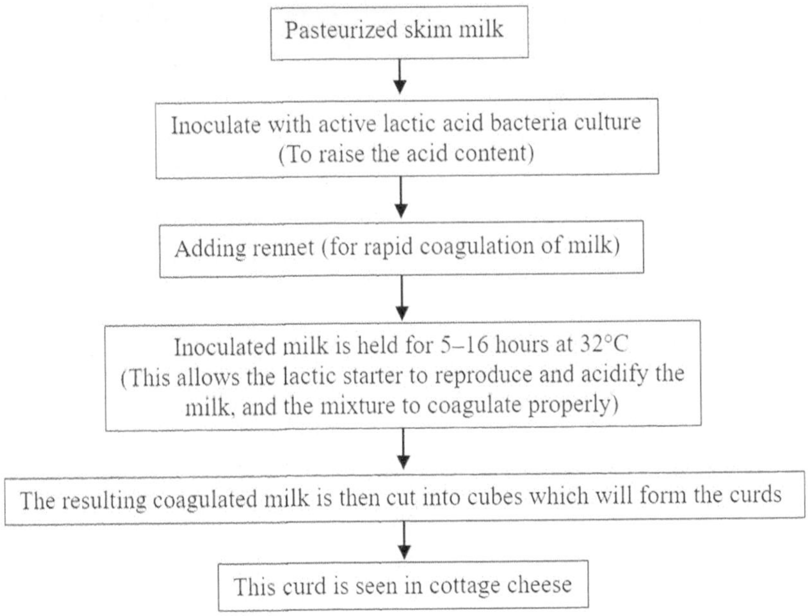


FIGURE 4.13 **Flow chart of the Cottage cheese manufacturing process.**

### 4.15.4 Swiss Cheese

According to the Federal Register, Swiss cheese is a product made from cow's milk using the Swiss cheese process (**Figure 4.14**). All over the cheese, it has produced holes or eyes. Swiss cheese originated in the European country of Switzerland and is known as the "King of Cheeses." In addition to Switzerland, the

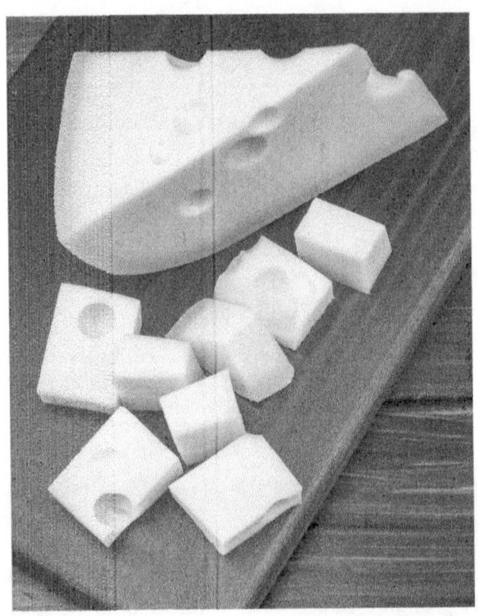

FIGURE 4.14 **Image of Swiss cheese.** Swiss cheese refers to any cheese that resembles Emmental cheese, a yellow, medium-hard cheese that originated in the Emmental region of Switzerland.

United States, Finland, and Denmark are important players in the production of this cheese. The cheese is known as Emmentaler cheese in its own country and Swiss cheese in other countries.

Real Swiss cheese has a flavor and aroma that other cheesemakers have struggled to replicate. Cheesemakers typically attribute this excellence to the smell of specific alpine grasses that is given to the milk and so forms a component of the cheese flavor. However, the exact duplication of all of the countless factors involved in production and ripening would most likely result in Swiss cheese with a flavor similar to Emmentaler.

#### 4.15.4.1 Manufacture of Swiss Cheese

The diagram for how Swiss cheese is made is shown in **Figure 4.15.**

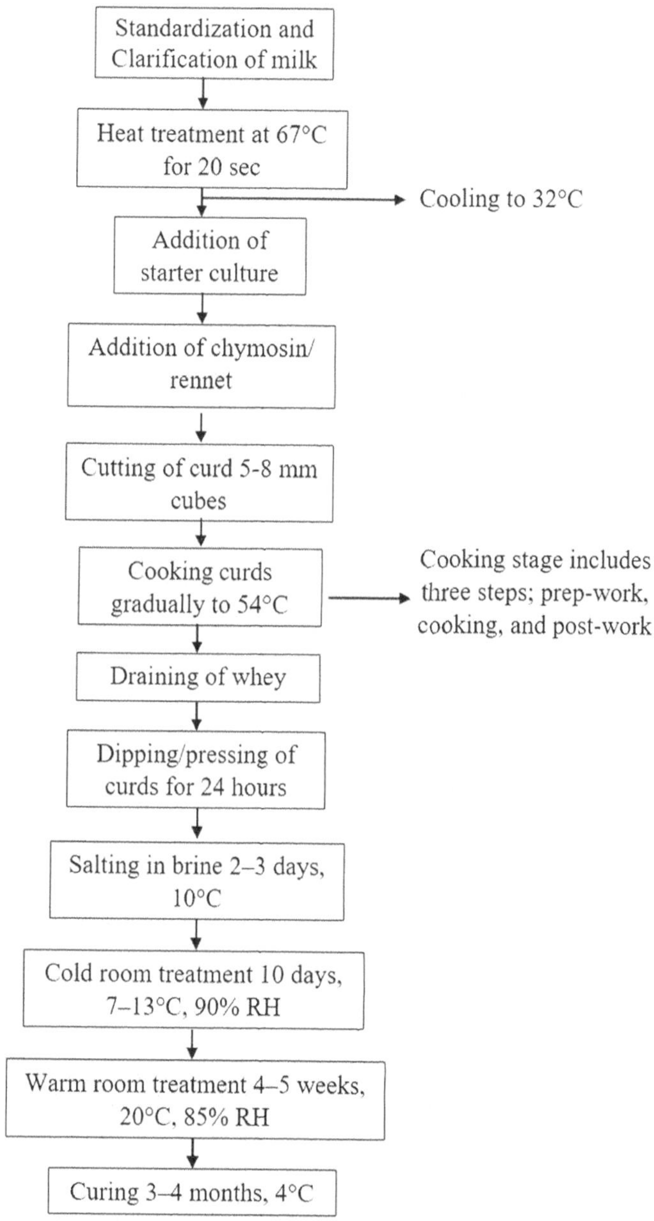


**FIGURE 4.15 Flow chart of the Swiss cheese manufacturing process.**

#### 4.15.4.2 How Does Swiss Cheese Form Its Holes?

Gas-producing bacteria are introduced during the curing process and produce bubbles inside the curd. This makes it taste and look different from other cheeses.

### 4.15.5 Brick Cheese

Brick cheese is a sweet-curd cheese, made from fresh sweet milk (**Figure 4.16**). It is mild and sweet in flavor and lacks the sharpness of cheddar and the strong flavor of Limburger, despite processing something of the flavors which distinguish these well-known varieties. It is softer than cheddar cheese. It's used for sandwiches and for cooking purposes and functions because it slices without crumbling and melts quickly and smoothly once it is heated. It keeps for weeks at 55°F after it's properly cured and ready to be used.

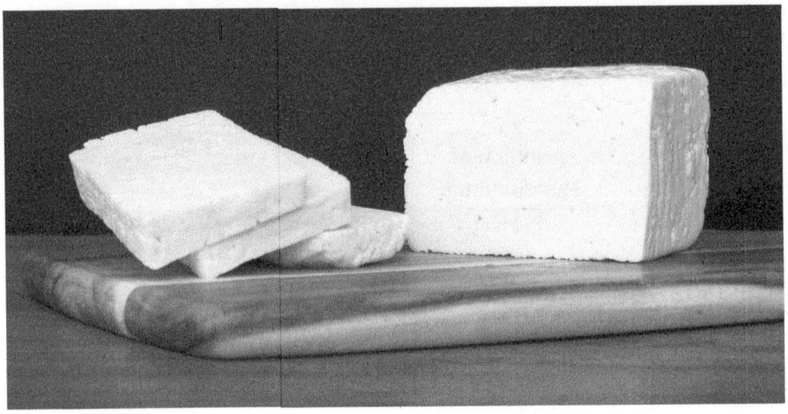

FIGURE 4.16 **Image of Brick cheese.** It gets its name from the fact that the cheeses are crushed with bricks during aging.

#### 4.15.5.1 Manufacture of Brick Cheese

The diagram of how Brick cheese is made is shown in **Figure 4.17.**

### 4.15.6 Cheddar Cheese

Cheddar cheese is one of the most popular cheeses in the world (**Figure 4.18**). This cheese was invented in the village of Cheddar in Somerset, in the southwest of England. It is categorized as hard cheese. Cheddar cheese must have a minimum of 50% fat content and a maximum moisture level of 39% to meet its identification standards. Cheddar cheese is rennet coagulated and can take up to 2 years to mature (aging) before being consumed (Phadungath, 2019).

#### 4.15.6.1 Manufacture of Cheddar Cheese

The diagram of how Cheddar cheese is made is shown in **Figure 4.19.**

- Starting ingredient: pasteurized whole milk.
- Setting the milk.
  - While stirring, heat to 31°C.
  - Add lactic acid-producing starter cultures 0.5–1%.
  - Add $CaCl_2$ (0.02%).
  - Add natural color (3 g/1000 g).

    - Add rennet to coagulate caseins and form curds (3 g/1000 g).
    - Stop stirring and let set.
- Cut the curd.
    - Increase surface area.
    - Release the whey.
- Cooking (38°C for 30 minutes).
    - Removes more whey.
    - Increases growth and acid production of cultures.

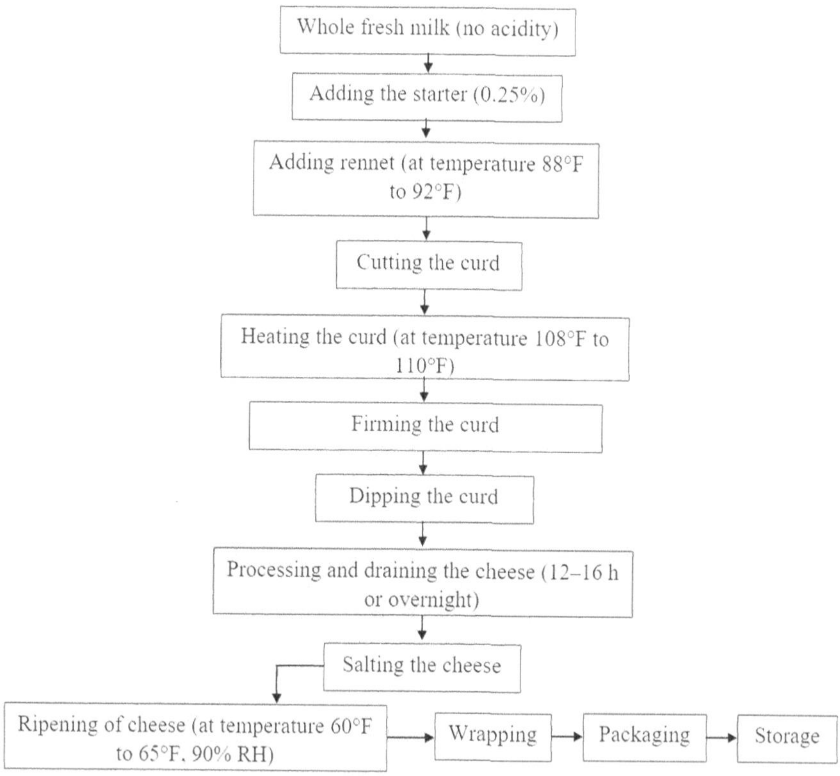


**FIGURE 4.17 Flow chart of the Brick cheese manufacturing process.**

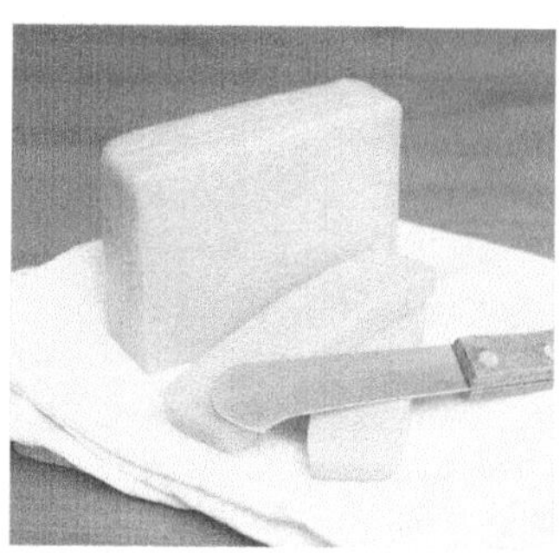

**FIGURE 4.18 Image of Cheddar cheese.** Cheddar cheese is normally ripened for 6–9 months.

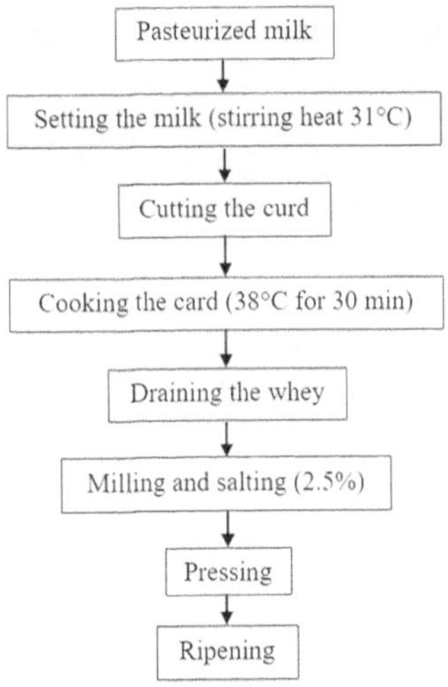


**FIGURE 4.19 Flow chart of Cheddar cheese manufacturing process.**

- Draining whey and matting the curd.
    - Remove excess whey.
    - Form curds into a slab.
    - Cheddaring: cutting curd slab into blocks to allow excess whey to drain and allow acidity to increase.
- Milling and salting.
    - Cut curds into small pieces.
    - 2.5% salt is added: drains whey, inhibits spoilage organisms, and adds flavor.
- Pressing to remove more whey.
    - Moisture content will affect bacterial growth and texture.
    - Ripening: bacteria develop flavor and texture over time.

### 4.15.7 Mozzarella Cheese

Mozzarella, a soft, unripened cheese variety belonging to the *pasta filata* family, originating in the Italian Battipaglia region (**Figure 4.20**). Traditionally, buffalo milk was used to make Mozzarella cheese. However, it is produced in Italy, several European nations, and the United States using cow milk, which needs suitable alterations. Mozzarella is derived from the Neapolitan

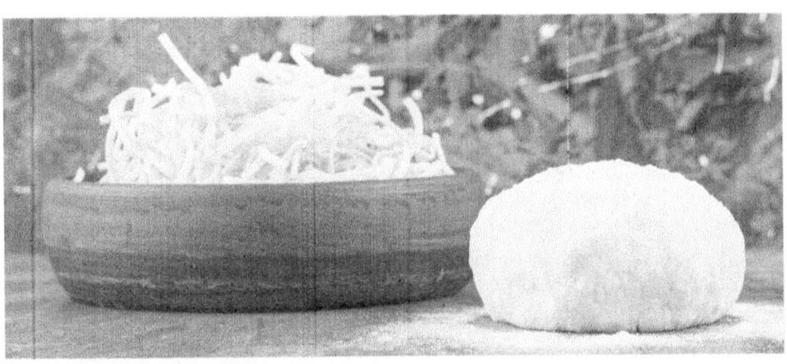

**FIGURE 4.20 Image of Mozzarella cheese.** Mozzarella originated in Southern Italy and was initially produced from water buffalo milk. The word "*mozzarella*" is derived from the Italian verb "*mozzare*," which means "to separate."

dialect spoken in Compania—the original from, *mozzal*, means to cut. It is a very popular cheese that may be used in a range of cuisine preparations. It is mostly used in the production of Italian foods and pizzas to enhance the texture features and organoleptic appeal of melted cheese. It is accessible as a soft-to-firm cheese depending on the technique of preparation and the moisture content preserved in the final product (Jana & Mandal, 2011). Mozzarella cheese is consumed fresh; it has a mild flavor and is pale yellow in color due to the lack of aging (Arora et al., 2019).

#### 4.15.7.1 Manufacture of Mozzarella Cheese

The diagram for how Mozzarella cheese is made is shown in **Figure 4.21.**

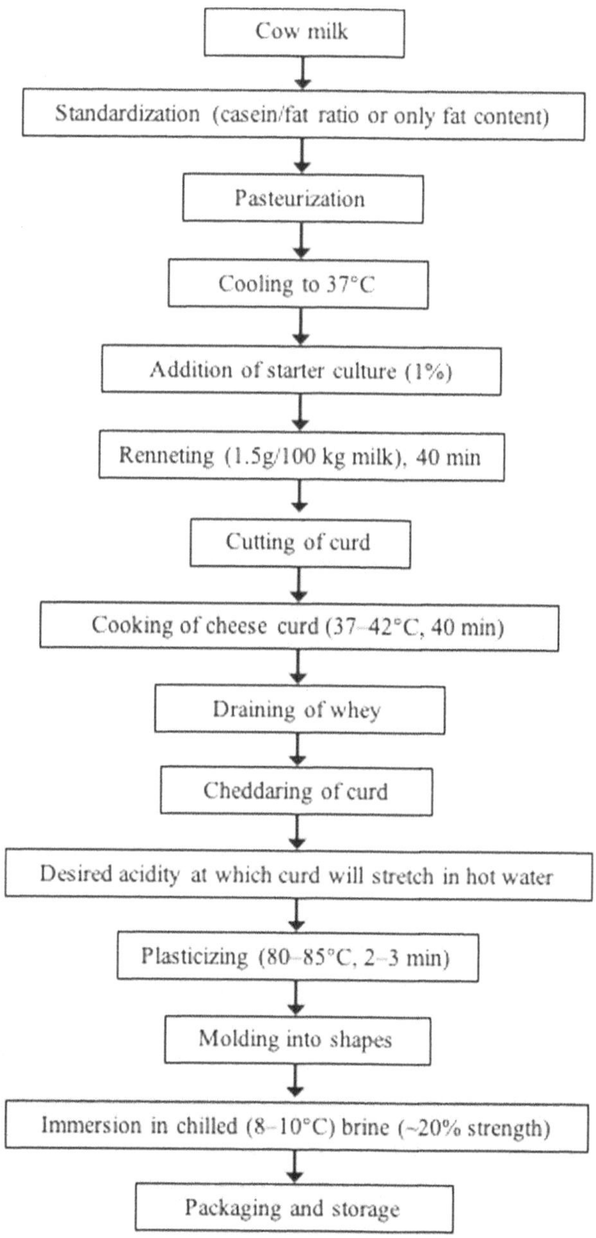


**FIGURE 4.21** Flow chart of the Mozzarella cheese manufacturing process.

## 4.16 CHEESE, NATURAL VS. PROCESSED

Natural cheeses are made in conventional ways. Natural cheese that has been crushed, blended, and pasteurized is referred to as processed cheese. The heat used during this procedure prevents the cheese from aging, increasing its shelf life and stabilizing flavor changes. Emulsifiers are used to prevent fat separation, resulting in a product with ideal slicing and melting properties. Processed cheese has a somewhat different taste and appearance from natural cheese. Natural Swiss cheese, for example, has holes in it, but processed Swiss cheese does not. Natural cheese is usually more expensive than processed cheese (Hickey, 2011).

## 4.17 CHEESE ADDITIVES AND PRESERVATIVES

### 4.17.1 Salts Inhibitory to Undesirable Organisms

To stop the growth of undesirable bacteria, salts such as potassium nitrate, sodium carbonate, calcium carbonate, mono-sodium dihydrogen phosphate, and nisin are used. These are typically added to some less acidic curd cheeses, such as Edam, Gouda, etc., primarily to prevent the growth of organisms that produce gas and lead to blown cheese defects (Kanawjia & Khetra, 2016). Nitrate has been used along with salt to inhibit the growth of bacteria that produce propionic acid in potable water while simultaneously controlling gas-producing butyric acid bacteria. However, there are two key factors that limit the usage of nitrates in cheese:

i. Certain amino acids cause color defects when they combine with nitrite.
ii. Nitrosamines, which are carcinogenic, are produced.

### 4.17.2 Salts to Refurbish the Calcium Balance in Milk

Calcium is present in soluble, colloidal, and complex forms that are in a delicate balance in milk. Successful coagulation depends on this balance of calcium. Sometimes the balance among the three different forms is disturbed because of heat treatment, cooling, or disturbances in the milk itself (colostrum, late lactation, mastitis). In these circumstances, it has been standard practice to add calcium salt, usually $CaCl_2$, to milk (Kanawjia & Khetra, 2016). This is frequently required, especially when using a variety of vegetable or microbial coagulants. Calcium lactate and calcium hydroxide are two more calcium salts that can be added in the form of a solution.

### 4.17.3 Use of Common Salt (NaCl)

Typically, salt is added to curds at a rate of around 2% of their weight. Salt is added to cheese in order to:

i. Prevent the development of undesirable microorganisms
ii. Support the physicochemical changes in the curd
iii. Prevent the development of lactic acid and other types of undesirable microorganisms
iv. Give the cheese a tasty flavor

### 4.17.4 Acidulants

The most common acidulant used in the manufacture of cheese is lactic acid, which is produced in situ by lactic acid bacteria naturally found in milk. While vinegar (0.03%) is used to make Mozzarella cheese, glacial acetic acid (12.5% concentrated acid and 2.7% of milk) is used to make Queso Blanco cheese. Lime juice is used in India to make Bandal cheese, paneer, and channa. Heat causes D-glucono-delta-lactone to create acid, which has been utilized to make acid in milk and curd (Kanawjia & Khetra, 2016). The cheese made using this acidulant is tasteless and bland because no enzymes are formed during this process. Phosphoric acid (4 L) is diluted to 10% strength in 40 L of water and then added to 1000 L of milk with vigorous stirring.

### 4.17.5 Bleach and Coloring Agents

It is usual practice to add additional color to light-colored milk to give the cheese an appealing and delicious appearance. Carotenoids and riboflavin are the key factors for the colors of milk. Riboflavin tends to give the curd a greenish tint and is yellow in solution with a green-yellow fluorescence. However, since riboflavin is water soluble, the majority of its color is lost in whey. Therefore, its impact as color in cheese is little. Carotenoids are more significant for the deep yellow-orange color. Colors are added to cheese in order to achieve uniform color because there is a significant seasonal variance in the color of milk.

### 4.17.6 Smoke

Some cheeses are thought to have a smoke-charged environment for the formation of smoky flavors. It causes fat to melt and escape from the surface of the cheese block, but no moisture to evaporate. The introduction of smoke vapors containing phenolic compounds has a protective effect as well as imparting a characteristic flavor to the cheese. Cheese is periodically coated with liquid condensed smoke.

### 4.17.7 Flavors, Spices, and Herbs

There are two categories of flavoring ingredients that are added to cheese: (i) those that are added to give the cheese taste (herbs and spices) and (ii) flavors that are already present in the cheese but only serve as a soft coating (ham, meats, etc.). These flavors are themselves nutritious foods. Cheese curds can be flavored and scented with chopped herbs, their juices, or dried crust semi-powders.

### 4.17.8 Cheese Bases

The use of a bland cheese base with herbs, vegetables, and cooked meats mixed in is likely inspired by the use of processed cheese in a similar way. The usual combinations use cheese as the main ingredient, and they also include lettuce, chives, onions, spinach, potatoes, carrots, chopped ham, and so on.

### 4.17.9 Addition of Beverages

Alcoholic drinks, wines, beers, and liquors are either added to the raw cheese curd or the entire cheese is submerged in the liquid. The combination of flavors, vegetables, spices, meat, and so on appears to deviate from tradition in order to considerably meet the taste of modern society for snack foods.

## 4.18 STORAGE OF CHEESE

Here are some points of agreement helping to decide on the method of storing cheese that works best:

- A re-sealable plastic bag can be utilized; however, it's not the perfect storage solution for cheese. The most effective way to wrap leftovers really depends on the particular type.
- Whatever the kind of cheese, storing it in the vegetable crisper of the refrigerator, wherever the temperature is cold and stable, will give longer protection from microbes.
- Use a fresh piece of plastic wrap or wax paper to rewrap the cheese after every use.
- The length of time for keeping cheese also differs according to the variety; normally, the harder the cheese, the longer it'll last (Felfoul et al., 2021).

**Hard, aged cheeses** (Parmigiano Reggiano, aged Gouda): First wrap in wax or parchment paper, and then add a layer of plastic wrap.
**Blue cheeses** (Gorgonzola, Roquefort): Cover with plastic wrap.
**Semi-hard and hard cheeses** (Cheddar, Swiss, and Gruyere): Wrap in plastic wrap.
**Soft, semi-soft, and stinky cheeses** (Goat, Camembert, Brie, Limburger): Place in a resealable plastic container.
**Fresh cheeses in water** (Mozzarella or Feta): Leave the cheese in the original packaging, changing the water every couple of days.

## 4.19 CHEESE ANALOGUES

A cheese analog is a dairy cheese alternative that resembles milk cheese in terms of composition, appearance, traits, and even intended purpose. In cheese analogues, vegetable proteins (such as peanut and soybean proteins) and vegetable fats and oils (such as partly hydrogenated vegetable fats like soybean, palm, and so on) are used to partially or entirely substitute milk protein and milk fat (**Figure 4.22**). According to market and consumer demands, cheese analogs are created and produced with the desired nutritional, functional, and storage qualities. It is possible to develop cheese substitutes that are nutritionally beneficial. Analog pizza cheese, which is used in baking as a topping on pizza and as slices in stuffed burgers, is made in a manner similar to that for processed cheese. The production procedure is often the same as that for processed cheese, keeping in mind that the protein is rennet casein rather than a combination of cheeses (Guinee, 2011). In order to achieve the required level of casein hydration/aggregation and fat emulsification in the analog formulation, the degree of calcium sequestration and paracasein aggregation must be adjusted. In terms of perceived viscosity and free oil, casein-based analog pizza cheeses were functionally more stable during chilled storage than natural Mozzarella cheese. An analogues of cheese made from soybeans with a spreadable, creamy consistency is "*sufu*." The items that are designed to partially or completely replicate cheese and in which milk fat, milk protein, or both are partially or completely substituted by non-milk-based alternatives, primarily of vegetable origin, are referred to as cheese substitutes or imitation cheese. Pizza's additional ingredients, such as tomato sauce, sausage, peppers, spices, anchovies, etc., provide taste; the essential qualities required of cheese analogues used in pizzas are meltability and stretchability. By incorporating cheese flavors created by biological or chemical processes, one should be able to create cheese analogues of other cheeses (Fox et al., 2015). A cheese substitute shouldn't have fewer nutritional benefits than the cheese it's

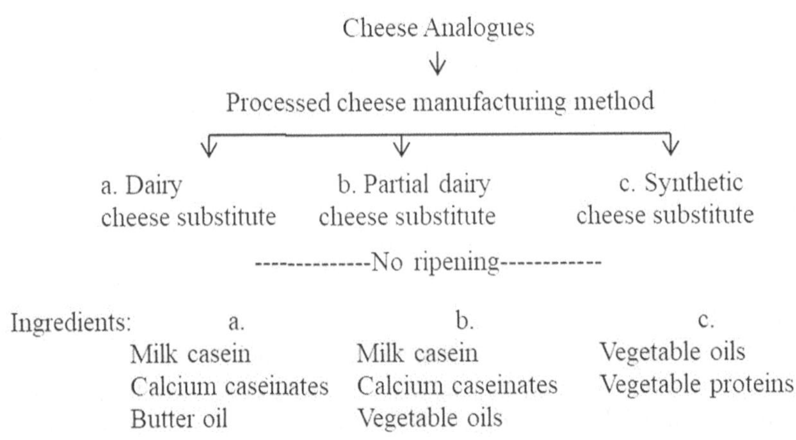


**FIGURE 4.22 Classification of cheese analogues with manufacturing ingredients.** Cheese analogues can alternatively be classified as dairy, partial dairy, or non-dairy, depending on whether the fat and protein components are derived from dairy or vegetable sources.

meant to imitate. Instead, promoters of imitation cheese suggest that it has nutritional advantages over real cheese, such as higher levels of unsaturated fatty acids, zero cholesterol, and fewer calories (Tamime, 2011).

## 4.20 QUALITY JUDGING OF CHEESE

The Hedonic Type scale is used to assess cheeses' sensory qualities (Nelson & Trout, 1951) The Hedonic Type scale is illustrated in **Table 4.7**.

**TABLE 4.7**
**Score Card for Sensory/Organoleptic Evaluation of Cheese**

| Name | Sample no: | | | Date |
|---|---|---|---|---|
| Color | Very good<br>9–8 | Good<br>7–6 | Average<br>5–3 | Not good<br>2–1 |
| Texture | Very good<br>9–8 | Good<br>7–6 | Average<br>5–3 | Not good<br>2–1 |
| Taste and aroma | Very good<br>9–8 | Good<br>7–6 | Average<br>5–3 | Not good<br>2–1 |
| Strange taste and aroma | No<br>9–8 | Very few<br>7–6 | Sensible<br>5–3 | A lot<br>2–1 |
| Salt content | Normal<br>9–8 | A little salty<br>7–6 | Salty<br>5–3 | Very much salty<br>2–1 |
| General acceptance | Very good<br>9–8 | Good<br>7–6 | Average<br>5–3 | Not good<br>2–1 |

## 4.21 FACTORS AFFECTING CHEESE QUALITY

The quality of cheese is influenced by its composition, particularly moisture content, sodium chloride concentration, pH, moisture content of non-fat components, and percentage of fat in dry matter (**Figure 4.23**). Cheese is the final product of a lengthy and complex process that can take 2 or more

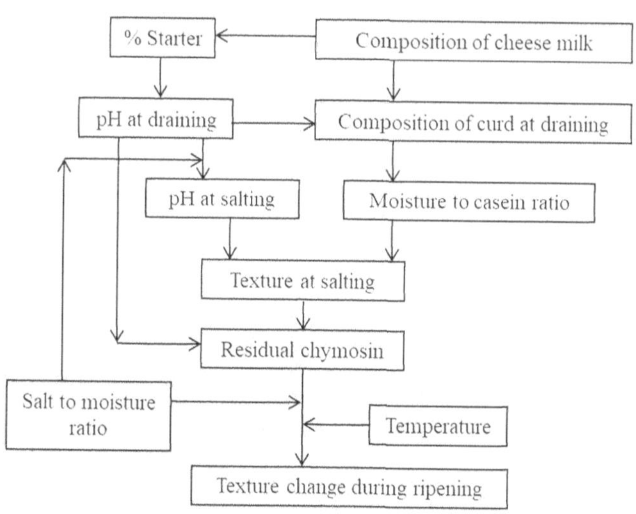


**FIGURE 4.23 Factors affecting changes in the texture of cheese during ripening**. A cheese's texture is mostly dictated by its pH and the ratio of intact casein to moisture.

years; thus, the quality of the product depends on a variety of conditions, some of which are generally relevant and some of which are variety specific (Mbye et al., 2022). The most significant are:

i. The composition, microbiological quality, standardization, heat treatment, and uniformity of the supplied milk
ii. The bacterial cultures that are utilized to acidify and play important roles during ripening
iii. The primary proteolytic agent—rennet—that is used to coagulate milk during ripening
iv. The non-starter bacteria that either naturally exist in milk or that enter milk or cheese during production from the environment (Daly et al., 2010)
v. Ingredients of the cheese
vi. Temperature and duration of the ripening of cheese curd

## 4.22 DEFECTS IN CHEESE

Defects related to texture, body, and flavor include crumbly, curdy, weak, gassy, woody/tough, pinholes, sticky, short, and bitter flavors. Common defects of cheeses are enlisted as follows:

### 4.22.1 Body Defects

i. **Short/crumbly:** Usually from too much acid or salt.
ii. **Corky:** Carried on by excessive salt, poor fat, low moisture, or overcooking.
iii. **Mealy:** This flaw can be felt on the palate or by rubbing the cheese between the thumb and forefinger. Usually, it's connected to too much acidity.
iv. **Pasty:** Caused by excessive moisture, adheres to the fingers and palate.
v. **Weak:** Due to excessive fat or moisture, degrades too quickly when handled by hand.

### 4.22.2 Texture Defects

i. **Gassy holes:** Many types of cheese are chosen for having gas holes.
ii. **Coliform-induced early gas problems**: These resemble tiny, sparkling holes with a spherical shape.
iii. **Yeasty slits:** Caused by the growth of yeast.

### 4.22.3 Flavor Defects

i. **Acid flavor:** Linked to the acidic body defects.
ii. **Bitter flavors:** Typical cheese defect.

### 4.22.4 Color Defects

i. **Pink discoloration:** Caused due to oxidation.
ii. **Non-uniformity:** It indicates a manufacturing flaw but consumer prefer it.

### 4.22.5 Finish Defects

i. **Checked/cracked:** The surface is too dry.
ii. **Greasy:** Due to too high temperature during pressing or curing.

### 4.22.6 Causes of Cheese Defects

i. Insufficient moisture content

a. In relation to the amount of fat and casein in cheese or the aging process or storage conditions
b. Usually associated with insufficient casein, excessive fat, and excessive moisture (too pasty or weak) = excessive proteolysis

ii. An improper rate and level of acid development

Regarding the amount of protein in milk and the ideal physical qualities of cheese:

iii. Poor quality ingredients (flavor and body)
iv. Microbial contamination
v. Retail abuse

## 4.23 WHY IS CHEESE EXPENSIVE?

One pound of cheese can be produced from 10 pounds of milk (1.25 gallons), but it takes a lot of work. No wonder it costs so much! Most cheese is not fresh, so it needs some form of aging. It costs money to spend time in a sanitary temperature- and humidity-controlled setting. Cheese making is a capital-intensive business and there is not a lot you can do with the equipment apart from making cheese.

## 4.24 UTILIZATION OF CHEESE

The nutritive value, appearance, flavor, texture, and cooking characteristics of cheeses vary to different degrees. As a result, cheese is able to meet a variety of nutritional and sensory demands. Cheese's use as a food element highlights the need for distinct and consistent qualities, which should be reached with the right flavor that works in harmony with the cuisine (**Figure 4.24**). **Table 4.8** illustrates the comparative cheese utilization levels in several food products. To satisfy a variety of tastes, cheese producers can create cheese with a variety of flavors, textures, and compositional

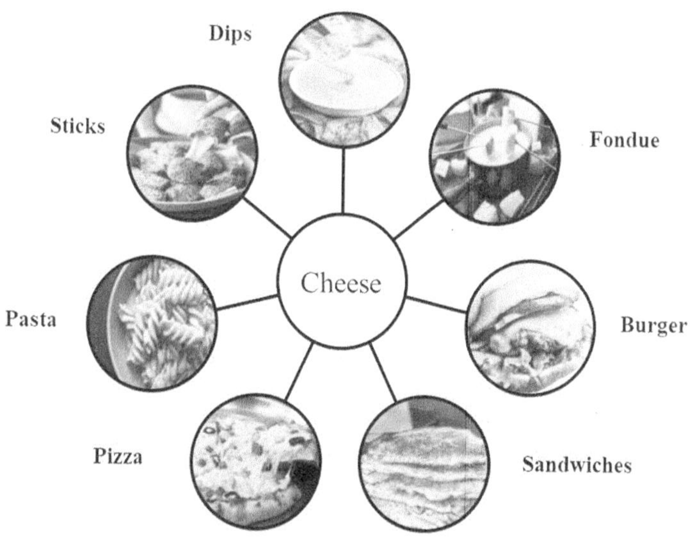


FIGURE 4.24 **Cheese utilization.** Cheese has grown in commercial importance in the food business over the last several decades due to its usage as an ingredient, notably as a topping on pizza, filler in appetizers, slices on hamburgers, and sauces in pasta meals.

**TABLE 4.8**
**The Use of Cheese in Various Food Products**

| Different food products | Usage (as % of total usage) |
|---|---|
| Pizza | 26 |
| Snack foods | 17 |
| Soups/sauces/dressings | 15 |
| Frozen entrees | 14 |
| Baked goods | 11 |
| Appetizers | 7 |
| Pet foods | 6 |
| Rice/noodle mixes | 3 |
| Shelf-stable entrees | 1 |

*Source:* Kanawjia & Khetra, 2016

characteristics (Guinee, 2011). It requires an understanding of its capabilities that can be successfully used for the consumers' benefit (Kanawjia & Khetra, 2016).

## 4.25 HEALTH BENEFITS OF CHEESE

Cheese serves as one of the good sources for essential nutrients, such as calcium and many other nutrients (proteins, phosphorous, zinc, selenium, vitamins A, D, K, $B_2$, and $B_{12}$, etc.). It improves the health advantages by generating specific peptides and free amino acids, which have a variety of bioactive qualities, including antimicrobial, anticarcinogenic, antithrombotic, and other capabilities. Some physiologically active lipids contained in cheeses, such as milk fat globule membrane (MFGM) and conjugated linolenic acid (CLA), have also been discovered to have positive health effects. As a result, it is a highly important function of a person's diet, but because it contains saturated fat, cholesterol, and salt, it has a bad reputation in terms of nutrition. By making low-fat or cholesterol-free cheese and including specific useful living materials, such probiotic bacteria, it can be overcome. The non-starter lactic acid bacteria (NSLAB) utilized within the cheeses is found to be bioactive, such as the inactivation of antigenotoxins and generation of gamma-aminobutyric. **Figure 4.25** illustrates the key potential health benefits of cheese.

### 4.25.1 Association of Cheese Consumption with Healthy Aging

Fermented dairy foods have enormous microbial biodiversity, making them a good source of metabolites that could reveal health benefits. Cardin et al. (2021) demonstrated that freeze-dried raw goat milk cheese and its extracts induced the activation of the DAF-2/DAF-16 pathway (DAF-16 is notable for being the primary transcription factor required for the profound lifespan extension observed upon mutation of the insulin-like receptor DAF-2), resulting in increasing longevity. At the same time, the cheese lipid extricate and the dried extricate W70, obtained with water, were able to decrease reactive oxygen species (ROS) generation in human leukocytes. The transcription factor DAF-16 has been demonstrated to regulate downstream genes that influence longevity and may be induced in the mechanism of activity of the cheese extracts in expanding the lifespan.

### 4.25.2 Association of Cheese Consumption with Gut Health

Creamy cheeses such as mozzarella are packed full of beneficial bacteria, helping the gut microbiome, which results in overall wellness and even improves mental health, are summarized in **Figure 4.25.**

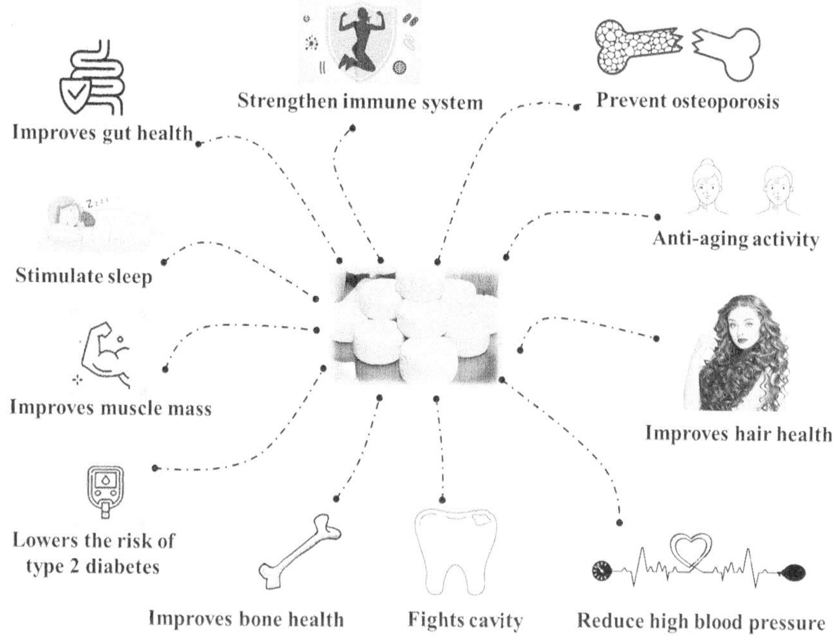


FIGURE 4.25 **Key potential health benefits of cheese.** Cheese is high in calcium, which is important for bone and tooth health, blood coagulation, wound healing, and maintaining normal blood pressure.

### 4.25.3 Association of Cheese Consumption with Bone Health

Cheese contains a lot of calcium and vitamin B, both of which are essential for fortifying bone and cartilage. Vitamin B aids in the body's distribution and absorption of calcium. Calcium-rich cheeses like Gouda and Blue cheese aid in increasing bone density (especially in older age).

### 4.25.4 Association of Cheese Consumption with Obesity Prevention

It might seem counterintuitive because cheese is full of fats; however, cheese such as Feta contains high levels of linoleic acid, which can help speed up the metabolism, resulting in faster fat burning.

### 4.25.5 Association of Cheese Consumption with Dental Health

Cheese's high calcium content also helps to keep teeth healthy and prevent cavities. The calcium and phosphorus in cheese not only strengthen bones, but the casein and whey protein in cheese can also help form enamel on teeth. A stronger and thicker enamel protects against the damaging effects of sugars, acids, and plaque on teeth. Chewing cheese can also increase saliva flow, which helps to treat cavities by washing away carbohydrates and germs. Cheese also has no staining characteristics, so there is no need to worry about losing a brilliant smile if it sticks to teeth.

### 4.25.6 Association of Cheese Consumption with Healthy Skin

Cheese, an essential part of a balanced diet, is also beneficial to skin health due to its high vitamin and mineral content. Cheese is high in vitamin $K_2$. This vitamin interacts with other vitamins and minerals, including calcium and vitamin D. It supports skin health by delivering and depositing these necessary vitamins and minerals. Cheese eating, according to experts, is another technique to get healthy and shining skin.

### 4.25.7 Association of Cheese Consumption with Healthy Hair

Cheese is particularly beneficial for hair development since it includes a lot of vitamin B. Furthermore, natural proteins such as casein and whey aid in hair development and keep the hair supple for a healthy natural glow.

### 4.25.8 Association of Cheese Consumption with Healthy Blood Pressure

Cheese's vitamin B has been discovered to help lower high blood pressure. Cheese assists in preventing malnutrition in the elderly. Basiricò et al. (2022) discovered that eating Parmigiano Reggiano cheese reduced blood pressure in rats.

### 4.25.9 Association of Cheese Consumption with Immune System Health

Some kinds of cheese aid in the development of a robust immune system, which aids the body in combating illness and infection. Blue vein cheese offers additional health advantages in addition to its delicious flavor and appealing appearance. It is a rich nutrient source that strengthens the immune system.

### 4.25.10 Association of Cheese Consumption with Cancer Prevention

Cheese contains sphingolipids and conjugated linolenic acid (CLA), both of which are crucial in the prevention of cancer. According to Wajszczyk et al. (2021), Cottage cheese consumption is linked to a lower risk of breast cancer in both premenopausal and postmenopausal women.

### 4.25.11 Association of Cheese Consumption with Great Sleep

Cheese has been shown in studies to help sleep. Calcium, present in cheese, assists the brain in using the tryptophan (an amino acid found in cheese that helps reduce stress and stimulate sleep) contained in dairy to produce sleep-inducing melatonin. Calcium also helps control muscular movements, which means fewer sleep disruptors like cramps or restless legs.

### 4.25.12 Food Value of Cheese

Cheese is a very nutritious food that contains protein, calcium, phosphorus, and vitamin A. Cheese and other dairy foods are important sources of good protein for vegetarians. It is suggested that people aged nine and older need to have three servings of low-fat and fat-free dairy foods, such as cheese, as part of their healthy diet. Cheese can provide important dairy nutrients for people who cannot digest lactose well. Cheeses like Cheddar, Mozzarella, and Swiss are not high in lactose and can usually be eaten without causing stomach problems. **Table 4.9** describes the food value of some varieties of cheese.

## 4.26 CHEESE INNOVATIONS

According to recent studies, cheese is becoming more and more popular as a snack around the world. This has impacted the cheese industry's innovation, with several notable cheese inventions emphasizing natural, healthful, extremely nutritious, and transparent ingredients and processing methods. Despite recent innovations, non-dairy and functional cheeses enhanced with enzymes and bioactive components are valued by customers for their nutritional value, demand, and sensory qualities (**Figure 4.26**).

**TABLE 4.9**
**Food Value of Some Varieties of Cheese**

| Cheeses | Calories | Fat (g) | Protein (g) | Calcium (mg) | Sodium (mg) |
|---|---|---|---|---|---|
| Cheddar | 114 | 9 | 7 | 204 | 176 |
| Parmesan | 111 | 7 | 10 | 336 | 454 |
| Blue | 100 | 8 | 6 | 150 | 395 |
| Brie | 95 | 8 | 6 | 52 | 178 |
| Goat (soft) | 76 | 6 | 5 | 40 | 104 |
| Mozzarella | 85 | 6 | 6 | 143 | 178 |
| Feta | 60 | 4 | 5 | 60 | 360 |
| Swiss | 100 | 9 | 5 | 150 | 170 |
| Cottage | 111 | 4.9 | 13 | 93.8 | 321 |
| Brick | 104 | 8 | 7 | 188.7 | 156.8 |

## 4.27 PERSPECTIVE OF THE GLOBAL CHEESE INDUSTRY

Cheese is a dairy product developed in a wide variety of flavors, textures, and shapes by coagulating the milk protein casein, typically derived from cow, buffalo, goat, or sheep's milk. Fast food restaurants are among the top cheese consumers in the world, and the fast food sector is expanding at a steady rate as a result of global urbanization and increased disposable incomes. The fast food industry's high growth is expected to lead to increased cheese consumption shortly. The cheese market will be worth around $105.93 billion by 2026, and it will grow by 6.81% every year from 2021 to 2026. The world made a lot of money from selling cheese in 2020—$72.26 billion. In 2020, the world made more cheese than the year before. They made 21.69 million MT of cheese, which is higher than the 20.98 million MT made in the previous year. In 2020, the EU made the most cheese out of all regions, producing 10.35 million metric tons. In 2019, Germany made the most cheese in the European Union, with 2.27 million metric tons, and France came in second with 1.92 million metric tons. Italy, Poland, the Netherlands, Argentina, and Russia are some big cheese-making countries.

The food and beverage industry is experiencing an increase in demand for mozzarella cheese because pregnant women are becoming more and more biotin deficient. Feta is sold in the biggest marketplaces across the world and shipped globally. Customers of Greek Feta manufacturers include big supermarkets, local stores, wholesalers, and food suppliers. The Parmesan cheese industry is presented with new growth chances by the ongoing developments and expansions of significant market companies.

Making cheese is an art—there are various competitions held globally, one of the famous ones being the World Championship Cheese Contest. Cheese consumption is a cultural phenomenon. While some people never have cheese on their plates, cheese is a common component of many people's daily diets. The difference is in the culture. With such global acceptance of this delicious ingredient, the sky is the limit to excel in the cheese business.

## 4.28 CHEESE YIELD

The amount of cheese made per 100 kg of processed milk is referred to as the yield. Cheese yield is affected by milk composition, final cheese moisture level, and the amount of recovery protein in the curd throughout the cheese-making process. The amount and type of fat in milk has an impact on both cheese quality and yield (Yiadom-Farkye, 1984).

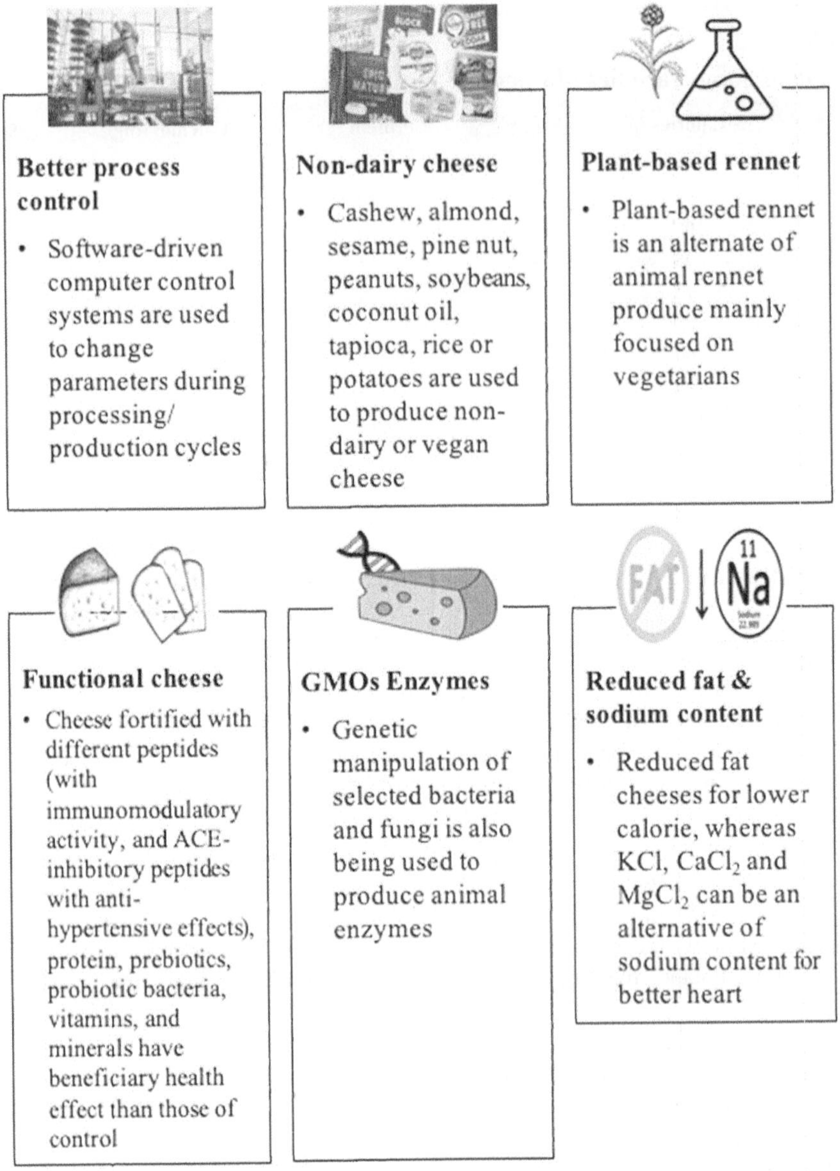


**FIGURE 4.26** Cheese innovations from production to nutrition and health attributes.

To calculate cheese yield, the following formula can be used:

$$\text{Cheese yield} = 2.3 \times \text{fat} + 1.4$$

This method is satisfactory for milk containing about 4% fat.

As a result, with 4% fat milk, the estimated output is: $(2.3 \times 4) + 1.4 = 10.6$ kg/100 kg milk.

This equation estimates cheese yield and is most commonly used for Cheddar cheese (Kayagil, 2006).

## 4.29 CONCLUSIONS

Cheese is a fascinating dairy food that has provided a means of nourishment, a way to preserve milk protein, and hedonic experiences to humankind from time immemorial. From unique raw material—milk—a wide variety of cheese flavors, textures, and shapes has evolved through the ages as a result of human craftsmanship. Today, the world of cheeses needs science to offer new insights and provide new opportunities. The chemistry, biochemistry, microbiology, and physical events that give rise to the majority of cheese variations; the roles played by its microbiota in these phenomena; and the effects of cheese microbes on consumer health have all been extensively studied over the past few decades. However, much remains to be exposed, and many exciting current publications in this area leave several questions unsettled. Moreover, cheese is inextricably linked to the culture of the society that manufactures and consumes it, with numerous artisan varieties throughout the world acting as a valuable cultural element and source of revenue for local communities. Ensuring the sustainability of premium quality cheese production is, therefore, also important to help these traditions cope with the challenges of the current competitive markets. In-depth research is crucial if this goal is to be accomplished.

## REFERENCES

Abou-Soliman, N. H. I., Awad, S., & El-Sayed, M. I. (2020). The impact of microbial transglutaminase on the quality and antioxidant activity of camel-milk soft cheese. *Food and Nutrition Sciences*, *11*(03), 153.

Alavi, F., & Momen, S. (2020). Aspartic proteases from thistle flowers: Traditional coagulants used in the modern cheese industry. *International Dairy Journal*, *107*, 104709.

Arora, S., Sindu, R., & Rekha. (2019). Production and processing methodology of mozzarella cheese. Research & reviews. *Journal of Dairy Science and Technology*, *8*(1), 30–34.

Basiricò, L., Morera, P., Evangelista, C., Galaverna, G., Sforza, S., Prandi, B., Bernabucci, U., & Nardone, A. (2022). Effect of parmigiano reggiano consumption on blood pressure of spontaneous hypertensive rats. *Dairy*, *3*(2), 364–376.

Cardin, G., Poupet, C., Bonnet, M., Veisseire, P., Ripoche, I., Chalard, P., Chauder, A., Saunier, E., Priam, J., Bornes, S., & Rios, L. (2021). A mechanistic study of the antiaging effect of raw-milk cheese extracts. *Nutrients*, *13*(3), 897.

Daly, D. F., McSweeney, P. L., & Sheehan, J. J. (2010). Split defect and secondary fermentation in swiss-type cheeses–A review. *Dairy Science & Technology*, *90*(1), 3–26.

El-Salam, M. A., & El-Shibiny, S. (2011). A comprehensive review on the composition and properties of buffalo milk. *Dairy Science & Technology*, *91*, 663–699.

Felfoul, I., Bouazizi, A., Tourki, I., Guesmi, C., & Attia, H. (2021). Effect of storage conditions on physicochemical, sensory, and structural properties of dromedary and cow's skim milk soft-brined cheese. *Journal of Food Processing and Preservation*, *45*(11), e15970.

Fox, P. F., Guinee, T. P., Cogan, T. M., & McSweeney, P. L. (2017). Fundamentals of cheese science (pp. 121–183). Springer US.

Fox, P. F., Uniacke-Lowe, T., McSweeney, P. L. H., & O'Mahony, J. A. (2015). Chemistry and biochemistry of cheese. *Dairy Chemistry and Biochemistry*, 499–546.

Guinee, T. P. (2011). Cheese analogues. *Encyclopedia of Dairy Sciences*, 814–821.

Hickey, M. (2011). Current legislation for cheeses. *Encyclopedia of Dairy Sciences*, 643–855.

Jacob, M., Jaros, D., & Rohm, H. (2011). Recent advances in milk clotting enzymes. *International Journal of Dairy Technology*, *64*(1), 14–33.

Jana, A. H., & Mandal, P. K. (2011). Manufacturing and quality of mozzarella cheese: A review. *International Journal of Dairy Science*, *6*(4), 199–226.

Kanawjia, S. K., & Khetra, Y. (2016). *Cheese technology. DT-5: Lesson 21*. Cottage Cheese.

Kayagil, F. (2006). *Effect of traditional starter cultures on quality of cheese* [Master's thesis, Middle East Technical University].

Lucey, J. A. (2011). Cheese | acid- and acid/heat coagulated cheese. *Encyclopedia of Dairy Sciences*, 698–705.

Mbye, M., Ayyash, M., Abu-Jdayil, B., & Kamal-Eldin, A. (2022). The texture of camel milk cheese: Effects of milk composition, coagulants, and processing conditions. *Frontiers in Nutrition*, *9*, 868320.

Moncel, B. (2019). *How has cheese changed through history?* The Spruce Eats.

Nelson, J. A., & Trout, G. M. (1951). *Judging dairy products* (p. 480). The Olsen Publishing Co. Milwaukee 12.

OECD-FAO. (2016). Agriculture in Sub-Saharan Africa: Prospects and challenges for the next decade. *OECD-FAO Agricultural Outlook*, *2025*(181), 1–39.

Phadungath, C. (2019). Cheddar cheese review: I cheese manufacture. *Koch Cha Sarn Journal of Science*, *37*(1), 1–17.

Rankin, S. A., Bradley, R. L., Miller, G., & Mildenhall, K. B. (2017). A 100-year review: A century of dairy processing advancements-Pasteurization, cleaning and sanitation, and sanitary equipment design. *Journal of Dairy Science*, *100*(12), 9903–9915.

Sevenich, R., Rauh, C., & Knorr, D. (2016). A scientific and interdisciplinary approach for high pressure processing as a future toolbox for safe and high quality products: A review. *Innovative Food Science & Emerging Technologies*, *38*, 65–75.

Skeie, S. (2010). *Milk quality requirements for cheesemaking. Improving the safety and quality of milk* (pp. 433–453). Woodhead Publishing.

Surono, I. S., & Hosono, A. (2011). Fermented milks | starter cultures. *Encyclopedia of Dairy Sciences*, 477–482.

Tamime, A. Y. (2011). *Processed cheese and analogues*. John Wiley & Sons.

Wajszczyk, B., Charzewska, J., Godlewski, D., Zemła, B., Nowakowska, E., Kozaczka, M., Chilimoniuk, M., & Pathak, D. R. (2021). Consumption of dairy products and the risk of developing breast cancer in polish women. *Nutrients*, *13*, 4420.

Wang, Y., Wu, J., Lv, M., Shao, Z., Hungwe, M., Wang, J., & Geng, W. (2021). Metabolism characteristics of lactic acid bacteria and the expanding applications in food industry. *Frontiers in Bioengineering and Biotechnology*, *9*, 612285.

Yiadom-Farkye, N. A. (1984). *Effect of casein/fat ratio on milk fat recovery in cheddar cheese*. [Master's thesis, Utah State University].

# 5 Fat-Rich Dairy Food—Cream

## 5.1 LEARNING OBJECTIVES

By the end of the chapter, the reader will be able to:

- Understand the classification and composition of the cream
- Understand the basic principles and different ways of separating cream from milk
- Gain knowledge of cream production and processing
- Understand the physicochemical alterations that occur during the processing of cream and their impacts on its functionality
- Learn how to judge and improve the quality of the cream
- Make cream enterprises profitable
- Understand the key potential health benefits of cream
- Discover cream innovations from production to nutritional and health attributes

There is immense and hidden complexity in cream. The combination of different elements in cream results in a suitable flavor and texture. When cream is exposed to heat and shear flow, it undergoes reactions that change its physical stability as an emulsion. These can be employed to create a multitude of cream variations, each offering unique flavors and textures, suitable for use in recipes.

## 5.2 INTRODUCTION

Dairy cream, a yellowish substance with lots of fat globules, will naturally float to the top when milk is allowed to stand for a period of time. It's a fat-rich dairy food. The fat content of cream products varies from about 10–50% (**Figure 5.1**). Cream is mechanically separated in the dairy business. Cream homogenization shrinks the size of the fat globules, making the final product less whippable (Deosarkar et al., 2016; Kwak et al., 2013).

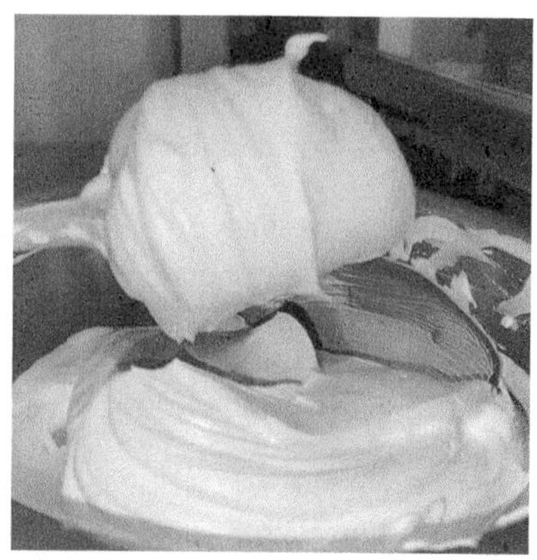

**FIGURE 5.1 Image of dairy cream.**

### 5.2.1 Definition

Cream can be defined as the portion of milk that is rich in milk fat or that has been gathered and which contains a large portion of milk fat. Cream can be produced when milk fat is condensed into a small amount of the original milk (Deosarkar et al., 2016; Hoffmann, 2002; Walstra et al., 2006).

The PFA Rules of 1976 state that cream should be derived from either cow milk, buffalo milk, or a blend of both, and it must possess a minimum of 25% milk fat, where sterilized cream is not included in this regard (PFA, 1976).

## 5.3 HISTORY OF CREAM

Cream is believed to have originated during the early stages of animal domestication in the Paleolithic era. It was favored by both the Celts and the Vikings. During the Middle Ages, people often had cream on their dining tables with vegetables and fresh cheeses (Deosarkar et al., 2016).

## 5.4 TYPES OF CREAM

Cream can be found in many forms and varieties, and is a common ingredient for a variety of cuisines. According to the federal Food and Drug Administration, cream may be classified as follows (Deosarkar et al., 2016; Walstra et al., 2006):

i. Light/coffee/table cream (18–30% fat)
ii. Whipping cream
  - Light whipping (30–36% fat)
  - Heavy whipping (36–38% fat)
iii. Sour cream/cultured sour cream (Acidity around 0.2%)
iv. Sour half-and-half cream (Acidity more than 0.2%)
v. Half-and-half cream (Mixing of milk and cream, containing 10.5% fat)
vi. Plastic cream (65–80% fat)

According to the Australia New Zealand Food Standards Code, cream may be classified as follows (Deosarkar et al., 2016; Walstra et al., 2006):

i. Extra light cream (12–12.5% fat)
ii. Light cream (18–20% fat)
iii. Thickened cream (35–36.5% fat)
iv. Single cream (35% fat)
v. Double cream (48–60% fat)

According to the standards of the United Nations Food and Agriculture Organization (Codex Alimentarius, 2006), cream is classified as follows based on fat content (Deosarkar et al., 2016; Walstra et al., 2006). Standards for the fat content of cream in some countries are illustrated in **Table 5.1.**

i. Cream: 18–26%
ii. Light cream (or coffee cream): >10%
iii. Whipping cream: >28%
iv. Heavy cream: >35%
v. Double cream: >45%

Various types of cream exist due to different methods of preparation. The steps involved in cultured cream (**Figure 5.6**), whipping cream (Shim et al., 2003) (**Figure 5.7**), UHT-treated cream (IDF, 1996) (**Figure 5.8**), and sterilized cream (**Figure 5.9**) preparation are shown in the flow diagram respectively.

**TABLE 5.1**
**Standards for the Fat Content of Cream in Some Countries**

| Country | Cream type | Fat content (g/100 g) |
|---|---|---|
| Australia and New Zealand | Cream | 18–40 |
| France | Light cream | 12–30 |
| | Cream | 30–40 |
| Germany | Coffee cream | 10–30 |
| | Whipping cream | 30–40 |
| The Netherlands | Cream | 10–30 |
| | Whipping cream | 30–40 |
| United Kingdom | Half cream | 12–18 |
| | Single cream | 18–35 |
| | Whipping cream | 35–48 |
| | Double cream | 48–55 |
| United States | Half-and-half cream | 10–18 |
| | Light cream | 18–30 |
| | Light whipping cream | 30–36 |
| | Heavy cream | 36–45 |

*Source:* Deosarkar et al., 2016; Walstra et al., 2006

### 5.4.1 Cream Liqueur

Cream liqueur is an alcoholic beverage containing emulsified milk fat (Banks & Muir, 1988). The basic principles involved in the manufacture of cream liqueurs are illustrated in the flow diagram in **Figure 5.10**.

## 5.5 NUTRITIONAL FACTS

Dairy cream is rich in nutrients (**Table 5.2**) and is a versatile dairy food. As a dairy product, heavy cream contains nutrients such as protein; vitamins A, D, E, and K; and minerals such as calcium and phosphorus.

**TABLE 5.2**
**Nutritional Composition of Cream**

| Ingredients | Light cream (%) | Whipped cream (%) |
|---|---|---|
| Fat | 18 | 36 |
| Protein | 2.94 | 2.2 |
| Lactose | 4.05 | 3.15 |
| Mineral | 0.6 | 0.46 |
| Moisture | 73.41 | 58.19 |

*Source:* Deosarkar et al., 2016; Hoffmann & Buchheim, 2006; Walstra et al., 2006

## 5.6 WORLDWIDE CREAM PRODUCTION AND CONSUMPTION TRENDS

The global fresh cream market size reached 8.5 million metric tons in 2021. Global cream production is projected to reach 10.8 million metric tons by 2027, with a CAGR of 4.07% from 2021–2027. In 2021, the worldwide fresh cream market was 8.5 million metric tons (MMT) in size. The market is predicted to grow and reach 10.8 MMT by 2027. This would mean a compound annual growth rate (CAGR) of 4.07% between 2021 and 2027. Germany, Russia, Canada, France, and Poland are the top fresh cream-consuming countries in the world.

## 5.7 PARTS OF A CREAM SEPARATOR

### 5.7.1 MECHANICAL CREAM SEPARATOR

The cream separator is the primary machine employed in mechanical cream separation, which can be operated by hand or power (**Figure 5.2**).

The parts are:

i. A bowl with a spinning rate (5000–6000 rotations per minute) using gears and a power transmission mechanism
ii. Establishing a system for transferring milk into the bowl
iii. Eliminating the cream and skim milk
iv. Driving the machine

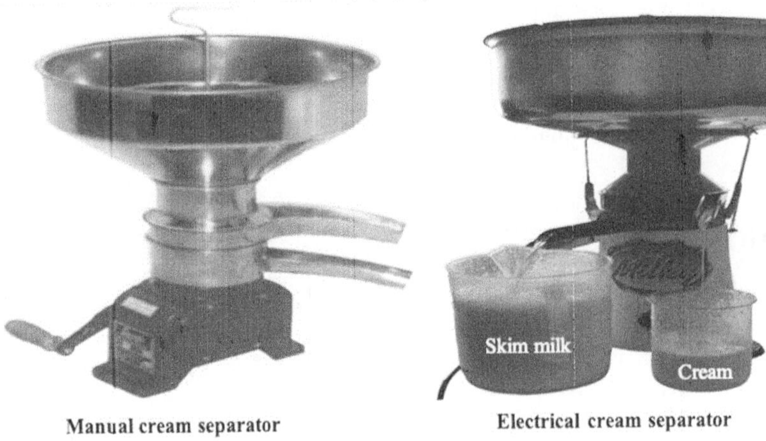


FIGURE 5.2 Cream separator

#### 5.7.1.1 Bowl Parts

- **Rubber ring or gasket:** It fits in the bottom of the bowl and stops it from leaking.
- **Distributor:** It spreads the milk evenly in three notches around the edge at the bottom.
- **Bottom disc:** This part of the disc is distinct from the rest. The exterior and interior of this item feature elevated portions and have three holes. It can also be named as separating disc.
- **Intermediate discs:** Their number ranges from six to seven. They are like the bottom disc but without any projection on the inside and only a projection on the outside. There

are three holes in these disks. More discs enhance the effectiveness of the separation process.

- **Top disc:** This is a very important part of the bowl. This is also called a separating or dividing disc. The connection between the skim milk and skim milk outlet is made possible by this disc. The disc has an outlet for the cream in its neck. During separation, the cream near the axis of the bowl oozes out from the cream outlet. This disc has a screw at its neck. The thickness of the cream can be adjusted by adjusting this screw.
- **Bowl hood:** It is placed on the top, covering the entire bowl.
- **Bowl spanner:** Its function is to make the bowl nut tighter.

#### 5.7.1.2 Arrangement for Supplying Milk to the Bowl

- **Supply can:** It holds the milk to be separated.
- **Faucet:** It is used to allow the flow of milk from the supply can into the bowl. This enables milk to flow from the supply can into the bowl.
- **Regulator:** It controls the milk flow that gets into the bowl.
- **Float:** It permits only a limited portion of milk through the regulator and into the bowl.

#### 5.7.1.3 Removing Cream or Skim Milk

- **Skim milk outlet:** The skim milk from the bowl moves between the dividing disc and the inside wall of the bowl. At the top, space is provided between to disc and bowl hood, which connects with the skim milk outlet. The skim milk is let out through this cover.
- **Cream outlet:** The cream coming out from the cream screw located on the top disc is trapped in the cream cover and is let out.

#### 5.7.1.4 Driving the Machine

- **Spindle rod:** The bowl rests on the spindle rod. The spindle rod has a suitable gear that is engaged with the crank gear.
- **Crank handle:** The machine is revolved with the crank handle at the speed indicated by the manufacturers. Generally, 60–70 revolutions per minute are sufficient to develop the speed.

i. **Clarification**
ii. **Separation**

### 5.7.2 Purpose of Cream Separation

i. To get a fat-free or low-fat milk
ii. To concentrate milk fat for the production of high-fat products
iii. To standardize milk's fat content
iv. To recover fat from milk

## 5.8 METHODS OF CREAM SEPARATION

### 5.8.1 Separation Processes

The basic steps involved in cream production are shown in the flow diagram in **Figures 5.3, 5.4, and 5.5**. There are two methods of cream separation:

- Gravity method
- Centrifugal method

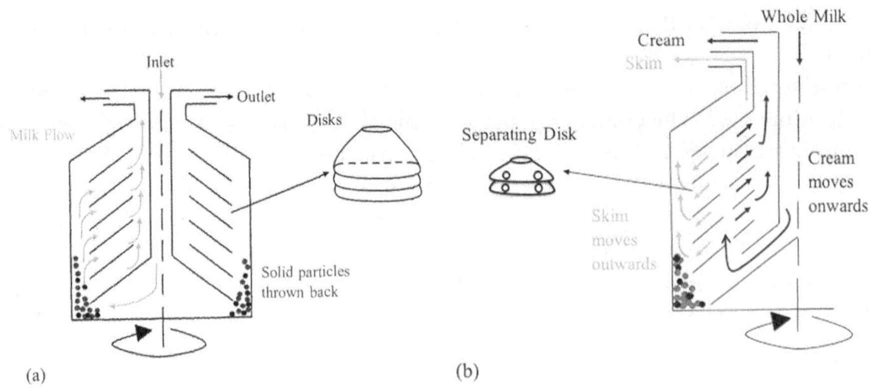


**FIGURE 5.3** (**a**) Schematic diagram of the clarification process. (**b**) Schematic diagram of a self-cleaning separator.

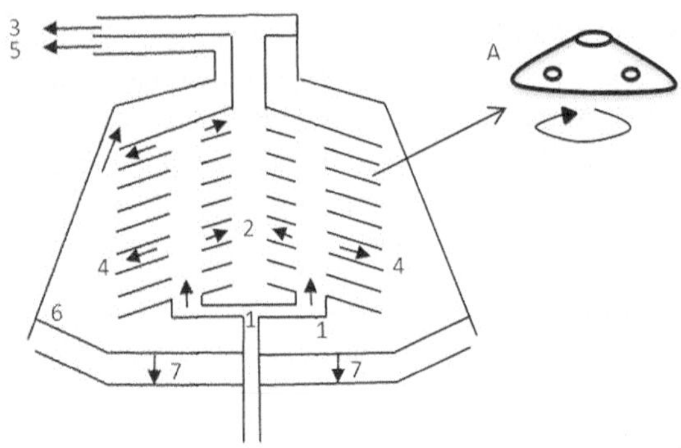


**FIGURE 5.4 Flow diagram of the centrifugal cream separation process.** A) Conical disk, from stack, showing top opening and milk distribution channels. Disk stack is rotating in separator. 1) Whole milk enters the disk distribution channel from below. 2) Fat globules move inward, carried by some skim milk to form the cream. 3) Cream outlet port. 4) Skim milk devoid of fat globules moves outward and upward, over the solid disk at the top. 5) Skim outlet port. 6) Sediment collects. 7) Momentary periodic release of bowl pressure causes sediment cavity to open, releasing sediment.

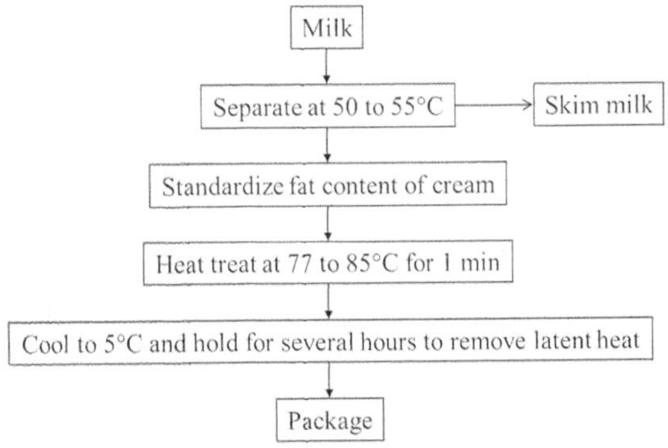


**FIGURE 5.5 Flow diagram of basic principles of cream separation.**

### 5.8.2 Cream Separation by Gravity Method

When milk is allowed to stand undisturbed for some time, there is a tendency for fat to rise.

The velocity, or rate, at which the fat globules rise is described by the following equation, which is known as Stoke's Law:

$$V = \frac{2G(d_s - d_f)r^2}{9\eta}$$

Where,

V = Rate of rise of fat globule in millimeters per second
r = Radius of fat globule
G = Force of gravity (981 dynes)
$\eta$ = Viscosity of skim milk
$d_s$ = Skim milk density
$d_f$ = Density of fat globule

According to Stoke's law, it is observed that, theoretically, velocity increases with the:

i. Increasing the radius of the fat globule
ii. Increasing difference in densities of skim milk and fat
iii. Decreasing viscosity of skim milk

However, in practice, the factors affecting the rate of rise of fat in the gravity method of separation are:

- **Size of fat globules:** The rate at which fat rises also increases with an increase in fat globule size. Larger fat globules rise faster than smaller ones. Because the fat globules in buffalo milk are larger than those in cow milk, gravity creaming happens faster in buffalo milk.
- **Temperature:** As temperature increases, viscosity decreases.
- **Clumping:** A clump or cluster works similarly to a single globule when it comes to moving through skim milk. Therefore, the effective "r" is increased, which in turn increases velocity.

There are five various methods for separating the cream using the gravity method:

i. **Shallow pan method:** Milk is allowed to stand in a pan of 10 cm depth and 45–60 cm diameter at 7°C for 24 h. The cream rises to the top during this period.
ii. **Deep pan method:** Milk is left to stand for 24 h at 10°C in a pan with a 20′ depth and 8–12′ diameter. These tall cans have glass on one side of the can and a faucet placed near the bottom. Skim milk is drawn through the faucet.
iii. **Water dilution method:** Milk is diluted with water and allowed to stand for 12 h at 37.7°C. Water reduces the milk's viscosity, allowing the fat globules to rise more easily.
iv. **Scalding method:** Heating and cooling of milk slowly causes the formation of the cream layer at the surface of the milk.
v. **Jersey creamery method:** In a jacketed vat, milk is heated to a temperature of 40°C using hot water and then cooled to a temperature of 10°C using chilled water in place of the hot water. The cream will be separated rapidly on cooling, immediately after heating the milk, by increasing the difference in densities of milk fat and serum. The gravity method is very slow; it is no longer used commercially for cream separation.

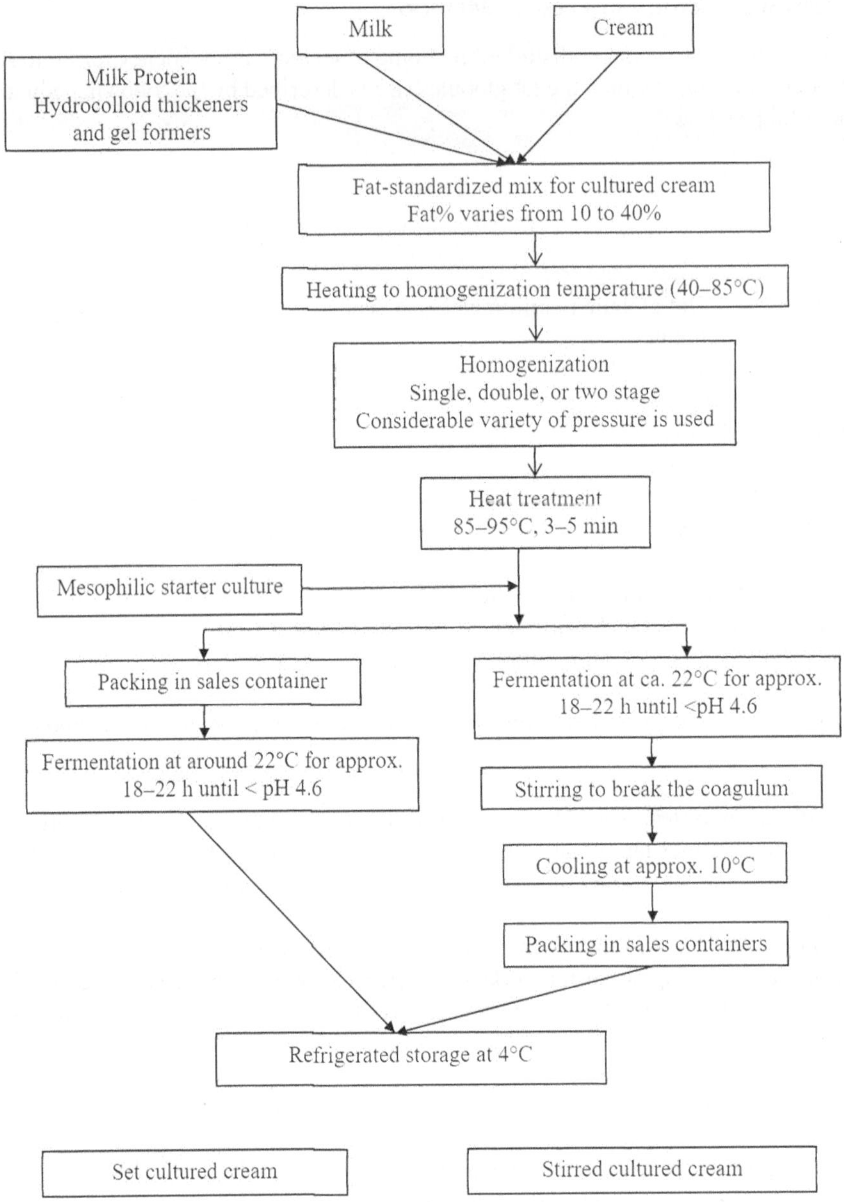


**FIGURE 5.6 Flow diagram of the cultured cream manufacturing process.**

### 5.8.3 Cream Separation by Centrifugal Method

Separation and clarification can be done at the same time in one centrifuge process (**Figures 5.3 and 5.4**). Milk is fed to the machine through a flow regulator. Milk comes to the regulating chamber from the milk basin by the milk faucet. When the milk enters the revolving bowl through the milk regulator of the machine, it is subjected to gravity and centrifugal force. Centrifugal force is about 3000 to 6000 times more than the gravitational force. Fat (0.93) and skim milk (1.037) are different in their specific gravity. When fat and skim milk are subjected to centrifugal force, the difference in density affects the fat, and skim milk (i.e., the heavier portion) is affected more intensely than the fat (lighter portion). So, skim milk is forced to the periphery and the fat portion (cream) moves toward the center. Cream and skim milk form separated vertical walls within the bowl and go out through separate outlets near the axis of rotation. In comparison to the skim milk outlet, the cream

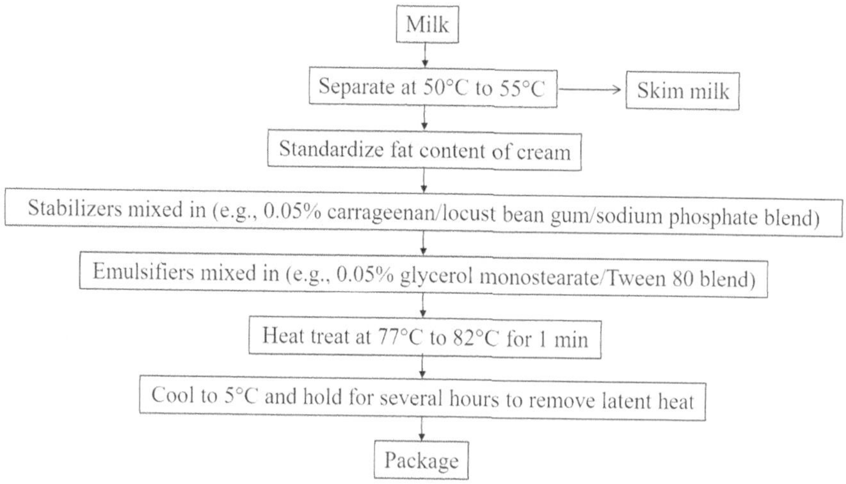


**FIGURE 5.7 Flow diagram of the whipping cream manufacturing process.**

outlet is located higher. The rate of movement of a fat globule in the machine is estimated by following Stoke's equation:

$$\mathbf{V = r^2 \times ((d_s—d_f)/n) \times N^2 \times R \times K}$$

Where,

$V$ = Rate of movement of a single fat globule
$r$ = Radius of fat globule
$d_s$ = Density of skim milk
$d_f$ = Density of fat
$N$ = Revolution per minute of bowl
$R$ = Distance of fat globule from the axis of rotation.
$K$ = Constant
$n$ = Viscosity of skim milk

## 5.9 FACTORS AFFECTING THE RICHNESS OF CREAM

The following factors influence the fat percentage in cream (Smiddy et al., 2009; Huppertz & Kelly, 2006; Scott et al., 2003):

i. **Positioning of the cream or skim milk screw:** Each machine has a device for regulating the richness of the cream. This is done by changing the proportion of material coming out of the cream and skim milk opening, either by changing the pressure on either of the two or by changing the size of the opening. In most machines, the richness of the cream is regulated using a cream screw and in a few by a skim milk screw. When the cream screw is turned in closure to the center of the bowl, the pressure is decreased and less flows through, making a richer cream. Closing the size of the opening has the same effect as enlarging the opening, and turning the cream screw out lowers the richness of the cream by increasing the amount. In a machine having skim milk screws the richness of the cream is affected oppositely.

ii. **Speed of the machine:** Separators are made to skim cream at a rated speed. As the speed of the separator is increased, the fat content of the cream produced is increased and the amount is less; the taste of the skim milk is unaffected.

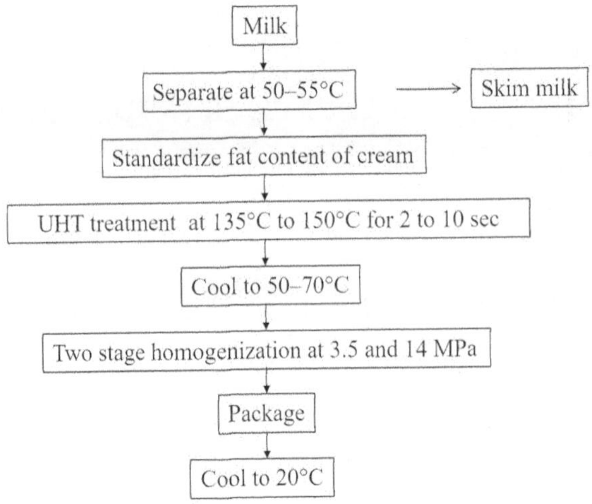


**FIGURE 5.8 Flow diagram of the UHT-treated cream manufacturing process.**

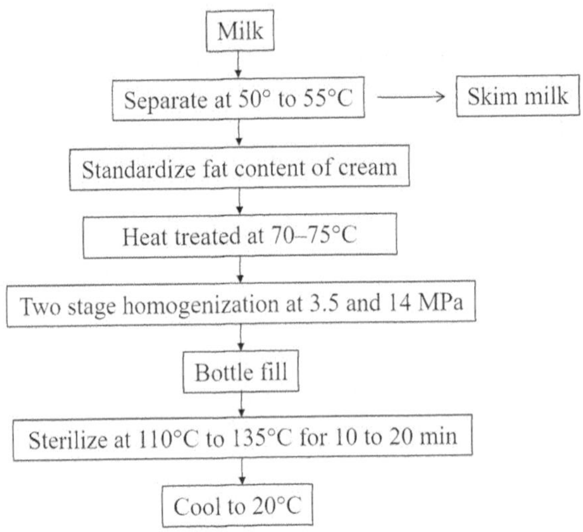


**FIGURE 5.9 Flow diagram of the sterilized cream manufacturing process.**

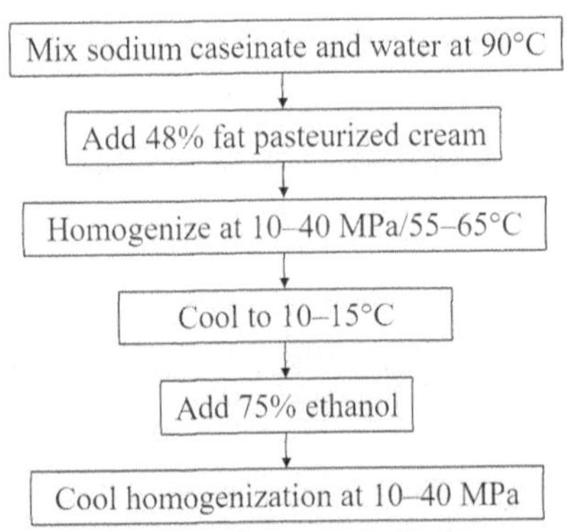


**FIGURE 5.10 Flow diagram of the cream liqueur manufacturing process.**

iii. **Temperature of the milk:** Milk that is too cold gradually will clot up the cream outlet, resulting in less and richer cream and lighter-tasting skim milk. This is because, with lower temperatures, cream becomes denser and more resistant to flow. Milk heated to a higher temperature than normal when separated will produce cream of a lower fat content because at high temperatures, cream is more fluid. The effect of low temperatures on the fat content of the cream varies with different machines. If the cream contains 30% fat when separated at 100°F, a fat percentage of 45% may be expected in milk separated at 75°F.
iv. **Rate of inflow:** As the inflow of milk is regulated by float or valve, there is little danger of feeding the machine. If the supply tank fault or valve is not open wide enough, the machine will be underfed; this means a higher taste of cream because the small amount of force is acting on a smaller amount of milk, and the skim milk taste is not affected.
v. **Richness of the milk:** With any increase in the fat content of milk, the fat content of the separated cream will also increase. If the separator is set with 40% cream when skimming a 6% fat milk, it will skim approximately 20% cream with a 3% fat milk. The cream becomes richer and more viscous, thus offering more resistance to flow, and as a result, less cream is produced and there is a corresponding increase in fat percentage.
vi. **Vibration of the bowl:** If the machine is not set the level, the bowl has been handled so roughly that it is out of balance, or if the bearings are worn, the bowl will vibrate and will not skim cream. This means a lower taste in the cream and a higher taste in skim milk.
vii. **Cleanliness of the bowl:** The machine should be washed each time it is used; otherwise, milk left in the bowl may sour and clog up the cream opening so that the machine does not skim milk. A dirty machine will not do good work.
viii. **The amount of flashing:** When the last milk has passed into the separator, the bowl is still. The cream part of its content is cream and the other part is skim milk. To get all the cream out of the bowl, it is customary to flush milk with either water or skim milk. To force all the cream out of the bowl, enough water or skim milk must be used in flushing to cause a dilution of the cream. The extent of dilution will depend upon the amount of either skim milk or water used in flushing and the amount of cream separated.

## 5.10 QUALITY JUDGING OF CREAM

To judge, the following guidelines should be performed, mostly for cream in glass containers: Bacterial count, viscosity, flavor, acidity, body and texture, color, sedimentation, container and closure, cream plugs, and serum separation. The following factors influence the quality of cream (Smith et al., 2000; Ozer et al., 2000):

i. The quality of the milk will last longer if it is produced cleanly by the animals, but it is also crucial to get milk of high caliber. Cream with a short shelf life is a result of poor raw milk quality, particularly when spore and thermoduric microbe counts are high.
ii. To stop the growth of psychotropic bacteria, which cause different taints in cream during storage, the milk purchased from the farmers needs to be cooled right away.
iii. Another aspect that influences the quality of cream is the separation and hygienic processing of the milk. If not cleaned thoroughly, cream separators are an important source of germs.
iv. Transport of cream to the dairy under lower temperature.
v. Cream should be promptly cooled and stored at a cooler temperature.
vi. Incorrect temperature selection for heat treatment.

## 5.11 DEFECTS IN CREAM

Several flavor defects that have been associated with cream are acid, cooked, malty, musty, utensil, weed, bitter, and oxidized/rancid. A few common defects in dairy cream are included in **Table 5.3**.

**TABLE 5.3**
**Defects in Cream with Their Possible Causes and Remedies**

| Name of the defect | Causes | Remedies |
|---|---|---|
| Cooked | Excessive heating during pasteurization of cream. | Proper heating of cream during pasteurization. |
| Highly acid/sour | i. Using sour milk for separation<br>ii. Acid development in cream | i. Using fresh, sweet milk for preparation<br>ii. Neutralization of cream |
| Oxidized/oily/ metallic/tallowy | Fat oxidation brought on by direct contact with milk with copper or iron, sunshine exposure, etc. | i. Milk or cream holding vessels should be properly tinned, and contact surfaces should be made of stainless steel or aluminum alloy.<br>ii. Vacuum pasteurization of cream |
| Rancidity | In milk or cream, fat hydrolysis occurs due to lipase action. | Proper pasteurization of milk and cream can inactivate the lipase activity. |

## 5.12 STORAGE OF CREAM

i. Half cream, single cream, and sour creams are stored at a temperature of 2–4°C (**Table 5.4**). These creams are not stored at freezing temperatures (IDF, 1982).
ii. Double cream and whipping cream are stored at freezing temperatures.
iii. If unwhipped cream is stored at freezing temperature, we have to add 10% sugar to the cream to make it stabilize.

## 5.13 HEALTH BENEFITS OF CREAM

Cream contains lots of vitamins, minerals, and other components. Some of the vitamins that cream has are vitamin A, vitamin C, vitamin D, vitamin E, vitamin K, vitamin $B_6$, vitamin $B_{12}$, choline, betaine, folate, niacin, thiamin, riboflavin, and pantothenic acid. Cream also contains omega-3 fatty acids, omega-6 fatty acids, sodium, and potassium, which have lots of health benefits. Apart from this, cream also has some minerals such as calcium, iron, magnesium, phosphorus, zinc, and selenium (Arab et al., 2006). **Figure 5.11** describes the key potential health benefits of dairy cream.

### 5.13.1 Association of Cream Consumption with Energy Boosting

One of the most important health benefits of cream is an energy boost. Cream is very high in calories; the consumption of 230 grams of cream can provide 455 calories of energy; due to this cream

**TABLE 5.4**
**Safe Storage Time of Various Creams**

| Types of cream | How to store | On refrigerator shelves 35–40°F (2–4°C) | In freezer 0°F or below, properly packaged |
|---|---|---|---|
| Sweet cream | i. In the original container, immediately refrigerate.<br>ii. Keep the container shut. | i. 30 days period for unopened boxes<br>ii. For a week, once open | Do not freeze. (Change in texture and body appearance, separation of fat) |
| Whipped topping | Keep covered | i. 3 months in aerosol can<br>ii. 3 days prepared from mix | Do not freeze |
| Sour cream | i. Refrigerate immediately in original container.<br>ii. Keep container closed. | 2 weeks | Upto 6 months |

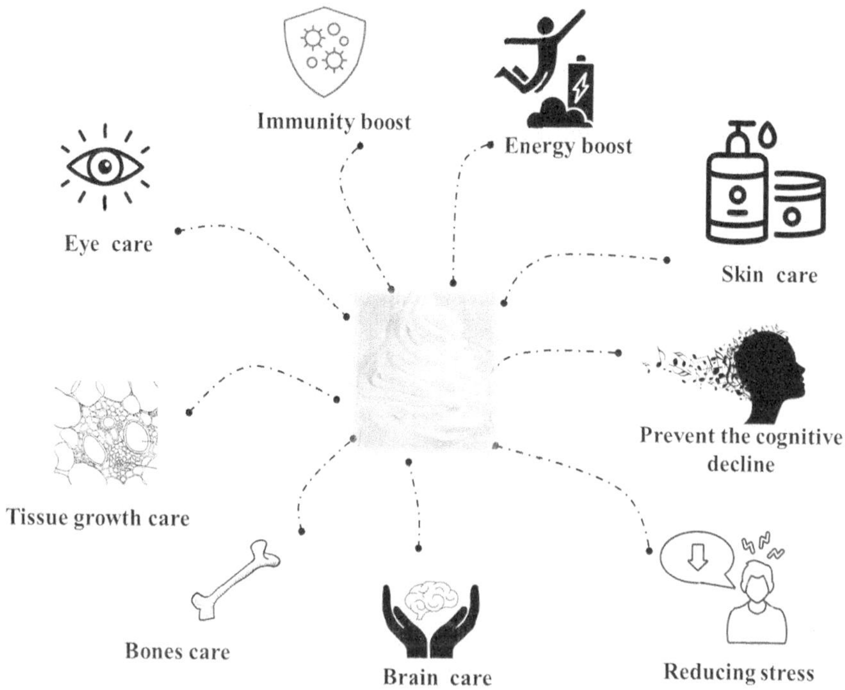


FIGURE 5.11 **Key potential health benefits of cream.** Heavy cream contains calcium, which is necessary for strong bones and teeth. Fat-soluble vitamins promote good eyesight and immunological function. Heavy cream's creamy texture and rich flavor may enhance the flavor of a variety of foods.

is an excellent energy booster (Park & Pariza, 2007; Pavoine & Pecker, 2009; Jones et al., 2008; Bhattacharya et al., 2006).

### 5.13.2 Association of Cream Consumption with Eye Health

Cream is very rich in different kinds of antioxidants such as vitamin A, and it is very useful to protect the retina from oxidative damage caused by harmful free radicals. Apart from these antioxidant properties, cream helps to neutralize free radicals and prevent oxidative damage to our ocular cells; oxidative damage is the primary cause of macular degeneration, which can lead to blindness. Studies have demonstrated that those who eat cream regularly in moderate amounts in their daily diet have less chance of suffering from various types of eye problems, such as cataracts.

### 5.13.3 Association of Cream Consumption with Growth

Vitamin $B_2$ is a vital component of cream that contributes greatly to tissue growth and development, for example, the eyes, skin, mucous membranes, connective tissue, immune system, nervous system, and reproductive organs. Moreover, it enhances the strength of the skin, hair, and nails.

### 5.13.4 Association of Cream Consumption with Bone Health

Because of the large amount of calcium and phosphorous present in cream, it is very beneficial for our bone health. Calcium and phosphorus help to improve our bone density and keep our bones stronger and healthy. Studies have proven that those who consume cream regularly have less chance of being affected by bone diseases such as osteoporosis (Hur & Park, 2007).

### 5.13.5 Association of Cream Consumption with Stress Management

The pantothenic acid present in cream is very useful for reducing stress and various mental problems such as depression, lack of concentration, and anxiety. It controls the hormones, which are the reason for these psychological conditions (Benjamin & Spener, 2009).

### 5.13.6 Association of Cream Consumption with Cognitive Function

Vitamin $B_6$, which is contained in cream, is a vital part of the focal sensory system. It improves cerebrum function and enhances the intellectual capacity. Apart from this, cream is highly rich in zinc, which is very beneficial in preventing cognitive decline. Studies have proven that those who consume zinc-rich foods such as cream daily have less chance of being affected by cognitive decline issues (Kumar, 2023).

### 5.13.7 Association of Cream Consumption with Immunity

Cream is highly rich in antibacterial and antiseptic properties, which are very beneficial for preventing certain types of bacterial infections in our body. Studies have proven that the consumption of cream can prevent various types of bacterial infections such as bronchitis, meningitis, and tuberculosis. Besides this, cream contains a high amount of antioxidants, such as vitamin A, which is very good for the immune system, protects our body from free radicals that do oxidative damage to our cells, and helps to protect our body from macular degeneration and various types of cancer (Evans et al., 2010).

### 5.13.8 Association of Cream Consumption with Brain Health

Your mind is exceptionally dependent on omega-3 fats. So, the consumption of omega-3 fatty acid-rich foods such as cream has appeared to beneficially affect a wide range of brain-related conditions. These can be as far-reaching as mood and stress reduction, treating learning issues in kids, lessening headaches, bringing down the danger of Alzheimer's, and enhancing the nature of your rest. Apart from this, cream is also highly rich in vitamin A that is good for brain health and improves neuron activity in the brain.

### 5.13.9 Association of Cream Consumption with Blood Cell Health

Red blood cells (RBCs) are the one of vital components in the human body. RBCs are the reason your body is working ideally because the metabolism system could work since hemoglobin in the RBCs conveys the supplements and oxygen to the cells. Iron and different minerals are fundamental to the formation of red cells, and fortunately, cream is rich in specific minerals and vitamins.

### 5.13.10 Association of Cream Consumption with Skin Health

Cream is highly rich in vitamin A, some B family vitamins, and minerals such as phosphorous and zinc, which are very good for our skin health. Vitamin A fights against free radicals and prevents oxidative damage to our skin cells, which is the main cause of various types of skin issues, such as wrinkles, acne, dark spots, etc. (Belury et al., 2007).

### 5.13.11 Association of Cream Consumption with Beneficial Nutrients

i. **Vitamin A (retinol):** Good for thyroid, adrenal, and cardiovascular health.
ii. **Essential fat:** Omega-3s improve hormone optimization and reduce inflammation.
iii. **Butyrate:** Reduces inflammation (Hamer et al., 2008).

iv. **Conjugated linoleic acid:** Protects against cancer, supports muscle growth, and reduces belly fat (Halade et al., 2010).
v. **Vitamin D and $K_2$:** Vitamin D helps bone growth and development, and vitamin $K_2$ reverses arterial calcification.

## 5.14 CREAM INNOVATIONS

The cream industry is influenced by changes in what consumers want, advancements in technology, and new laws. These are the main reasons why innovations in the cream industry happen. Intensive research means studying new ways to keep dairy products fresh and healthy for longer periods. Microfluidization, a two-stage separation method, an innovative approach using dissolved $CO_2$, UV light treatment, ultrasound, and ohmic heating are different ways to process or treat something. UV light treatment uses ultraviolet light to kill or deactivate harmful microorganisms. Ultrasound refers to using sound waves to clean or manipulate something. Ohmic heating is a method that uses electric current to heat something quickly and evenly. Many researchers are studying ways to protect the taste and nutrients in dairy products and make sure they are safe from harmful bacteria. Various sizes of milk fat droplets will help create new and unique dairy products. A way to control or change manufacturing processes is by using a two-step separation method and $CO_2$-enhanced crystallization. **Figures 5.12 and 5.13** illustrate powdered milk innovations from production to nutritional and health attributes (Dhungana et al., 2020; Schipper et al., 2016).

## 5.15 CREAM YIELD

The yield of cream from milk can be calculated by the following formula:

Quantity of cream = (Fat percent in milk – Fat percent in skim milk)/(Fat percent in cream – Fat percent in skim milk) × Quantity of milk

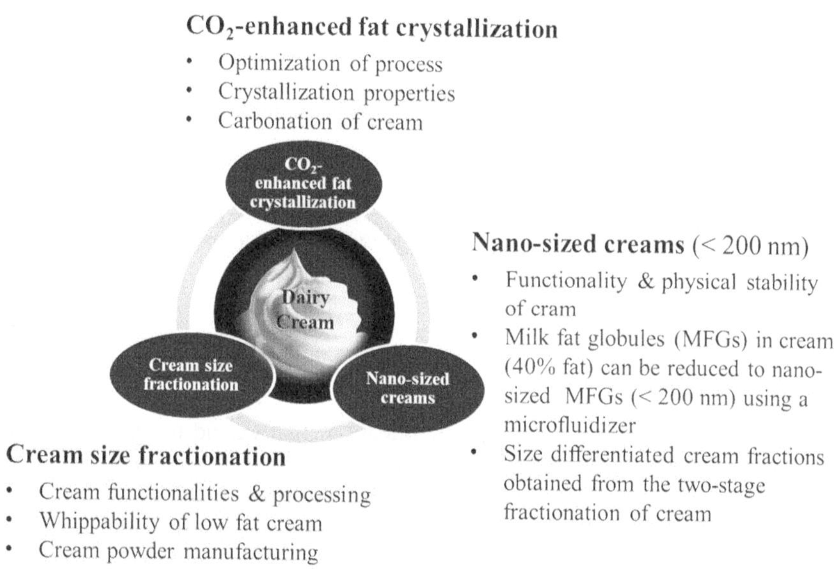


FIGURE 5.12 **Cream innovations in production attributes.**

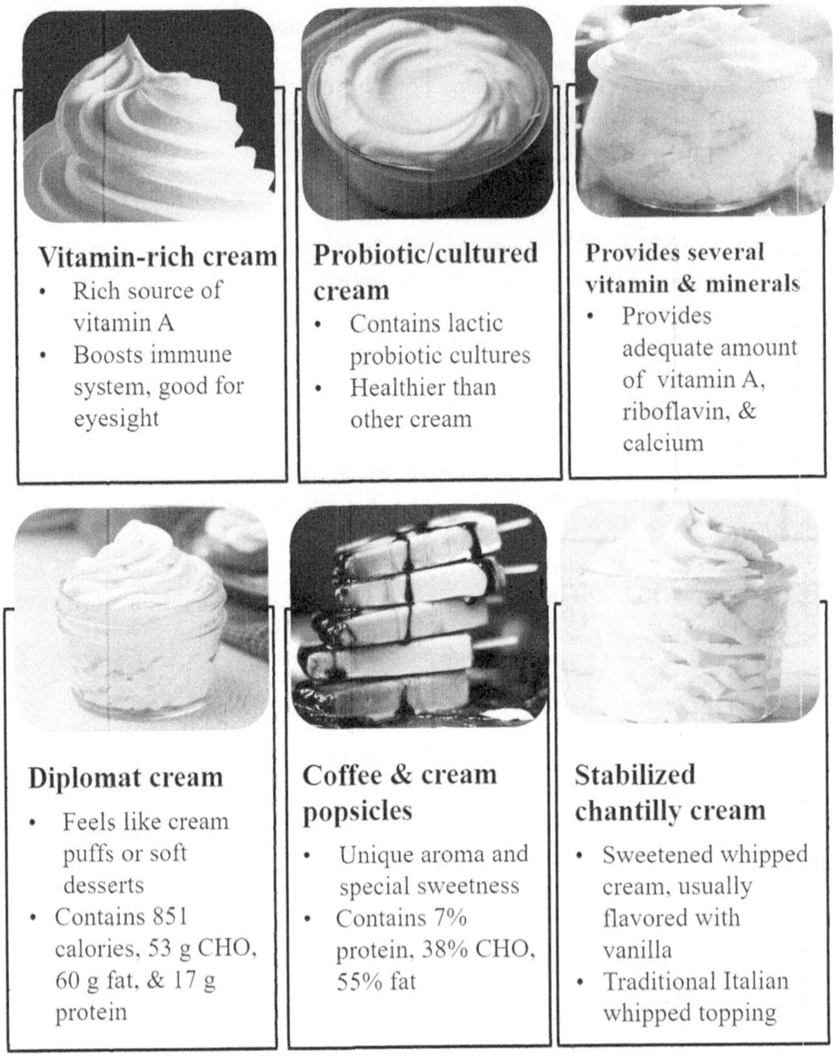


**FIGURE 5.13 Cream innovations in nutritional and health attributes.**

Normally, cow milk contains about 4% fat. So, about 100 ml of cream will be produced by 1 liter of milk.

## 5.16 CONCLUSIONS

Cream is an extremely versatile product with applications that extend far beyond the dairy sector (Hoffmann, 2011). Cream products have been traditionally regarded as luxury products, and their popularity may be affected in the current climate by consumer concerns about high fat intake. With recent advances in our understanding of cream constituents and their interactions with other ingredients, the development of reduced-fat cream products with properties equivalent to their traditional high-fat counterparts should be possible (Ha et al., 2010). According to research, crosslinking β-cyclodextrin with adipic acid helps to eliminate over 90% of cholesterol until the eighth time of reuse. The entrapped constituents are insignificant, and the remaining β-cyclodextrin was only a tiny quantity in cream following cholesterol removal by crosslinked β-cyclodextrin (Ha et al., 2010). This suggests that more research on cholesterol and saturated fat reduction in cream, as well as their novel bioactive components, is required to promote human health and well-being.

The entrapped ingredients are negligible, and the residual β-cyclodextrin was a trace amount in cream during cholesterol removal by crosslinked β-cyclodextrin (Ha et al., 2010). This means that in the future, butter, ghee, and cream with the cholesterol removed will be great health-beneficial foods with no loss of beneficial components. More research is needed on cholesterol and saturated fat lowering in butter, ghee, and cream, and on their new bioactive components to benefit human health and well-being.

## REFERENCES

Arab, K., Rossary, A., Soulere, L., & Steghens, J. P. (2006). Conjugated linoleic acid, unlike other unsaturated fatty acids, strongly induces glutathione synthesis without any lipoperoxidation. *British Journal of Nutrition*, *96*(5), 811–819.

Banks, W., & Muir, D. D. (1988). Stability of alcohol-containing emulsions. In E. Dickinson & G. Stainsby (Eds.), *Advances in food emulsions and foams*. Elsevier Applied Science.

Belury, M. A., Kavanaugh, C. J., & Liu, K. L. (2007). Conjugated linoleic acid modulates phorbol ester–induced PPAR-δ and K-FABP mRNA expression in mouse skin. *Nutrition Research*, *27*(1), 48–55.

Benjamin, S., & Spener, F. (2009). Conjugated linoleic acids as functional food: An insight into their health benefits. *Nutrition & Metabolism*, *6*(1), 1–13.

Bhattacharya, A., Banu, J., Rahman, M., Causey, J., & Fernandes, G. (2006). Biological effects of conjugated linoleic acids in health and disease. *The Journal of Nutritional Biochemistry*, *17*(12), 789–810.

Codex Alimentarius. (2006). *Codex standard for milk fat products*. Codex Stan 280–1973 Rev 1–1999. FAO, WHO.

Deosarkar, S. S., Khedkar, C. D., Kalyankar, S. D., & Sarode, A. R. (2016). Cream: Types of cream. In B. Caballero, P. Finglas, & F. Toldrá (Eds.), *The encyclopedia of food and health* (Vol. 2, pp. 331–337). Academic Press.

Dhungana, P., Truong, T., Bansal, N., & Bhandari, B. (2020). Effect of fat globule size on the physicochemical properties of dairy cream powder produced by spray drying. *Drying Technology*, *39*(15), 1–13.

Evans, N. P., Misyak, S. A., Schmelz, E. M., Guri, A. J., Hontecillas, R., & Bassaganya-Riera, J. (2010). Conjugated linoleic acid ameliorates inflammation-induced colorectal cancer in mice through activation of PPARγ. *The Journal of Nutrition*, *140*(3), 515–521.

Ha, H. J., Lee, J. E., Chang, Y. H., & Kwak, H. S. (2010). Entrapment of nutrients during cholesterol removal from cream by crosslinked β-cyclodextrin. *International Journal of Dairy Technology*, *63*(1), 119–126.

Halade, G. V., Rahman, M. M., & Fernandes, G. (2010). Differential effects of conjugated linoleic acid isomers in insulin-resistant female C57Bl/6J mice. *The Journal of Nutritional Biochemistry*, *21*(4), 332–337.

Hamer, H. M., Jonkers, D. M. A. E., Venema, K., Vanhoutvin, S. A. L. W., Troost, F. J., & Brummer, R. J. (2008). The role of butyrate on colonic function. *Alimentary Pharmacology & Therapeutics*, *27*(2), 104–119.

Hoffmann, W. (2002). Cream products. In H. Roginski, P. F. Fox, & J. W. Fuquay (Eds.), *Encyclopaedia of dairy sciences* (pp. 551–557). Academic Press.

Hoffmann, W. (2011). Cream. In J. F. Fuquay, P. F. Fox, & P. L. H. McSweeney (Eds.), *Encyclopedia of dairy sciences* (2nd edn). Academic Press.

Hoffmann, W., & Buchheim, W. (2006). Significance of milk fat in cream products. In P. F. Fox & P. L. H. McSweeney (Eds.), *Advanced dairy chemistry* (3rd ed., Lipids, Vol. 2, pp. 365–375). Springer.

Huppertz, T., & Kelly, A. L. (2006). Physical chemistry of milk fat globules. In P. F. Fox & P. L. H. McSweeney (Eds.), *Advanced dairy chemistry* (3rd ed., Lipids, Vol. 2, pp. 173–212). Springer.

Hur, S. J., & Park, Y. (2007). Effect of conjugated linoleic acid on bone formation and rheumatoid arthritis. *European Journal of Pharmacology*, *568*(1–3), 16–24.

IDF. (1982). *Technical guide for the packaging of milk and milk products*. International Dairy Federation, Document no. 143.

IDF. (1996). *UHT cream*. International Dairy Federation, Document no. 315, pp. 4–34.

Jones, P. J., Jew, S., & AbuMweis, S. (2008). The effect of dietary oleic, linoleic, and linolenic acids on fat oxidation and energy expenditure in healthy men. *Metabolism*, *57*(9), 1198–1203.

Kumar, S. (2023). *Unexplored benefits of zinc: 9 foods to add.* www.onlymyhealth.com/health-benefits-of-zinc-and-foods-to-add-1688728888.

Kwak, H. S., Ganesan, P., & Mijan, A. M. (2013). Butter, ghee, and cream products. *Milk and Dairy Products in Human Nutrition: Production, Composition and Health*, 390–411.

Ozer, B., Kirim, B., & Atamer, M. (2000). Effect of hydrogen peroxide treatment on the quality of raw cream. *International Journal of Dairy Technology*, *53*(3), 83–86.

Park, Y., & Pariza, M. W. (2007). Mechanisms of body fat modulation by conjugated linoleic acid (CLA). *Food Research International*, *40*(3), 311–323.

Pavoine, C., & Pecker, F. (2009). Sphingomyelinases: Their regulation and roles in cardiovascular pathophysiology. *Cardiovascular Research*, *82*(2), 175–183.

PFA. (1976). Commentary on the prevention of food adulteration act.

Schipper, L., Van Dijk, G., Broersen, L. M., Loos, M., Bartke, N., Scheurink, A. J., & van der Beek, E. M. (2016). A postnatal diet containing phospholipids, processed to yield large, phospholipid-coated lipid droplets, affects specific cognitive behaviors in healthy male mice. *Journal of Nutrition*, *146*, 1155–1161.

Scott, L. L., Duncan, S. E., Sumner, S. S., Waterman, K. M., & Kaylegian, K. E. (2003). Influence of emulsifying component composition on creams formulated with fractionated milkfat. *Journal of Agricultural and Food Chemistry*, *51*(20), 5933–5940.

Shim, S. Y., Ahn, J., & Kwak, H. S. (2003). Functional properties of cholesterol-removed whipping cream treated by β-cyclodextrin. *Journal of Dairy Science*, *86*(9), 2767–2772.

Smiddy, M. A., Kelly, A. L., & Huppertz, T. (2009). Cream and related products. In A. Y. Tamime (Ed.), *Dairy fats and related products* (pp. 61–85). Wiley-Blackwell.

Smith, A. K., Kakuda, Y., & Goff, H. D. (2000). Changes in protein and fat structure in whipped cream caused by heat treatment and addition of stabilizer to the cream. *Food Research International*, *33*(8), 697–706.

Walstra, P., Wouters, J. T., & Guerts, T. J. (2006). Cream products. In *Dairy science and technology* (2nd ed., pp. 447–466). CRC Press.

# 6 Fat-Rich Dairy Food—Butter

## 6.1 LEARNING OBJECTIVES

By the end of the chapter, the reader will be able to:

- Understand the classification and composition of the butter
- Learn the procedure of butter making
- Interpret the technique of optimum use of milk fat during churning, thereby lowering the loss of fat in buttermilk
- Understand how to judge and improve the quality of the butter
- Make butter enterprises profitable
- Know the key potential health benefits of butter
- Discover butter innovations from production to nutritional and health attributes

Researchers have developed a new and natural way to remove cholesterol from butter to fulfill consumer demand. The low-cholesterol butter (reduction of 44%) was obtained from cream fermented with *L. paracasei*. Low-cholesterol butter was rated well in sensory tests. Present scientific data do not support the dietary consumption to reduce or avoid full-fat dairy foods like butter, as they seem to be positive or neutral to cardiovascular health.

## 6.2 INTRODUCTION

Butter is one of the oldest dairy foods, made by churning fresh or fermented cream. It is typically used as a spread, a condiment, and in cooking processes like baking, preparing sauces, and frying. Butter (**Figure 6.1**) is a water-in-oil emulsion formed by inverting cream, which is an oil-in-water emulsion; the emulsifiers are milk proteins. When chilled, butter doesn't change; it stays solid. At room temperature, it becomes spreadable, and at 32–35°C, it melts into a thin liquid. Its color ranges from deep yellow to almost white but is often pale

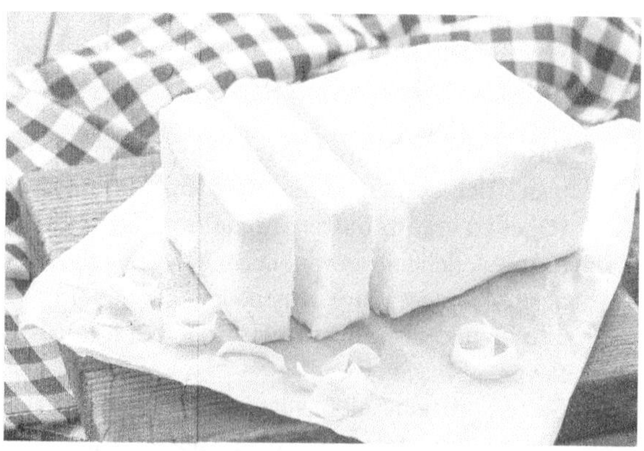

**FIGURE 6.1 Image of butter.** It has been a staple of human diets for thousands of years.

DOI: 10.1201/9781003397786-6

yellow. Its natural color depends on the feed given to the animals, and during industrial production, food colorings, most frequently annatto or carotene, are used to alter the color. Milk and/or items derived from milk should be used as the raw ingredients. To address public health concerns and enhance the properties of butter, various butter products, such as reduced-fat and low-fat butter (spreads), have been developed and commercialized and are currently being sold alongside regular butter. Market Watch (2020) estimates that the global butter market had a turnover of over $54 billion in 2020 and is expected to exceed $60 billion by 2026, growing at a rate of 3% annually.

### 6.2.1 Definition

A mixture of water-in-oil emulsion, milk fat, or cream can be used to make butter, which is a soft, solid product that typically has a minimum fat content of 80% and a maximum moisture content of 16% (Lee et al., 2018). It includes a small amount of the components found in natural milk, whether salt and colorings are added or not.

## 6.3 HISTORY OF BUTTER

The Latin word "*butyrum*" is a Latinization of the Greek word "*bouturon,*" where the term "butter" originates from (through Germanic languages). Butter is mentioned in the Old Testament as well. Butter has been utilized in a variety of ways throughout history. The ancient Greeks recognized butter as a complete food. It was also utilized as a beauty lotion by the ancient Romans. In 1848, the first butter factory was established near Goshen, New York. After the successful introduction of cheese factories a decade earlier, the first factories arose in the United States in the early 1860s.

## 6.4 TYPES OF BUTTER

There are numerous varieties of milk butter on the market. However, cultured cream butter and sweet cream butter are the most widely used. Sweet cream butter has a sweeter taste compared to other butter because of its pH. Cultured cream butter has a more acidic pH due to the inclusion of lactic acid bacteria (LAB) during the fermentation process. In this phase, bacteria serve as the raw material that produces butter's distinctive flavor, aroma, and texture. Due to the production of the diacetyl compound, these microorganisms are responsible for producing the distinctive "butter scent" of cultured cream butter. Another type of butter made through cream fermentation is sour cream butter. However, particular LAB strains, typically from the genus *Lactococcus*, such as *L. lactis* and *L. paracasei*, are utilized here. The inclusion of nitrogen gas during the cream churning process gives whipped butter sufficient spreadability, another variety of sour cream butter sold on the market (Budhkar et al., 2014; Lorenzen et al., 2013; Caballero et al., 2015). Here is a summary of a few different types of butter:

i. **Pasteurized cream butter:** Usually made from pasteurized sweet cream. This butter tastes lighter than butter made from similar cream that has not been pasteurized.
ii. **Ripened cream butter:** Made from cream that has been ripened before churning to give a pleasant, delicate aroma (i.e., inoculating the cream with a starter culture and holding it at the desired temperature). Ripened cream butter has a delicate flavor when produced properly.
iii. **Unripened cream butter:** Made from unripened cream. Such butter usually has a light flavor.
iv. **Salted butter:** Salt has been added to the butter.
v. **Unsalted butter:** Contains no added salt.
vi. **Sweet cream butter:** The acidity of the churned cream is less than 0.20%.
vii. **Sour cream butter:** Made from cream which has more than 0.20% acidity.

viii. **Fresh butter:** Such butter hasn't been kept in cold storage. (Fresh butter shouldn't typically be kept for longer than 3 weeks.)

ix. **Cold storage butter:** This butter has been stored at a temperature of about −18°C (0°F) for some time (When supplied for retail trade, butter from cold storage is typically 1 to 6 months old).

x. **Dairy butter (USA):** This is farm-produced butter. It is typically produced from unpasteurized, non-acidity-standardized sour cream. Due to the high acid content of the cream, this butter typically has a sour flavor.

xi. **Creamery butter:** This is creamery or dairy factory-produced butter. Compared to dairy butter, its quality is more consistent.

## 6.5 NUTRITIONAL FACTS

Butter has a high nutritional content and health-promoting characteristics, as well as excellent flavor and aroma values. A major portion of nutrients and calories comes from the fat content of butter (**Table 6.1**), where saturated fatty acid holds the highest amount with 51 g/100 g (**Table 6.2**). A few minerals can also be obtained from butter (**Table 6.3**).

## 6.6 STRUCTURE OF BUTTER

Butter has a remarkably complex chemical composition. The varying content of milk fat and maturation are major determinants of the size and extent of crystal networks, both within globules and within non-globular phases. The quantity of physical work performed on the butter after

**TABLE 6.1**
**Nutritional Composition of Salted Butter and Indian Butter**

| Constituent | Normal salted butter (%) | Indian butter (%) |
|---|---|---|
| Fat | 80–82 | 80 |
| Moisture | 15.6–17.6 | 16 |
| Salt | About 1.2 | 1.6–1.7 |
| Curd | 1.0 | 1.0 |
| Protein | About 1.2 | 1.0 |
| Fat-soluble vitamins A, D, E | Trace | Trace |

*Source:* Lee et al., 2018

**TABLE 6.2**
**Fatty Acid Composition of Butter**

| Fatty acids | Average (g/100 g) |
|---|---|
| Unsaturated fatty acids | 49 |
| Monounsaturated fatty acids | 21 |
| Palmitoleic acid | 0.961 |
| Oleic acid | 19.961 |
| Polyunsaturated fatty acid | 3.043 |

**TABLE 6.2** *(Continued)*
**Fatty Acid Composition of Butter**

| Fatty acids | Average (g/100 g) |
|---|---|
| Linoleic acid | 2.728 |
| Linolenic acid | 0.961 |
| Saturated fatty acid | 51 |
| Butyric acid | 3.226 |
| Caproic acid | 2.007 |
| Capric acid | 2.529 |
| Caprylic acid | 1.19 |
| Stearic acid | 9.999 |
| Lauric acid | 2.587 |
| Myristic acid | 7.436 |
| Palmitic acid | 21.697 |

*Source:* Lee et al., 2018

**TABLE 6.3**
**Nutritional Composition of Butter**

| Components | Amount/100 g |
|---|---|
| Iron (mg) | Trace |
| Copper (mg) | 0.01 |
| Zinc (mg) | 0.1 |
| Chloride (mg) | 994 |
| Selenium (μg) | Trace |
| Manganese (mg) | Trace |
| Iodine (μg) | 38 |
| Niacin (mg) | Trace |
| Vitamin $B_6$ (mg) | Trace |
| Vitamin $B_{12}$ (μg) | 0.3 |
| Folate (μg) | Trace |
| Pantothenate (mg) | 0.05 |
| Retinol (μg) | 958 |
| Carotene (μg) | 608 |
| Calcium (mg) | 18 |
| Magnesium (mg) | 2.0 |
| Potassium (mg) | 27 |

*Source:* Lee et al., 2018

churning also plays a significant role in determining how much fat is globular versus non-globular (Kwak et al., 2013). It is divided into two stages: continuous and dispersed. A water-in-oil emulsion is when water acts as a dispersed phase in oil, which is a continuous phase in the emulsion, and an oil-in-water emulsion is when oil acts as a dispersed phase in water, which is a continuous phase in the emulsion, as demonstrated in **Figure 6.2.**

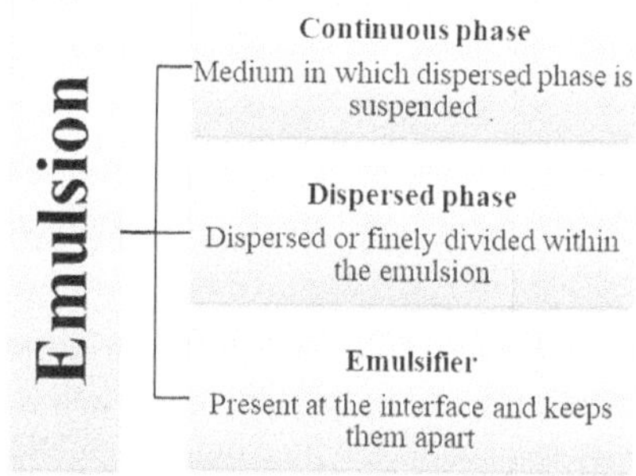


FIGURE 6.2 **Different phases (constituents) of an emulsion.**

## 6.7 WORLDWIDE BUTTER PRODUCTION AND CONSUMPTION TRENDS

India is the world's largest butter producer around the globe. **Table 6.4** illustrates butter production in various countries of the world. The International Dairy Federation estimates that New Zealand holds the title for the most butter consumed per year per capita, but Belarus boasts a close second. **Figure 6.3** illustrates butter consumption per capita in 2021 with information from various countries of the world.

TABLE 6.4
**Butter Production in Various Countries of the World in 2021**

| Rank | Country | Production (1000 MT) |
|---|---|---|
| 1 | India | 6,700 |
| 2 | EU-27 | 2,040 |
| 3 | USA | 975 |
| 4 | New Zealand | 475 |
| 5 | Russian Federation | 280 |
| 6 | Mexico | 245 |

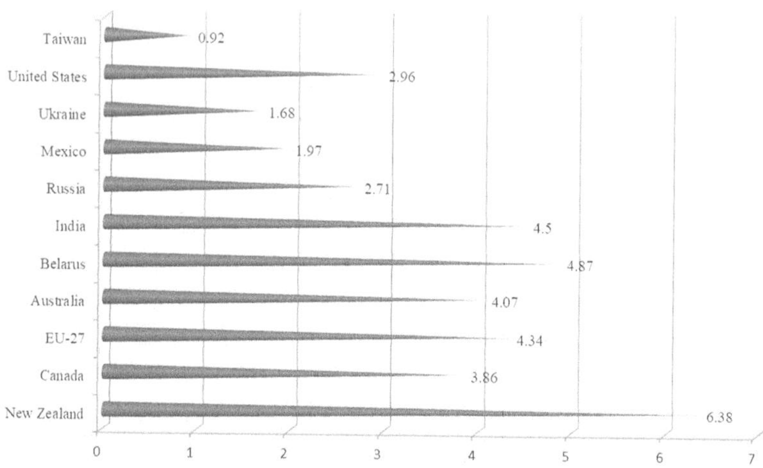


FIGURE 6.3 **Worldwide butter consumption per capita (in kg) in 2021.**

## 6.8 PRINCIPLES OF BUTTER MAKING

The process of manufacturing creamery butter is fundamental for making the majority of concentrated milk fat products. So, it might be informative to look into the science and technology underlying the process (Fearon, 2011). The following list summarizes the primary procedures involved in producing creamery butter, whether they are carried out in a batch or continuous butter maker:

- Making cream through the centrifugal separation of liquid milk with a normal fat content of about 40%.
- Using a specific temperature regime, cream aging is used to enhance the crystallization of milk fat.
- Emulsion destabilization and phase inversion from an oil-in-water cream emulsion to a water-in-oil butter emulsion achieved by physical agitation (churning).
- Butter grains are physically worked to produce bigger granules, release buttermilk, distribute moisture, and produce a homogeneous butter mass.

## 6.9 MANUFACTURING PROCESS

Butter was still prepared in the nineteenth century from cream that had been left to stand and naturally sour (Hae-Soo et al., 2013). After that, the cream was removed from the milk's surface and placed into a wooden tub. Butter was traditionally made by hand in butter churns. However, the natural souring process is extremely delicate, and contamination with foreign microbes frequently ruins the outcome (Bylund, 2021). Commercial butter production nowadays is a result of knowledge and expertise acquired through time in areas like sanitation, bacterial acidification, and heat treatment, as well as the quick technological advancement that resulted in the advanced equipment now in use. By the middle of the twentieth century, the continuous churn had been commercialized, although the commercial cream separator had first been launched at the end of the nineteenth century (Caballero et al., 2015).

There are four different ways to make butter:

i. Traditional batch churning using milk fat (MF) cream with a 25–35% content
ii. Continuous flotation churning using milk fat cream with a 30–50% content
iii. The concentration procedure, which involves separating "plastic" cream at 82% MF from 35% MF at 55°C before turning this oil-in-water emulsion cream into a water-in-oil emulsion butter without further draining of buttermilk
iv. The anhydrous milk fat technique, which produces butter oil by emulsifying water, non-fat solids, and salt in a manner similar to making margarine

i. The butter manufacturing process preparation is shown in the flow diagram (**Figure 6.4**). A fluid milk dairy can supply the cream, or the butter producer can separate it from whole milk. The cream should be sweet (pH >6.6, titratable acidity = 0.10–0.12%), not rancid, and not oxidized.
ii. The whole milk is heated to the necessary temperature in a milk pasteurizer before being passed through a separator if the cream is separated by the butter producer. The cream is cooled before being transported to a storage tank, where the fat content is measured and, if necessary, adjusted to the correct value.
iii. Before being transferred to storage, the skim milk from the separator is pasteurized and cooled. It usually ends up being concentrated and dried.
iv. The cream is pasteurized at 95°C or above after leaving the intermediate storage tank. To prevent enzymes and microorganisms from affecting the butter's ability to retain, a high temperature is required.
v. Mixture cultures of both acid-producing organisms (*Lactococcus lactis*, *L. cremoris*) and flavor-producing organisms (*S. lactis* subsp. *Diacetylactis*, *Leuconostoc citrovorum*, and/or *Leuconostoc dextranicum*) (0.5 to 2.0% acidity) are employed to ripen cream to pH 5.5 at 21°C and then pH 4.6 at 13°C if ripening is desired for the production of cultured butter.

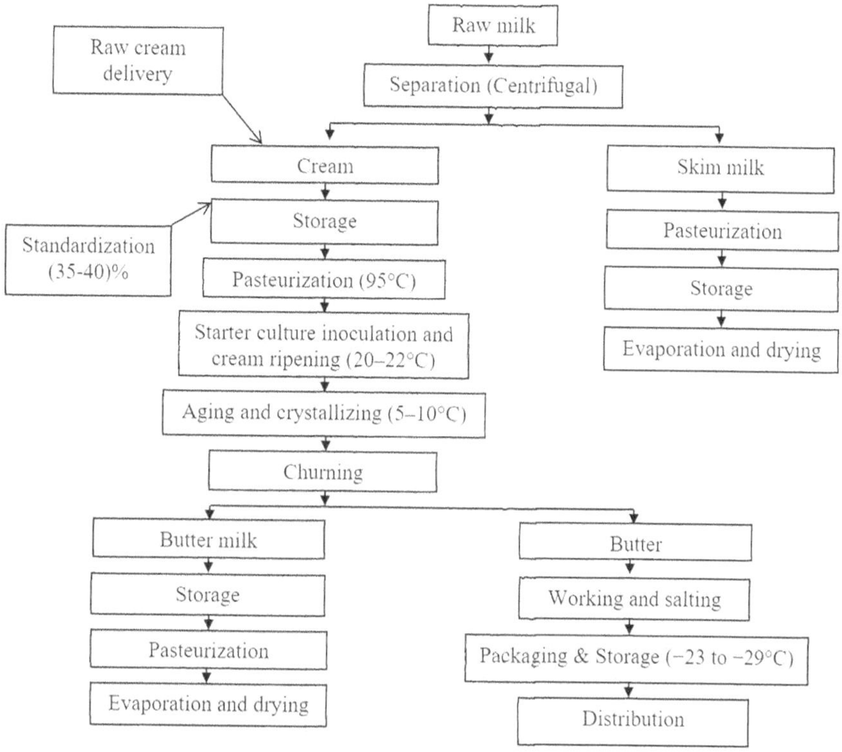


**FIGURE 6.4 Flow diagram of the butter manufacturing process.**

Most flavor development occurs between pH 5.5 and 4.6. The flavor develops more acid production at cooler ripening temperatures. Typically, ripened butter is neither salted nor washed.

vi. The cream is put through a controlled cooling program in the aging tank to give fat the necessary crystalline structure. The program is chosen to take into account several aspects, including the composition of butterfat, which is, for instance, stated in terms of the iodine value and is a measurement of the unsaturated fat content. Even though the treatment has a low iodine value, butter can still be produced with an acceptable consistency, i.e., when the unsaturated fat proportion is low. Aging typically takes 12 to 15 hours.

vii. The cream is transferred from the aging tank to the churn or continuous butter maker via a plate heat exchanger, which raises the temperature to the proper level. The cream is vigorously stirred during the churning process to break up the fat globules, which causes the fat to coagulate into butter grains while lowering the fat content of the remaining liquid, buttermilk. Thus, butter granules and buttermilk are divided into two fractions from the cream.

viii. In conventional churning, after the grains have reached a specific size, the machine stops, and the buttermilk is then drained out. Buttermilk is continuously drained when using a continuous butter maker. The butter is processed into a continuous fat phase with a finely dispersed water phase after draining. Washing the butter after churning to eliminate any leftover buttermilk or milk solids was a frequent process, but it is now much less common. Since salt is a preservative, it is utilized to increase flavor and shelf life. In the case of batch manufacturing, salt (1–3%) is distributed over the surface of the butter if it is to be salted. The butter is mixed with the salt slurry in the continuous butter maker.

ix. The packaged unit receives the prepared butter before sending it to cold storage.

## 6.10 THEORIES OF CHURNING

Using the proper mechanical adjustments, churning is the process of transforming cream into butter. The conversion of the oil-in-water (O/W) emulsion of cream into a water-in-oil (W/O) emulsion to form butter has been explained by various theories of churning. These are discussed as follows:

### 6.10.1 Foam Theory

This theory claims that the presence of foam is necessary for churning. It also postulates that there is a "foam-producing" substance present in cream (and milk) that gradually solidifies as the cream or milk is agitated. Foam is created during the churning period. The fat globules, due to surface tension effects, tend to concentrate and clump on the foam bubbles. When the foam-producing ingredient has a solid character, the foam disintegrates. Butter is produced when the fat globules combine.

**Drawback:** Some continuous processes for manufacturing butter don't involve foam generation (air formation).

### 6.10.2 Phase Reversal Theory

According to this theory, churning is a process of phase reversal, i.e., changing an oil-in-water type emulsion (such as cream) to a water-in-oil type emulsion (such as butter). When the cream is agitated during the churning process, fat globules cluster and clump together until ultimately the surface area to fat unit volume ratio decreases to the point where it is no longer able to hold all the buttermilk in a stable condition. The emulsion of oil-in-water abruptly breaks down, releasing butter granules and free buttermilk.

**Drawback:** Butter is not a true water-in-fat emulsion. According to microscopic analyses, some of the butter's fat globules are still present in the worked butter.

### 6.10.3 Modern Theory

The fat is formed as clusters of fat globules in chilled cream at churning temperature; inside each globule, it is present partially in solid and partially in liquid form. Churning breaks up the clusters and causes foam formation. The globules become concentrated to some extent. The emulsion-protecting surface of the phospholipid–protein complex gradually deteriorates due to the movement of the globules over each other in the foam layer. The globules subsequently stick together to create ever-larger particles. Those particles eventually emerge as butter grains (granules).

## 6.11 FACTORS AFFECTING THE CHURNING ABILITY OF CREAM

Churning is the process of shaking up cream or whole milk to make butter, usually in a butter churn. In other words, churning is the process of turning cream into butter utilizing the proper mechanical force.

The factors that affect how well cream churns can be divided into two categories:

i. The factors that affect the cream's basic characteristics
ii. The conditions throughout the manufacturing process

Factors related to the initial character of the cream include the chemical composition of the butterfat, the size of fat globules, the richness of the cream, and the viscosity of cream, while factors related to processing conditions are churning temperature, the fullness of the churn, speed of the churn, design of the churn, etc. The sections that follow cover each of these elements.

### 6.11.1 Factors Related to the Basic Character of the Cream

#### 6.11.1.1 Chemical Composition of Butterfat

The churnability of cream is greatly influenced by the proportion of soft fats (low melting points) and hard fats (high melting points). The level of fat solidification in the chilled cream is determined by this ratio. The churning time will be decreased, the butter will be less solid, and there will be more fat losses in the buttermilk if the proportion of soft fats is higher. It will take longer to churn the mixture if the quantity of soft fats is low.

#### 6.11.1.2 Richness of Cream

The churning will be finished more quickly in the case of richer cream. The cream is not sufficiently creamy to be so thick that it would stick to the inside of the churn and prevent agitation. If rich cream is churned at a high temperature, the butter will form in a remarkably short time, provided all other conditions are favorable. While rich cream is churned at a high temperature and the butter forms quickly (about 10 minutes), thin cream churns considerably more slowly and can be heated to a higher temperature than a thick cream; typically the butter will be greasy in body and will contain a little buttermilk, which will be more or less difficult to remove on washing.

#### 6.11.1.3 Viscosity of Cream

The length of time needed to finish the churning process increases with the viscosity of the cream. More viscosity reduces the fat globules' freedom of movement, minimizes their chance of being brought together, and delays coalescence, lengthening the churning process.

#### 6.11.1.4 Size of the Fat Globules

Cream that contains large fat globules (avg. diameter 4.6 μm) churns more quickly than cream with small globules. Cream with small fat globules (avg. diameter 3.4 μm) churns slowly and takes twice as long to break as cream with large globules. The butter made from such cream has short grains and a crumbly character.

### 6.11.2 Conditions in the Process of Manufacturing

#### 6.11.2.1 Fullness of the Churn

It has an impact on the churn's level of agitation. If the amount of cream in the churn is small, it may adhere to the wall of the churn and receive little or no agitation.

#### 6.11.2.2 Churning Temperature

Temperature stands as a significant determinant when it comes to the churnability of cream. The higher the temperature of the cream, the sooner the churning process will be completed. As the cream's temperature increases, the churning process concludes more rapidly. However, a churning temperature that is too high is not preferred. It makes the butter lumpy and mushy rather than flaky and granular. The quality of the butter is negatively impacted by this (Mallia et al., 2008). It causes, first, a greasy texture of butter, and second, it causes the incorporation of too much buttermilk in the butter. This buttermilk contains lactose, curd, and water, which, when present together in butter, are likely to sour and in other ways deteriorate the butter. Butter should be kept as free of curd and lactose as possible to prevent any potential bacterial growth. Even though it is preferable to have a slightly lower temperature than a higher one, too low a temperature is still undesirable.

#### 6.11.2.3 Speed of Churn

The cream is stirred by the speed of the churn. It depends on the centrifugal and gravitational forces. Churning time is dependent on the speed of churning and the starting temperature of the cream. If churning starts with cream at 65°F and churns at a speed of about 120–150 RPM, the total time of making butter is about 20–25 minutes.

## 6.12 FACTORS CAUSING INCREASED FAT IN BUTTER

### 6.12.1 Stage of Lactation

The butterfat test experiences a noticeable change throughout the lactation period. It has almost similar effects on milk protein and fat percentages. Colostrum, generated shortly after freshening, holds the greatest protein and fat concentrations in milk. Levels hit their minimum during the post-calving period of 25 to 50 days. Then, after 250 days, they reach the highest point as the amount of milk starts to decrease.

### 6.12.2 Age

The fat percentage shows a mild reduction as the animal ages, yet the overall decrease is quite minimal. Both milk fat and protein diminish as the animal grows older. Milk fat experiences an annual decline of approximately 0.2% from the initial to the fifth lactation, likely due to higher production and more udder infection.

### 6.12.3 Season

Milk fat is significantly influenced by the changing seasons. In the northeastern region, the fat content experiences a notable drop during the hot and humid months of July and August. During the fall season, milk's fat content progressively rises, and the highest level is usually seen in winter when the weather gets colder. As temperatures rise in the spring, the levels of milk components progressively diminish. These variations can serve as indicators of altered feed intake patterns, stemming from variations in weather and temperature during the summer months.

### 6.12.4 Mastitis Infection

The most typical illness in dairy cows is mastitis, an infection of the mammary gland that can be fatal. It reduces the fat content of milk. Additionally, the milk handler may lose quality premiums.

### 6.12.5 Genetics and Inheritance

Inheritance determines an animal's ability to produce a certain amount of butterfat relative to the amount of milk produced. Therefore, a dairy operator should choose cows based on their genetic capacity to produce the quantity and quality of milk desired. The genetic makeup of the cows determines the prospective average butterfat test of a herd, whereas environmental factors that will be considered later influence the daily variation.

### 6.12.6 Breeds of Cattle

There is a distinct difference in the fat content of milk from cows of different breeds. The average results of various breeds' butterfat tests are as follows: Guernsey, 5.0%; Holstein, 3.4%;

Brown Swiss, 4.0%; Jersey, 5.35%; and Ayrshire, 3.9%. In comparison to milk from herds mostly comprised of Holsteins, milk from herds composed primarily of Jersey and Guernsey will test higher.

### 6.12.7 Individuals within Breeds

Within breeds, the butterfat tests show huge variations as well. The minimum and maximum found in the low- and high-testing breeds are as follows: Holsteins, 2.6 to 6.0%; Jerseys, 3.3 to 8.4%. Consequently, significant breed-specific variations should be expected.

### 6.12.8 Milk Yield

Typically, the milk fat decreases as milk production increases. This is not always true.

### 6.12.9 Milking Practice

The "managed milking" or "rapid milking" technique should be used to achieve the highest possible butterfat and milk and to maintain the health of an udder.

### 6.12.10 Feeding

For a long time, it was generally accepted as a fact that the fat content of a cow's milk could not be increased or decreased for any length of time through feeding practices. Recent research indicates a clear correlation between feeding and butterfat test results, but no ration has yet been identified that will appreciably enhance milk's butterfat content throughout any duration. The milk's fat level has temporarily increased when certain oils have been fed, whereas it has been reduced when other oils have been fed. The butterfat test appears to be minimally affected or unaffected by high or low protein intake. The potential upper limits of the fat test appear to be determined by genetics.

## 6.13 PACKAGING, STORAGE, AND DISTRIBUTION OF BUTTER

Butter is sold either in blocks (wrapped in waxed paper or aluminum foil) with a net weight of 250 g or in bulk blocks (wrapped in waxed paper) with a net weight of 25 kg. The waxed paper and aluminum foil act as opaque and airtight packaging materials to protect the butter from a reduction in quality (Patel et al., 2017).

### 6.13.1 Packaging

Packaging is defined as the protection of materials of all/any kind using any packaging material designed to prevent damage to the contents by outside influences and also increase shelf life.

### 6.13.2 Characteristics of Packaging Materials Required

i. Prevent light passage
ii. Grease-proof
iii. Prevent oxygen transmission
iv. Shall offer resistance to microbial contamination
v. Shall offer good strength
vi. Low metallic contact; metals favor the oxidation of fat

### 6.13.3 Packaging Materials Used

i. Wood/timber
ii. Parchment paper/substitutes
iii. Aluminum foil/laminators
iv. Tin plate

### 6.13.4 Techniques of Packaging

i. **Hand molding and wrapping:** Slow and cumbersome.
ii. **Mechanical molding, patting, and wrapping:** Suitable for large-scale operations.
iii. **Fully automatic unit:** Mechanically molds and wraps. Reduces labor costs and handling losses, suitable for large-scale production.
iv. **Vacuum packaging:** Due to the oxygen included in butter being partially eliminated, it does not considerably improve its keeping quality.
v. **Canning:** It is not sterile.

### 6.13.5 Control Measures

The product can be contaminated by air when exposed during packaging; hence, air in the packing environment should be of good quality.

As butter is vulnerable to mold, secondary packing material (cardboard) must not be handled in the packing area but in another room.

Proper control of humidity is necessary during labeling and wrapping; otherwise, moisture may condense on the surface portion.

### 6.13.6 Storage

The temperature of commercial cold storage of butter ranges from –23°C to –29°C (–10°F to –20°F). While butter is kept in a commercial cold storage facility, its flavor will always deteriorate to some extent. As a result, salted acidic butter starts to taste fishy. Bacterial decomposition is minimal; however, chemical deterioration is the main factor.

### 6.13.7 Distribution

The wholesaler receives the butter in its original bulk packaging from the butter factory, and the retailer receives it as wrapped pats in cartons, boxes, or tin cans. Typically, the temperature over the entire distribution time should range from –18°C to –29°C. Deep-frozen or refrigerated butter boxes may also be used for retail sales.

### 6.13.8 Keeping the Quality of Stored Butter

The following parameters have an impact on this: storage temperature, copper and iron content, salt content, curd content, acidity content, air (oxygen) content, raw or pasteurized cream, light exposure, and packaging method.

## 6.14 BUTTER OVERRUN

Butter overrun is the term used to designate the amounts of butter made more than the weight of butterfat used for its manufacture. In other words, overrun in butter may be defined as the increase in the amount of butter made from an amount of fat. It is generally spoken of as a percent overrun.

Butter is produced in greater quantities when moisture, curd, salt, air, etc. are present. In general, creameries show an overrun of 24 to 24.5%. Applying the definition of percent overrun:

$$B = F + \frac{F}{100} Y \; or \; Y = \frac{B - F}{F} \times 100$$

B = Quantity of butter churned
F = Quantity of butterfat used for churning
Y = Percent overrun

### 6.14.1 Composition Overrun

% Churn overrun = (Kg butter made – Kg fat churned)/Kg fat churned × 100 %

% Composition Overrun = (100 – % fat in butter)/% fat × 100 %

### 6.14.2 Factors Affecting the Overrun in Butter

i. Inaccuracy in weight, the fat test of milk, cream, or butter.
ii. Fat decreases in skim milk or buttermilk.
iii. Unavoidable fluctuation in the fat content of butter.
iv. Fat losses due to mechanical operation.
v. During the handling process, fat losses affect the overrun.

### 6.14.3 Advantages of Overrun in Butter

i. From an economic aspect, this overrun process is a source of profit for the butter maker.
ii. From a product aspect, this process increases the amount of butter.
iii. This process also influences the sensory attribute of butter due to the high butter
iv. From a technical aspect, this process helps to check the efficiency of factory operation

### 6.14.4 Disadvantages of Overrun in Butter

i. This process requires a high initial cost because of the machinery.
ii. This process requires continuous observation.
iii. Highly skilled persons are required.

### 6.14.5 Defects in Butter by Overrun

a) **Volume:** Volume losses will result from a low overrun percentage.
b) **Bubbles:** When the overrun percentage is higher than the normal range, bubbles form into the butter.
c) **Consistency:** Butter's consistency is influenced by overrun.

## 6.15 QUALITY JUDGING OF BUTTER

Generally, sensory assessment is conducted utilizing a 5-point hedonic scale, ranging from 1, indicating dislike extremely, to 5, indicating like extremely. During this evaluation, panelists assess the sensory characteristics such as texture, color, flavor, taste, spreadability, and overall acceptability of butter. Both an individual and commercial perspective can be used to evaluate butter. The judge needs to familiarize themselves with the quality of the butter according to market standards. They should then evaluate the butter based on what most consumers want, not their preferences. A keen sense of taste and smell is crucial for accurately assessing butter quality. Despite having a sharp and sensitive sense of taste and smell, it still requires significant practice or experience. The majority of people can easily distinguish between a high-quality butter and an inferior one, yet it necessitates both skill and hands-on familiarity to tell apart two samples that exhibit similar levels of excellence. A crucial aspect of butter assessment lies in developing a comprehensive understanding of the ideal butter flavor; then, one will easily become proficient in assessing the butter by repeatedly comparing many butter samples to this one ideal flavor.

For the sensory evaluation of butter, a variety of scorecards are developed, with the highest marks given for each of the butter's sensory characteristics (**Table 6.5**).

**TABLE 6.5**
**Score Card for Sensory Evaluation of Butter**

| Name: | | Sample no: | | | Date: |
|---|---|---|---|---|---|
| **Sl. no** | **Color and appearance** | **Flavor** | **Body and texture** | **Overall acceptability** | **Total remarks** |
| 1 | | | | | |
| 2 | | | | | |
| 3 | | | | | |
| 4 | | | | | |
| 5 | | | | | |

| Rate | Organoleptic score |
|---|---|
| Like extremely | 5 |
| Like very much to like moderately | 4 |
| Like slightly to neither like nor dislike | 3 |
| Dislike slightly to dislike moderately or dislike very much | 2 |
| Dislike extremely | 1 |

i. **Packaging:** Should be appealing, neat, clean, and well-finished (smooth, attractive surface). All packages must be neatly and securely closed.
ii. **Salt:** It needs to be appropriately distributed and dissolved. Butter typically has a grainy effect when there is undissolved salt present.
iii. **Color and appearance:** Uniform, light, pale yellow color is liked most by the consumers.
iv. **Body and texture:** Butter should have a firm body with a unique waxy, tight-knit texture. When broken, the appearance of good-quality butter should present a somewhat jagged, irregular, wrought-iron-like surface. Butter should have smooth spreadability.
v. **Flavor:** It should have a taste and aroma that are light, sweet, clean, and pleasant. High-quality butter is characterized by its ability to stimulate the appetite and make one want more of the food.

## 6.16 DEFECTS IN BUTTER

A flaw or irregularity that affects the flavor, body, texture, color, or other properties of butter is referred to as a defect (**Figure 6.5**).

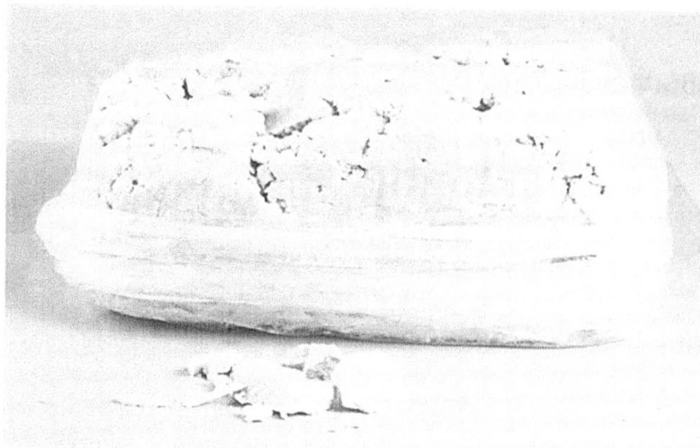

FIGURE 6.5 **Defects of butter.**

### 6.16.1 Types of Defects of Butter

There are mainly three types of defects of butter. These are:

i. Flavor defects (**Table 6.6**)
ii. Body and texture defects (**Table 6.7**)
iii. Color defects (**Table 6.8**)

Other defects include salt defects and packaging defects.

## 6.17 NEW MANUFACTURING TECHNIQUES TO LOWER CHOLESTEROL

Cholesterol is bound to milk fat and can be reduced by biological, physical, or chemical methods, including adsorption, extraction, fractionated crystallization, steam distillation, and enzyme reactions. Recently, cholesterol reduction in cow and buffalo butter was achieved to about 90% by β-cyclodextrin (Kumar et al., 2010). Research has shown that until the eighth time of reuse, the crosslinking of β-cyclodextrin with adipic acid in cream helps to remove over 90% of cholesterol (Han et al., 2007). When cholesterol was removed by crosslinked β-cyclodextrin, there were very few entrapped components and very little leftover β-cyclodextrin in the cream (Ha et al., 2010). This implies that in the future, foods like butter with reduced cholesterol will be excellent for health without losing any healthy elements.

## 6.18 HEALTH BENEFITS OF BUTTER

Butter has functional ingredients and has proven beneficial effects. The large body of scientific proof indicates that various bioactive compounds such as fat globule membranes (MFGM), MFGM polar lipids, conjugated linoleic acid (CLA), short-chain fatty acids (SCFAs), sphingolipids, and medium-chain fatty acids (MCFAs) in butter provide beneficial effects on various human diseases such as osteoporosis, cancer, atherosclerosis, and other degenerative disorders in humans. Some components are endowed with nutrients such as peptides, lipids, minerals, and vitamins (A, E, and K), which have bioactive properties along with beneficial effects, and

## TABLE 6.6
## Flavor Defects in Butter with Their Possible Causes and Remedies

| Name of the defects | Causes | Remedies |
|---|---|---|
| **Acid defects** (recognized by sour taste of butter on the tip of the tongue) | A result of using acidic or improperly neutralized cream. The fault can be accelerated by bacterial contamination or the presence of water, oxygen, light, enzymes, and some metals. | Use of fresh and sweet cream or properly neutralized cream can prevent this defect. |
| **Alkaline or neutralized flavor** | The use of over neutralized cream results in butter having the flavor of the neutralizer. | Can be reduced by employing the ideal amount of suitable neutralizers. |
| **Bitter flavor** (tastes somewhat like quinine; persists as a distinct lingering aftertaste even after the sample has been removed from mouth) | Caused by the usage of cream made from milk from cows or buffalo that had access to some bitter plants, or from milk that had not been sufficiently boiled to inactivate the lipase enzyme. | Lipase activity in milk is destroyed by heating it above 37°C, and cream is stored at 5°C to prevent the growth of bacteria that break down proteins during storage. |
| **Cheesy Flavor** (the flavor of butter resembles that of Cheddar cheese) | Caused by the growth of proteolytic microorganisms leading to the breakdown of casein that resembles the flavor of cheddar cheese. | Storage of cream at 5°C to control the growth of proteolytic bacteria can prevent this defect. |
| **Cooked flavor** | Caused by the overheating of cream or milk at any stage of processing. | Recommended time–temperature combination during processing can prevent this effect. |
| **Feed flavor** | Caused by the cream obtained from milk which gives flavor of hay or silage. | Grading of milk should be done carefully, and milk with this flavor defect should not be used for cream production. Pasteurization may inhibit this defect. |
| **Fishy flavor** | Develops in high-acid salted butter when copper and/or iron is present, and the scent is comparable to that of cod liver oil, fish flour, or codfish. | By using sweet cream to make butter instead of potential sources of metallic contamination, it can be avoided. |
| **Flat flavor** (Lacks characteristic buttery flavor) | Caused due to low diacetyl and low salt contents. | By ripening of cream with butter culture to proper acidity, using correct amount of salt. |
| **Rancid flavor** (pungent and very undesirable flavor) | Caused by lipolytic action in milk or cream, which hydrolyzes fat. It looks like rotting meat. | This can be avoided by inactivating the lipase enzyme by heating milk appropriately. |
| **Oxidized/metallic/tallowy flavor** | Caused by fat oxidation brought on by contamination with copper or iron and direct exposure of milk, cream, or butter to the sun. | Storage of milk, cream, and butter in opaque cans constructed of tin or aluminum alloy can stop it. |
| **Stale flavor** | Caused by keeping the butter at a low temperature for an extended period or a high temperature for a brief amount of time. | Avoiding storing cream or butter for longer periods and using the correct temperature of storage can prevent this defect. |
| **Yeasty flavor** | Use of old and yeasty cream for butter making that gives a typical fruity, vinegar-like aroma. | This flaw can be fixed by using fresh sweet cream and storing butter in hygienic conditions. |

TABLE 6.7
Body and Texture Defects of Butter with Their Possible Causes and Remedies

| Name of the defects | Causes | Remedies |
|---|---|---|
| **Crumbly or brittle body** (defects are indicated by a lack of cohesion, dryness, a rough surface, and difficulty in slicing (**Figure 6.4**)) | Caused by alterations in the fat composition due to the seasons, a sudden chill, or underworking the butter. | The best way to fix this defect is by correct butter processing, regulated cooling and aging of cream, and proper churning and washing of butter. |
| **Greasy body** (too smooth and quickly melts in the mouth) | Caused by overworking and high temperature of wash water. | The use of wash water at adequate temperature can prevent this. |
| **Gummy body** (in the mouth, butter does not easily melt) | Caused by butter's high concentration of high-melting triglycerides (solid fats) that do not melt readily in the mouth | Removing high-melting-point fats from the milking cows' diets to control the problem. |
| **Leaky body** (when a sample is obtained from butter, moisture droplets are visible) | Excessively high churning and wash water temperatures, excessive butter churning, insufficient cooling, and cream that hasn't been properly aged. | At various phases of manufacturing butter, the control methods include adequate working, optimal churning, and utilization of proper temperatures. |
| **Mealy body** (butter does not spread or cut well) | Incorrect oiling off of fat during the production of butter and the improper neutralization of high-acid cream with lime. | This can be avoided by following the right neutralization procedures, employing the right neutralizers, and using the right temperatures during the processing steps to avoid oiling off. |
| **Spongy/weak body** (characterized by butter's rapid melting and extreme suppleness) | Inadequate aging and cooling, a high churning temperature, and a large percentage of slowly melting fat. | This can be avoided by properly aging, cooling, and churning cream at the ideal temperature. |
| **Sticky body** (although it seems dry, butter adheres to the butter tester) | Overworking of butter. | Requires controlled working under proper temperature. |
| **Gritty body** | Presence of undissolved salt particles indicates gritty body of butter. | Proper salting method, using salt after grinding, and avoiding long storage of butter can prevent this defect. |

TABLE 6.8
Color Defects of Butter with Their Possible Causes and Remedies

| Name of the defects | Causes | Remedies |
|---|---|---|
| **Mottled color** (spots of butter in both lighter and darker shades of yellow serve as a sign) | Poor butter working, inappropriate salt inclusion, and inadequate butter washing. | The prevention strategies include thorough washing, accurate salt inclusion, and efficient butter processing. |
| **Streaky color** (butter has distinct waves that are various hues of yellow) | A result of the uneven and inefficient processing of two or more batches of butter. | It can be controlled by properly and evenly working the butter. |
| **Dull/pale color** | Overworking of butter causes this defect. The color of the exposed surface of butter darkens, indicating this color fault. | To prevent this defect, butter must be properly packaged so that the entire surface is covered. |
| **Mold discoloration** | A variety of colors are produced when mold grows on the surface of butter. | The problem can be controlled by properly packing and storing butter in spaces with controlled humidity and temperature. |

they lead to a long, healthy life. **Figures 6.6 and 6.7** illustrate the key potential health benefits of butter.

### 6.18.1 Association of Butter Consumption with Cancer Prevention

Cancer risks can be reduced by eating butter. Sphingolipid levels and the enzymes involved in metabolizing sphingolipids are found to be altered in cancer (Ryland et al., 2011). Additionally, a number of studies indicate that MFGM proteins may inhibit the development of human cancer cells (Evans et al., 2010). According to some research, high quantities of CLA in cow's milk and dairy products such as butter decrease the incidence and the number of breast tumors.

### 6.18.2 Association of Butter Consumption with Bactericidal Effects

Butter displayed prominent antibacterial activity that could potentiate the effect of fusidic acid on inhibiting bacterial growth (Elsewedy et al., 2022). Through mechanisms known as competitive inhibitory mechanisms, sphingolipids provide defense against specific strains of bacteria, viruses, and toxic substances (Kaida & Kusunoki, 2010).

### 6.18.3 Association of Butter Consumption with Diabetes Prevention

Consuming butter has been related to health advantages in diabetics. CLA in butter has antidiabetic effects (Huot et al., 2010; Jourdan et al., 2009). Also, sphingolipid metabolites act as both diabetes mellitus promoters and inhibitors. Reduced β-cell mass causes both types of diabetes mellitus, which eventually causes liver cells to proliferate less and perish more quickly (Hui et al., 2004).

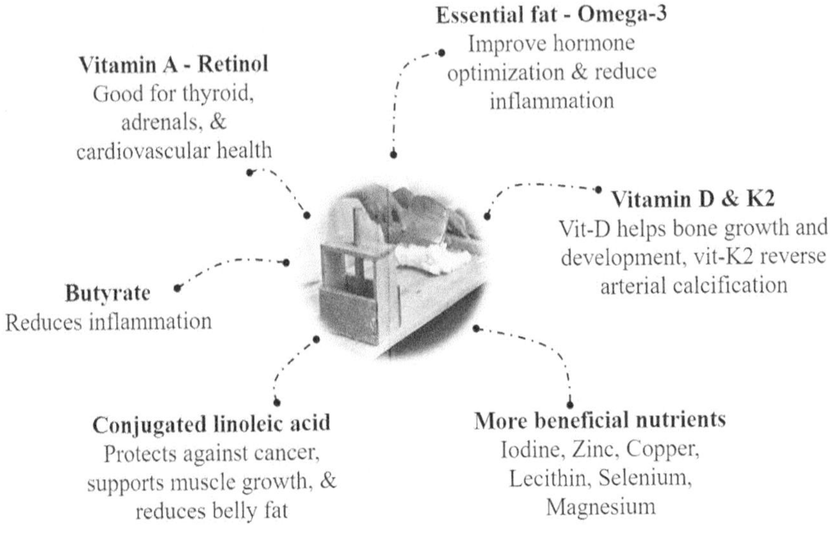


**FIGURE 6.6 Health-promoting properties of butter.** It's high in minerals like calcium, which helps strengthen bones, and it contains chemicals that have been linked to a decreased risk of obesity. Butter can also be used in a low-carbohydrate diet, which may help people maintain or lose weight faster than a low-fat diet.

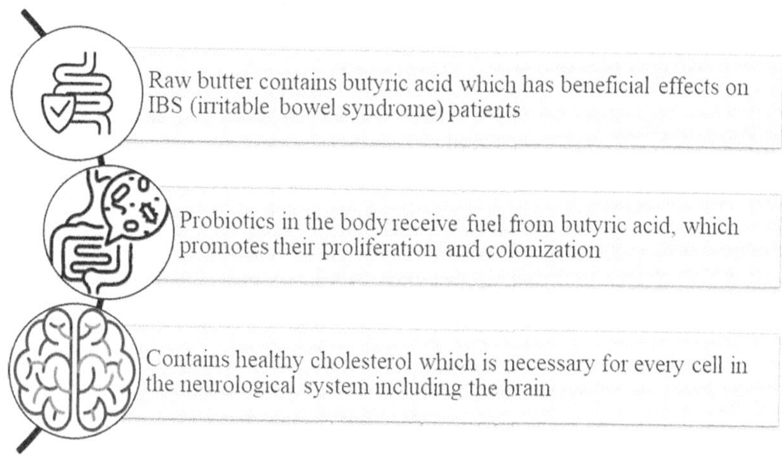


**FIGURE 6.7 Health benefits of butter.** Butyrate, a kind of short-chain fatty acid that has been linked to a number of health advantages, is abundant in butter. Butyrate is also created by beneficial bacteria in the gut and is utilized as an energy source by intestinal cells.

### 6.18.4 Association of Butter Consumption with Obesity Prevention

Weight could be reduced by eating butter. Butter includes short-chain fatty acids such as butyric acid that are beneficial to gut health and may aid in weight loss. It contains CLA, a fatty acid with anti-obesity effects. Some studies have shown that CLA consistently decreases body fat (Nagao et al., 2003).

### 6.18.5 Association of Butter Consumption with Immunity Enhancement

1. Butter contains CLA, but few studies have found that CLA increased the anti-inflammatory cytokine IL-10 while decreasing the pro-inflammatory cytokines tumor necrosis factor-alpha (TNF-$\alpha$) and interleukin (IL)-1. Recent research suggests that CLA may aid in the development of newborn immunity by increasing the production of antibodies (Ramírez-Santana et al., 2011).

### 6.18.6 Association of Butter Consumption with Brain Development

Butter contains functional ingredients such as MFGMs. MFGM proteins are found to have health benefits, for example, fatty acid binding proteins, xanthine dehydrogenase/oxidase (XDH/XO), butyrophilin, BRCA2, and BRCA1. MFGMs may potentially play roles in brain development and cognitive function, immunity, and cardiovascular health (Le et al., 2015). Butterfat contains healthy cholesterol, which is necessary for children's brain and nervous system development.

### 6.18.7 Association of Butter Consumption with Gut Health

Butter contains butyrate, a type of fat that may improve digestive health, decrease inflammation, reduce gut inflammation, and improve intestinal motility. Some studies report that feeding rats with sphingomyelin benefits neonatal gut maturation during nursing. Similarly, studies report that it prevents gastrointestinal infections in the very young or the elderly (Spitsberg, 2005).

### 6.18.8 Association of Butter Consumption with Cholesterol Reduction and Heart Disease Prevention

Butter meta-analyses examined the link between butter intake and several vascular disorders, and no significant impacts were found for cardiovascular disease (CVD) (Fontecha et al., 2019), coronary heart disease (CHD) (Gholami et al., 2017), and stroke (De Goede et al., 2016). Similarly, two studies (Gholami et al., 2017) revealed no significant influence of butter consumption on stroke risk. As a result, existing data suggest that consuming dairy products may not increase the risk of cardiovascular events (CVD, CHD, and stroke) and may even have a mild protective influence (Fontecha et al., 2019).

### 6.18.9 Association of Butter Consumption with Multiple Sclerosis

Multiple sclerosis could be reduced by eating butter. Sphingolipids and their metabolites are crucial to the development of the illness (Walter & Faßbender, 2010). They serve as sphingosine 1-phosphate (SP) mediators by helping them attach to the S1P1 and S1P4 receptors on lymphocytes. Different lymphocytes have different levels of expression; the lymph nodes exhibit higher levels, whereas the circulation has lower levels (Lo et al., 2005).

### 6.18.10 Association of Butter Consumption with Antibacterial and Anti-Adhesive Effects

Some scientific data suggest that many bioactive chemicals, such as MFGMs in butter, have antibacterial and anti-adhesive properties. MFGM proteins act as antibacterial and anti-adhesive agents in the gastrointestinal tract of humans (Fox & Wang, 2007).

## 6.19 BUTTER INNOVATIONS

Consumer interest in food products is changing. People used to just want tasty food, but now they also want food that is good for their health and good for the environment. However, in today's world, people from all over the globe have become aware of the positive impacts of dairy products on health. As a result, the production and consumption of dairy goods are predicted to increase steadily in the future, particularly in developing nations. This is mainly because there has been a lot of progress in the past 10 years in studying milk and dairy foods. For example, researchers have been working on reducing the amount of cholesterol in butter. **Figures 6.8, 6.9, and 6.10** illustrate butter innovations from production to nutritional and health attributes (Panchal et al., 2021; Gaba et al., 2023).

## 6.20 USES OF BUTTER

Butter is not only used in food; it may also be used:

- To treat wounds and as an anti-inflammatory agent (Fox & Wang, 2007).
- To avoid sunburn
- To treat dry skin, pimples, rashes, and wrinkles
- As a natural moisturizer
- To moisturize dry hair
- To guard against dental decay
- To guard against joint calcification via an anti-stiffness component

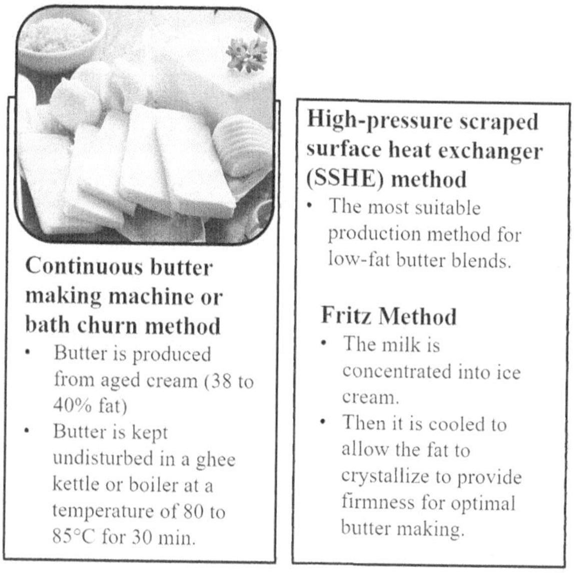


FIGURE 6.8 **Butter innovations in production attributes.**

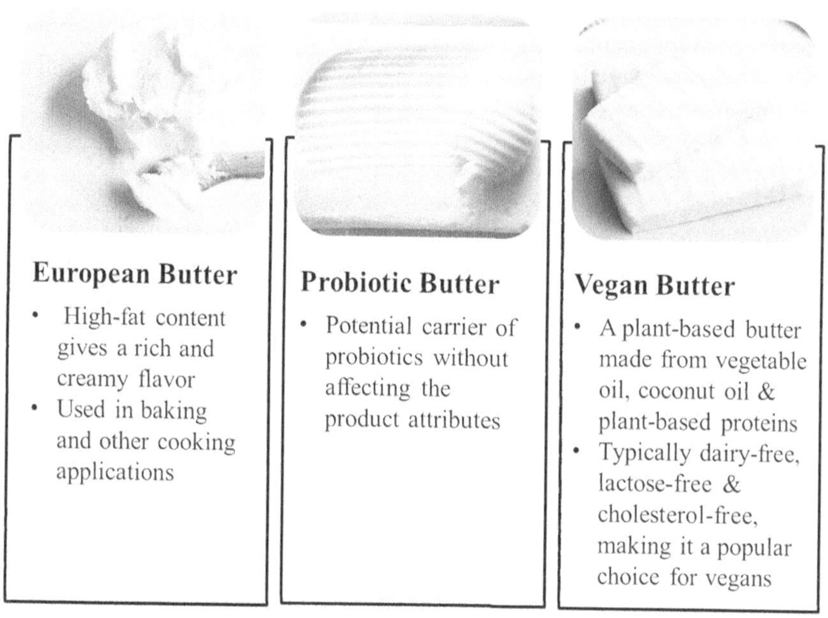


FIGURE 6.9 **Butter innovations in nutritional attributes.**

## 6.21 NEGATIVE PUBLICITY OF BUTTER

Even though butter has many health advantages, it mostly consists of fats, which if ingested in excess can lead to a variety of unpleasant issues. These include cancer, heart disease, high blood pressure, and obesity (Desroches et al., 2005). Butter contains 4% trans-fat and 50% saturated fat, according to the Australian Women's Weekly (2022). Consuming excessive amounts of saturated fat

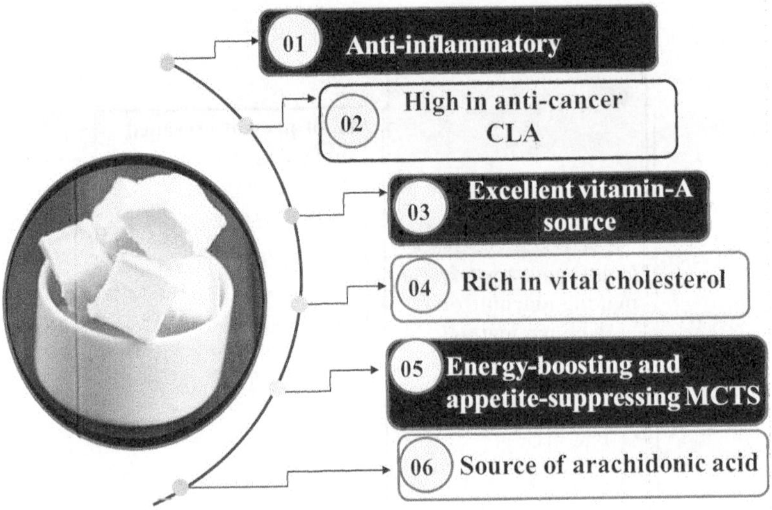


FIGURE 6.10 **Butter innovations in health attributes.**

**Abbreviations:** MCTS; medium-chain triglycerides, CLA; conjugated linoleic acid.

raises blood cholesterol, particularly bad (LDL) cholesterol (Jung et al., 2005). Type 2 diabetes may also develop as a result of continuously consuming large amounts of butter (Halade et al., 2010). People with high blood pressure or heart disease may need to carefully limit their butter intake or maybe stop eating it altogether for a while.

## 6.22 BUTTER YIELD

It depends on whether the milk originates from cows or buffalo, as the fat percentages differ between the two. Compared to buffalo milk, cow milk has a lower fat content. Cow milk comprises 4% fat while buffalo milk consists of approximately 6% fat. With 1 kg full-cream milk of 6% fat, there is 60 g fat for butter. Utilizing a cream separator, around 150 g of cream with 40% fat and 850 g of skim milk remains. Churning 150 g cream produces about 71.42 g white butter at 84% fat.

The formula for calculating butter yield is as follows:

$$\text{Butter Yield (BY)} = (F \times (100 + \%\ OR))/100$$

Where,

Y = Yield of butter
F = Fat content of cream (kg)
% OR = Percent overrun in butter

## 6.23 CONCLUSIONS

Butter is a fat-enriched dairy product with functional ingredients, and there is no doubt that a limited amount of butter taken regularly is highly beneficial for healthy aging. With butter's novel bioactive components, additional efforts are required to lower cholesterol, reduce saturated fat, and promote human health, aging, and well-being. In addition, new models including systemic inflammation biomarkers need to be investigated to elucidate the cardiovascular protective mechanisms of dairy fats.

## REFERENCES

Budhkar, Y. A., Bankar, S. B., & Singhal, R. S. (2014). Microbiology of cream and butter. In C. Batt & M. L. Tortorello (Eds.), *Encyclopedia of food microbiology* (Vol. 1, 2nd ed., pp. 728–737). Academic Press.

Bylund, G. (2021). *Dairy processing handbook*. Tetra Pak.

Caballero, B., Finglas, P., & Toldrá, F. (2015). *Encyclopedia of food and health*. Academic Press.

De Goede, J., Soedamah-Muthu, S. S., Pan, A., Gijsbers, L., & Geleijnse, J. M. (2016). Dairy consumption and risk of stroke: A systematic review and updated dose–response meta-analysis of prospective cohort studies. *Journal of the American Heart Association*, *5*(5), e002787.

Desroches, S., Chouinard, P. Y., Galibois, I., Corneau, L., Delisle, J., Lamarche, B., Couture, P., & Bergeron, N. (2005). Lack of effect of dietary conjugated linoleic acids naturally incorporated into butter on the lipid profile and body composition of overweight and obese men. *The American Journal of Clinical Nutrition*, *82*(2), 309–319.

Elsewedy, H. S., Shehata, T. M., & Soliman, W. E. (2022, June 16). Shea butter potentiates the anti-bacterial activity of fusidic acid incorporated into solid lipid nanoparticle. *Polymers* (Basel). *14*(12), 2436.

Evans, N. P., Misyak, S. A., Schmelz, E. M., Guri, A. J., Hontecillas, R., & Bassaganya-Riera, J. (2010). Conjugated linoleic acid ameliorates inflammation-induced colorectal cancer in mice through activation of PPARgamma. *The Journal of Nutrition*, *140*(3), 515–521.

Fearon, A. M. (2011). Butter and butter products. *Dairy Ingredients for Food Processing*, 199–223.

Fontecha, J., Calvo, M. V., Juarez, M., Gil, A., & Martínez-Vizcaino, V. (2019). Milk and dairy product consumption and cardiovascular diseases: An overview of systematic reviews and meta-analyses. *Advances in Nutrition*, *10*(Suppl. 2), S164–S189.

Fox, J. G., & Wang, T. C. (2007). Inflammation, atrophy, and gastric cancer. *The Journal of Clinical Investigation*, *117*(1), 60–69.

Gaba, K., Anand, S., & Syamala, A. (2023). Development of value-added butter by incorporating whey protein hydrolysate-encapsulated probiotics. *Microorganisms*, *11*(5), 1139.

Gholami, F., Khoramdad, M., Shakiba, E., Alimohamadi, Y., Shafiei, J., & Firouzi, A. (2017). Subgroup dairy products consumption on the risk of stroke and CHD: A systematic review and meta-analysis. *Medical Journal of the Islamic Republic of Iran*, *31*, 25.

Ha, H. J., Lee, J. E., Chang, Y. H., & Kwak, H. S. (2010). Entrapment of nutrients during cholesterol removal from cream by crosslinked β-cyclodextrin. *International Journal of Dairy Technology*, *63*(1), 119–126.

Hae-Soo, K., Palanivel, G., & Mohammad Al, M. (2013). Butter, ghee, and cream products. *Milk and Dairy Products in Human Nutrition: Production, Composition and Health*, 390–411.

Halade, G. V., Rahman, M. M., & Fernandes, G. (2010). Differential effects of conjugated linoleic acid isomers in insulin-resistant female C57Bl/6J mice. *The Journal of Nutritional Biochemistry*, *21*(4), 332–337.

Han, E. M., Kim, S. H., Kim, K. W., & Kwak, H. S. (2007). Morphological Change of Crosslinked β-cyclodextrin after recycling. *Journal of Milk Science and Biotechnology*, *25*(1), 9–13.

Hui, H., Dotta, F., Di Mario, U., & Perfetti, R. (2004). Role of caspases in the regulation of apoptotic pancreatic islet beta-cells death. *Journal of Cellular Physiology*, *200*(2), 177–200.

Huot, P. S., Sarkar, B., & Ma, D. W. (2010). Conjugated linoleic acid alters caveolae phospholipid fatty acid composition and decreases caveolin-1 expression in MCF-7 breast cancer cells. *Nutrition Research*, *30*(3), 179–185.

Jourdan, T., Djaouti, L., Demizieux, L., Gresti, J., Verges, B., & Degrace, P. (2009). Liver carbohydrate and lipid metabolism of insulin-deficient mice is altered by trans-10, cis-12 conjugated linoleic acid. *The Journal of Nutrition*, *139*(10), 1901–1907.

Jung, T. H., Kim, J. J., Yu, S. H., Ahn, J., & Kwak, H. S. (2005). Properties of cholesterol-reduced butter and effect of gamma linolenic acid added butter on blood cholesterol. Asian-Australasian *Journal of Animal Sciences*, *18*(11), 1646–1654.

Kaida, K., & Kusunoki, S. (2010). Antibodies to gangliosides and ganglioside complexes in Guillain–Barré syndrome and fisher syndrome: Mini-review. *Journal of Neuroimmunology*, *223*(1–2), 5–12.

Kumar, M., Sharma, V., Lal, D., Kumar, A., & Seth, R. (2010). A comparison of the physico-chemical properties of low-cholesterol ghee with standard ghee from cow and buffalo creams. *International Journal of Dairy Technology*, *63*(2), 252–255.

Kwak, H. S., Ganesan, P., & Mijan, A. M. (2013). Butter, ghee, and cream products. *Milk and Dairy Products in Human Nutrition: Production, Composition and Health*, *390*, 411.

Le, T. T., Phan, T. T. Q., Van Camp, J., & Dewettinck, K. (2015). Milk and dairy polar lipids: Occurrence, purification, and nutritional and technological properties. In *Polar lipids* (pp. 91–143). Elsevier.

Lee, C. L., Liao, H. L., Lee, W. C., Hsu, C. K., Hsueh, F. C., Pan, J. Q., Chu, C. H., Wei, C. T., & Chen, M. J. (2018). Standards and labeling of milk fat and spread products in different countries. *Journal of Food and Drug Analysis*, *26*(2), 469–480.

Lo, C. G., Xu, Y., Proia, R. L., & Cyster, J. G. (2005). Cyclical modulation of sphingosine-1-phosphate receptor 1 surface expression during lymphocyte recirculation and relationship to lymphoid organ transit. *The Journal of Experimental Medicine*, *201*(2), 291–301.

Lorenzen, P. C., Walte, H. G., & Bosse, B. (2013). Development of a method for butter type differentiation by electronic nose technology. *Sensors and Actuators B: Chemical*, *181*, 690–693.

Mallia, S., Escher, F., & Schlichtherle-Cerny, H. (2008). Aroma-active compounds of butter: A review. *European Food Research and Technology*, *226*, 315–325.

Market Watch. (2020). *Global butter market (2020). Industry trends and investigation growth rate, consumption by regional data, product & application segmentation, key companies a top countries analysis & top manufacturers, showing impressive growth by 2026*. Market Watch.

Nagao, K., Wang, Y. M., Inoue, N., Han, S. Y., Buang, Y., Noda, T., Kouda, N., Okamatsu, H., & Yanagita, T. (2003). The 10trans, 12cis isomer of conjugated linoleic acid promotes energy metabolism in OLETF rats. *Nutrition (Burbank, Los Angeles County, Calif.)*, *19*(7–8), 652–656.

Panchal, B., Truong, T., Prakash, S., Bansal, N., & Bhandari, B. (2021). Influence of emulsifiers and dairy ingredients on manufacturing, microstructure, and physical properties of butter. *Foods*, *10*, 1140.

Patel, H. G., Modha, H., & Ranganadham, M. (2017). *Packaging of dairy product*. Agrimoon.

Ramírez-Santana, C., Castellote, C., Castell, M., Moltó-Puigmartí, C., Rivero, M., Pérez-Cano, F. J., & Franch, À. (2011). Enhancement of antibody synthesis in rats by feeding cis-9, trans-11 conjugated linoleic acid during early life. *The Journal of Nutritional Biochemistry*, *22*(5), 495–501.

Ryland, L. K., Fox, T. E., Liu, X., Loughran, T. P., & Kester, M. (2011). Dysregulation of sphingolipid metabolism in cancer. *Cancer Biology & Therapy*, *11*(2), 138–149.

Spitsberg, V. L. (2005). Invited review: Bovine milk fat globule membrane as a potential nutraceutical. *Journal of Dairy Science*, *88*(7), 2289–2294.

The Australian Women's Weekly. (2022). *Nutrition*. www.womensweekly.com.au/health/nutrition/battle-ofthespreads-butter-versus-margarine-12998/.

Walter, S., & Faßbender, K. (2010). Spingolipids in multiple sclerosis. *Cellular Physiology and Biochemistry*, *26*(1), 49–56.

# 7 Fat-Rich Dairy Food—Ghee (Clarified Butter/Butterfat)

## 7.1 LEARNING OBJECTIVES

By the end of the chapter, the reader will be able to:

- Understand the classification and composition of ghee
- Gain knowledge of ghee production and processing
- Learn how to judge and improve the quality of the ghee
- Detect adulteration in ghee
- Make ghee enterprises profitable
- Learn about the key potential health benefits of ghee
- Discover ghee innovations from production to nutritional and health attributes

Ghee and butter have comparable nutritional profiles although ghee might be preferable for people with lactose or casein intolerance. Ghee is regarded as a healthy fat because of its anti-diabetic, anticancer, anti-stress, cardioprotective, and wound-healing attributes.

## 7.2 INTRODUCTION

Ghee (clarified butterfat) is termed as the most popular fat-rich dairy product in the Indian subcontinent. It is a class of clarified butter that is made from the milk of cows or buffalo. It originated from the Indian subcontinent and used in South Asian and Middle Eastern cuisines, traditional medicine, and religious rituals (**Figure 7.1**). It is considered the supreme cooking and frying medium because of its unique flavor and texture. The word ghee evolved from the Sanskrit word "*ghrta*." It stems from the old Sanskrit "*ghr*," which means bright. Ghee is also known as butteroil, butterfat, clarified butter, dehydrated butter, dry butterfat, etc. The ancient Ayurvedic literature and even recent research findings have highlighted ghee's nutritional and therapeutic value (Rajorhia, 1993).

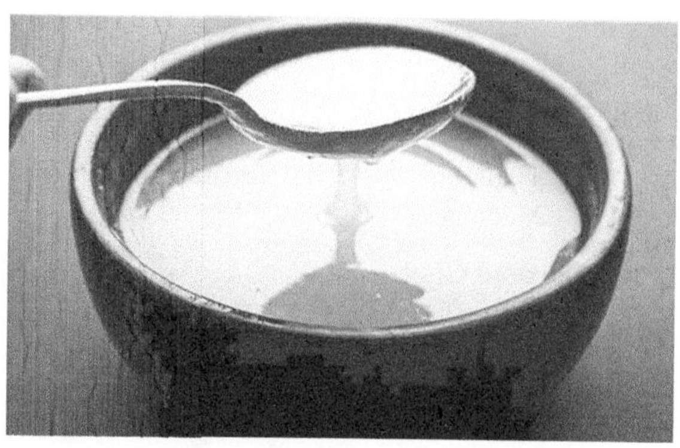

FIGURE 7.1 **Image of ghee.** Ghee is a traditional cooking fat that is widely utilized in the South Asian region.

DOI: 10.1201/9781003397786-7

### 7.2.1 Definition

Ghee is the pure butterfat left over after the milk solids and water are removed from butter (PFA, 2001). Ghee may be defined as clarified butterfat obtained from milk, cream, or butter from various animal species and consists of large milk fat crystals, clotting in liquid fat giving the product a coarse appearance via the removal of moisture and non-fat solids contents (Kumar et al., 2017).

Ghee is a complex lipid composed of mixed glycerides, free fatty acids, phospholipids, sterols and their esters, carotenoids, carbonyl compounds, hydrocarbons, charred casein, moisture, and trace amounts of metals such as copper and iron (Hazra & Parmar, 2014). For flavor, spices can be added. The quality of the butter, the type of milk used in the process, and the length of the boiling time all affect the ghee's texture, color, and flavor.

## 7.3 HISTORY OF GHEE

"*Ghṛta*" is the Sanskrit word from which the term "ghee" originates. Clarified butter, or ghee, has a long and distinguished history. Ghee, often known as "liquid gold" or "sacred fat," was created in ancient India when cows were first domesticated and butter was first consumed (1500–500 BC). Butter would frequently turn rancid before it was eaten in India because of the country's hot weather. So, in order to increase the shelf life of butter, they started clarifying it. Ghee has been used in Hindu religious rites, Ayurvedic procedures, and traditional Indian food for thousands of years. In addition to India, Pakistan, Bangladesh, and some regions of Southeast Asia and the Middle East consume ghee. In several places in East Africa, ghee is used in different forms.

## 7.4 TYPES OF GHEE

i. **White ghee**
   Used in:
   a. North Indian sweets
   b. Bakery items

ii. **Brown ghee/fully boiled ghee**
   Used in:
   a. Biriyani
   b. Rice
   c. Savory items

iii. **Cow ghee**
   Used in:
   a. Temples
   b. Traditional and religious rituals
   c. Medicine

iv. **Flavored Ghee**
   Used in different types of snacks

## 7.5 NUTRITIONAL FACTS

Ghee, a complex lipid, is made up of glycerides (mostly triglycerides), free fatty acids, phospholipids, sterols, sterol esters, fat-soluble vitamins, carbonyls, hydrocarbons, and carotenoids (only in ghee derived from cow milk). It is a complex biological dairy product composed of mainly milk fat and other minor components (Kumar et al., 2010; Kwak et al., 2013). The composition of ghee varies from species to species. Different compositions of ghee are shown in **Tables 7.1, 7.2, and 7.3.**

**TABLE 7.1**
**Nutritional Composition of Ghee**

| Components | Amount/100 g |
|---|---|
| Energy | 886 kcal |
| Milk fat | 99–99.5% |
| Free fatty acid | 0.1–0.3% |
| Protein | 0.3–0.4% |
| Moisture | 0.2–0.5% |
| Vitamins and minerals | Trace amount |
| Cholesterol | 260.8 mg |
| Omega-3 fatty acids | 1.447 mg |
| Omega-6 fatty acids | 2.247 mg |

*Source:* Mahakalkar et al., 2014; Sindhuja et al., 2020; Kwak et al., 2013

**TABLE 7.2**
**Fat Composition of Ghee**

| Parameter | Amount g/100 g |
|---|---|
| Total Fat | 99–99.5 |
| Saturated Fat | 75.10 |
| Monounsaturated fatty acids | 22.26 |
| Polyunsaturated fatty acids | 2.64 |

*Source:* Sindhuja et al., 2020; Kwak et al., 2013

### 7.5.1 Fatty Acid Composition of Ghee

At least 500 fatty acids and their derivatives with a carbon chain of 4–20 atoms or more are present in milk fat. The fatty acid typically has an even number of carbon atoms and can be saturated or unsaturated. The composition of fatty acids (butyric, caproic, capric, lauric, myristic, palmitic, stearic, oleic, linoleic, and linolenic acids) (Kumar et al., 2010) also varies between buffalo milk fat and cow milk fat.

Ghee is mostly made up of fatty acids, trans-fats, cholesterol, monounsaturated fats, polyunsaturated fats, saturated fats, omega fatty acids, and vitamins A, B, D, K, and E, with very little water (**Table 7.3**). Ghee contains essential fatty acids and fat-soluble vitamins that cannot be synthesized in our body. Ghee also provides the milk fat components, including CLA (conjugated linolenic acid), sphingomyelin, butyric acid, and other lipids with anticarcinogenic potential. In addition to other nutrients, including phospholipids, diglycerides, and triglycerides, it provides antioxidants like vitamin E and beta-carotene (600 IU) (Kwak et al., 2013; Akalln & Tokusoglu, 2003; Mahakalkar et al., 2014; Sindhuja et al., 2020).

## 7.6 MANUFACTURING PROCESS

Different methods are used to produce ghee, including the Desi method, which is mostly used in rural households. **Figure 7.2** illustrates the general procedure for ghee manufacturing. The

**TABLE 7.3**
**Major Vitamin and Mineral Composition of Ghee**

| Components | Amount/100 g |
|---|---|
| Iron | 1.1 mg |
| Potassium | 5 mg |
| Vitamin A | 0.78 mg |
| Vitamin E | 1.49 mg |
| Vitamin K | 8.6 μg |

*Source:* Mahakalkar et al., 2014; Sindhuja et al., 2020; Kwak et al., 2013

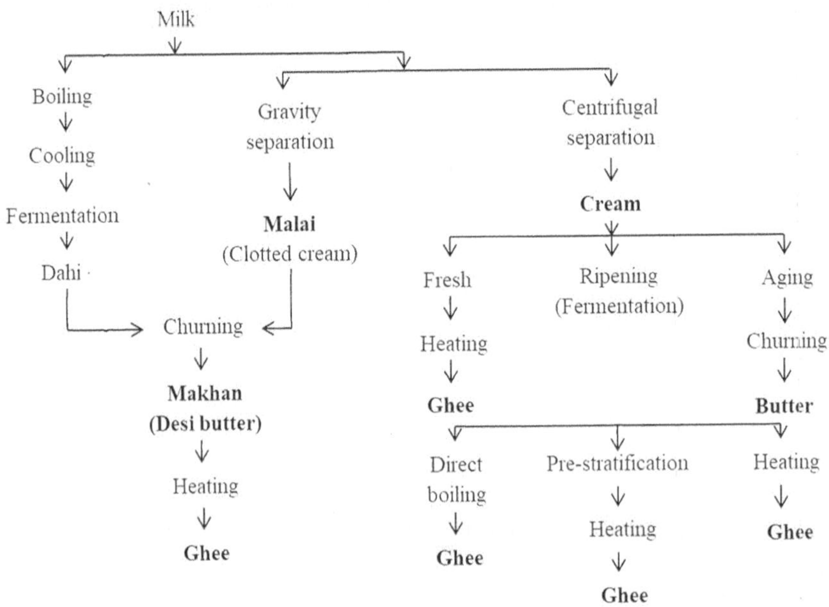


**FIGURE 7.2** **Flow diagram of the general manufacturing process of ghee.**

production process varies depending on the scale (small or large). The principles used to prepare ghee include: (i) concentration of milk fat (as cream or butter), (ii) heat clarification, reducing the amount of water to less than 0.5% by heating the portion of milk that is high in fat, and (iii) the removal of the ghee residue (the curd content).

There are five methods of ghee manufacture (Patel et al., 2006):

i. Desi or traditional method
ii. Direct cream method
iii. Creamery butter method
iv. Pre-stratification method
v. Continuous method

### 7.6.1 Desi or Traditional Method

This has been the custom in rural communities for ages when surplus milk is cultured and left overnight to ferment. The resulting curd is churned with hand-driven wooden beaters to separate the milk fat into Desi butter (**Figure 7.3**). Some follow slightly different methods wherein the milk is heated continuously to about 80°C, and the malai (creamy layer) that forms over the surface is collected manually. Over time, curd particles begin to settle and the clear fat is carefully decanted. There is only a 75–85% chance of recovering fat using this method.

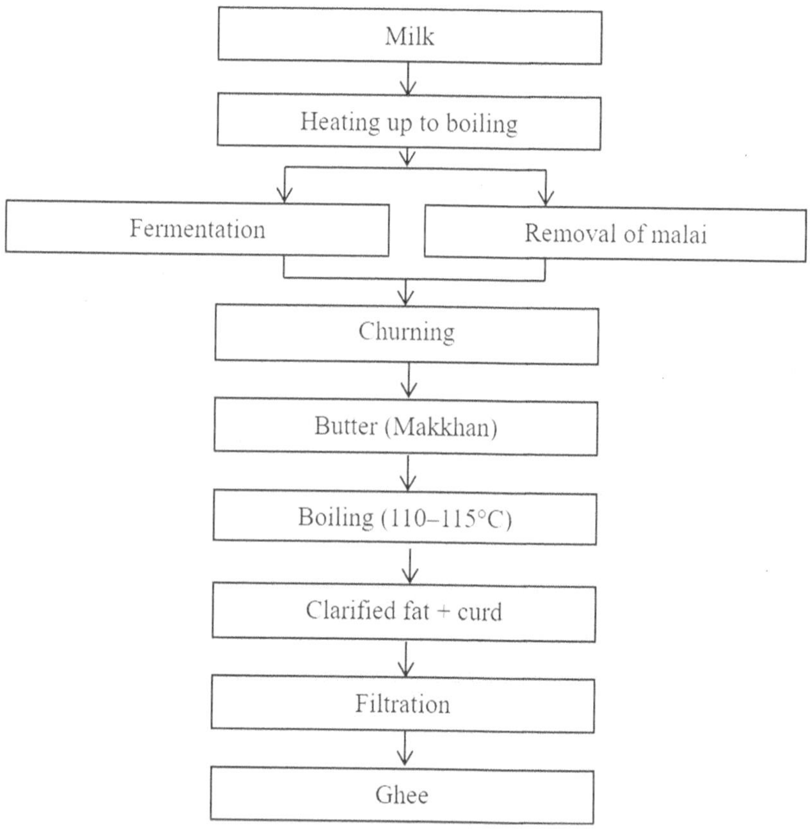


**FIGURE 7.3 Flow diagram of the Desi or traditional method for manufacturing ghee.**

### 7.6.2 Direct Cream Method

The direct cream method is reportedly the most economical method for preparing ghee and the product has better keeping quality. This process omits the need for the production of butter because the cream is directly converted into ghee. It is especially suitable for large-scale production (**Figure 7.4**). A kettle is needed to evaporate moisture. The kettle might be a standard gas-heated or steam-heated, double-jacketed stainless-steel kettle. The choice of the kettle is based on the scale of operation. In this process, a steam-heated jacketed ghee kettle is fitted with an agitator, steam control valve, pressure and temperature gauges, and a movable, hollow, stainless-steel tube.

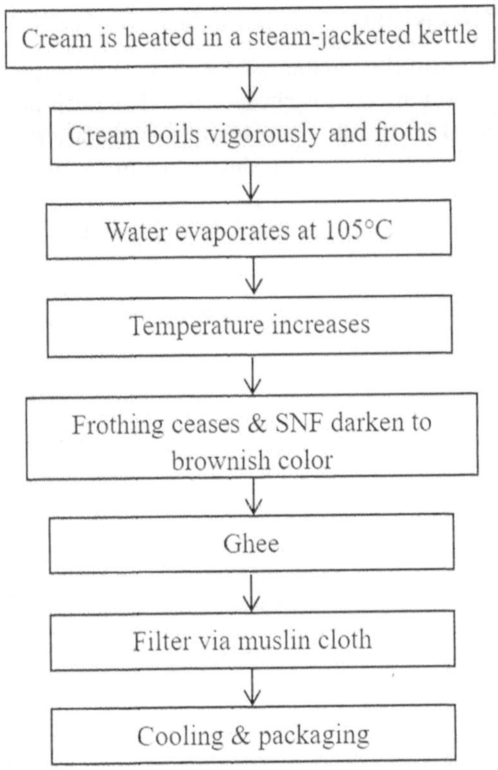


FIGURE 7.4 **Flow diagram of the direct cream method for manufacturing ghee.**

**Advantages:**

No need for butter production prior to manufacturing of ghee.

**Limitations:**

i. Long heating period to eliminate moisture.
ii. The high content of serum solids in the cream may also produce a highly caramelized flavor in the ghee.
iii. A 4–6% loss of milk fat in the ghee residue during handling procedures.
iv. To reduce fat loss and steam consumption, 70–80% fat cream is recommended.

### 7.6.3 Creamery Butter Method

It is suitable for commercial operations because less fat is lost. With industrial interest, the use of this method is increasing. The cream is separated from milk via a cream separator & churned into butter (**Figure 7.5**). Then, the butter is converted into ghee. This is its main principle. The cream is churned at 9°C in summer and 13°C in winter.

At first, fresh, clean milk is collected and pasteurized or boiled for about 10 minutes. The cream should be separated from the milk with the help of a centrifugal cream separator. If the acidity of the cream is more than 0.5%, it should be neutralized with dilute $Ca(OH)_2$ or $NaHCO_3$. The separated cream should be pasteurized at 63°C for 30 min or 77°C for 5 min. About 5–10%

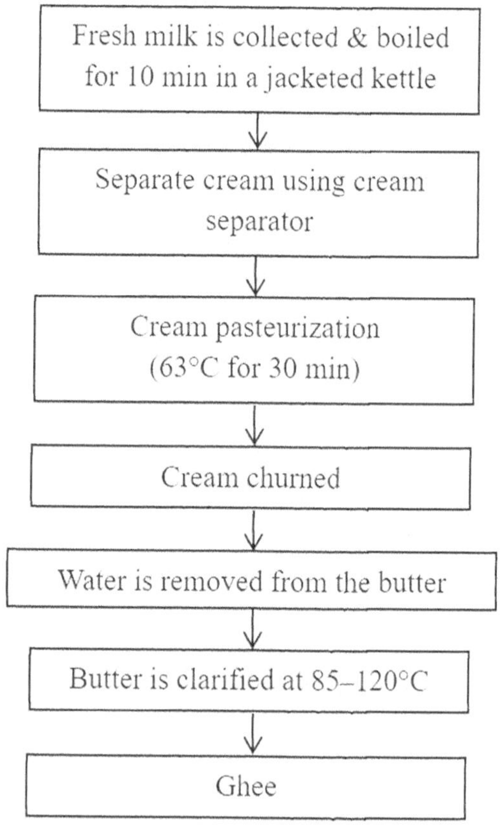


**FIGURE 7.5** **Flow diagram of the creamery butter method for manufacturing ghee.**

of proper starter culture is to be added with pasteurizing cream and should be held at 21°C until an acidity of 0.2–0.4% is developed. Churning should be continued until the butter granules are the size of a pea. At that stage, buttermilk should be drained out, and cold water needs to be added, followed by rechurning the butter until the water is clear. The collected butter should be worked out to remove as much water as possible. Finally, butter should be clarified to obtain ghee.

## Advantages:

i. Ghee made with this procedure is of extremely high consistency.
ii. The quantity of ghee residue is much less; hence, less fat loss.
iii. Less space is required for the storage of cooking butter, and raw material for this method.
iv. Energy requirements are lower than for direct cream and indigenous methods.
v. Longer-lasting quality compared to the traditional approach.

## Limitations:

i. The flavor of ghee prepared by the creamery butter method is criticized to be either flat/bland or cooked.
ii. Poor texture.

### 7.6.4 Pre-Stratification Method

Butter is made from aged cream that contains 38 to 40% fat using a batch churn or continuous butter making machine. The butter is then moved to the butter melter, where it is melted at 80°C. For 30 minutes, this molten butter is left undisturbed in a ghee kettle or boiler at a temperature of 80 to 85°C. The middle and upper layers are not disturbed as the bottom layer is then carefully removed (**Figure 7.6**). The middle layer largely consists of fat heated to 114±2°C along with a top layer of floating curd particles and denatured protein. This step is required to create the distinctive ghee aroma. Milder-flavored ghee can be produced since most of the curd content is removed before the final clarification temperature of the ghee.

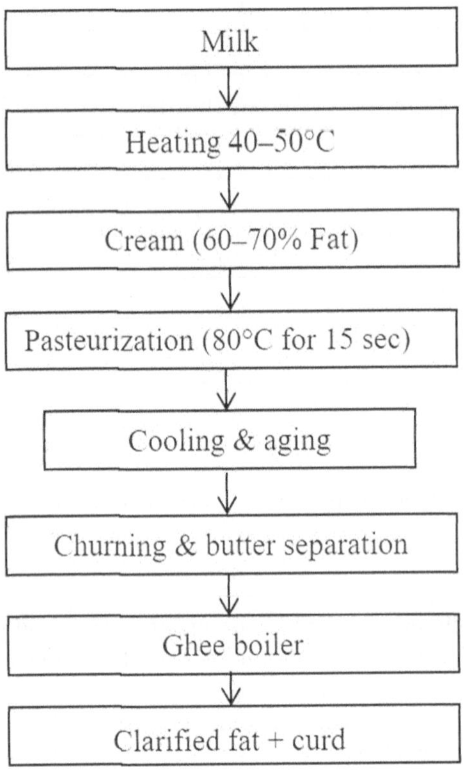


FIGURE 7.6 **Flow diagram of the pre-stratification method for manufacturing ghee.**

**Advantages:**

i. A 60% reduction in fuel usage when compared to direct clarification.
ii. Ghee has a lower acidity, which prolongs its shelf life.
iii. Shorter duration of high temperature exposure.
iv. There is a decrease in the development of residue.

**Limitations:**

i. Since it produces ghee in batches, it is not appropriate for continuous ghee production.
ii. Ghee has a very mild or bland flavor.

### 7.6.5 Continuous Method

The previously stated batch ghee manufacturing techniques are ideal for small- and medium-scale ghee production. With the increase in demand and scope for the export of ghee, some very large organized dairies prefer to adopt continuous ghee-making methods (**Figure 7.7**). The de-emulsification of cream fat from the oil-in-water phase to the water-in-oil phase is the basis for this method of producing ghee. During this procedure, milk is divided into 40% fat cream using a clarifixator and a centrifugal cream separator. This cream is further concentrated due to the centrifugal force-driven concentrator. The clarifixator and concentrator use mechanical means to de-emulsify fat. Flavor is produced, and the majority of the moisture from the fat concentrate is removed using a scraped surface heat exchanger. Ghee residue is removed by an oil clarifier, and any moisture that is left in the ghee is removed in a vapor separator (Abichandani et al., 1995; Kumar et al., 2017).

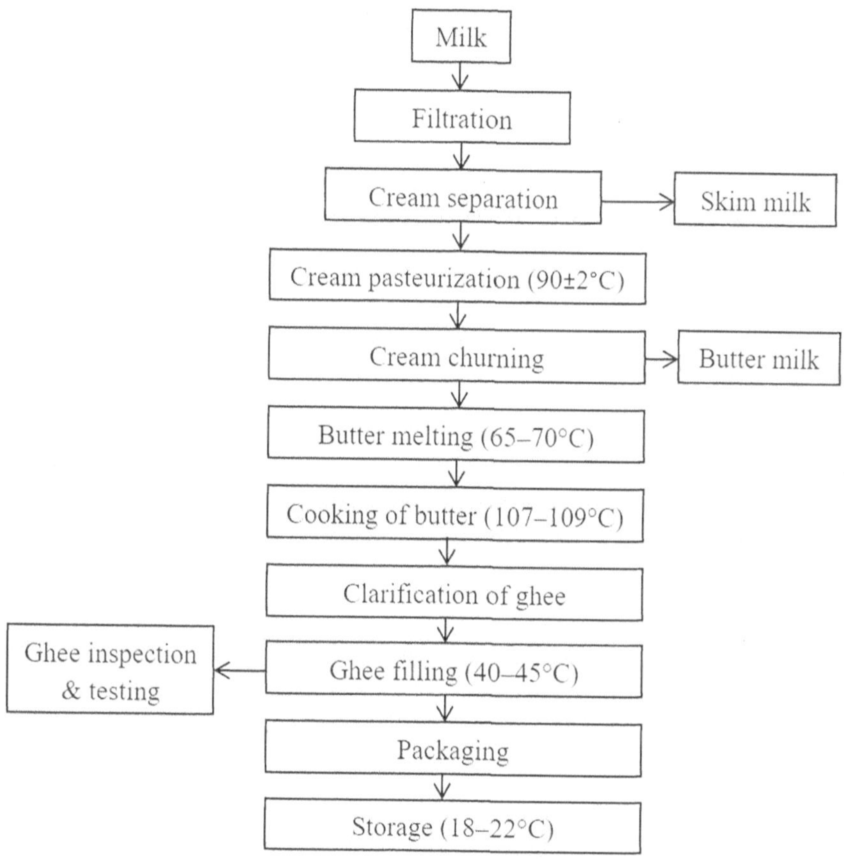


FIGURE 7.7 **Flow diagram of the industrial method for manufacturing ghee.**

**Advantages:**

i. Improved control over product quality.
ii. There is never a significant hold-up of raw materials in the facility, eliminating the possibility that the entire batch may get spoiled.
iii. Handler contamination can be removed entirely.
iv. It is feasible for CIP.
v. The product doesn't spoil while being produced.

**Limitations:**

i. Requires a lot of energy because the heat transfer coefficient is so low.
ii. Unsatisfactory equipment cleaning and sanitation.
iii. Equipment and processes are unsuitable for large volumes of production.
iv. Ghee spill causes the floor to become slippery.
v. Handling losses is more common.

### 7.6.6 Starter Culture in the Manufacture of Ghee

The pleasing flavor of ghee is different from the milk, cream, dahi, and butter from which it is made. The flavor of ghee is highly variable and depends on many factors; one of them is the starter culture that is used. For the ripening of cream for ghee making, two popular starter cultures (*Streptococcus lactic* and *Lactobacillus bulgaricus*) have been used. *Streptococcus lactis* subsp. *diacetilactis* DRC-l, *S. thermopiles*, *Leuconostoc citrovorum*, and *Leuconostoc dextranicum* are also used as starter cultures.

## 7.7 ADULTERATION OF GHEE

Ghee is a costly product, pricing three times as much as vegetable oils. Because of its expensive nature, ghee is susceptible to being adulterated with vegetable oil/mineral oil or animal body fat by unscrupulous manufacturers, traders, and vendors.

Major adulterants of ghee are as follows:

i. Vanaspati (hydrogenated vegetable oil). Because of how closely its texture resembles ghee, this is most frequently used as an adulterant.
ii. Refined (de-odorized) vegetable oil.
iii. Animal body fat.

For the detection of adulteration in ghee, a number of techniques have been developed, including the determination of analytical properties (RM, PV, SV, IV, BR, etc.), phytosterol acetate test, chromatographic methods, color reaction, etc.

### 7.7.1 Physiochemical Properties of Ghee

Physicochemical properties of ghee are required to determine the ghee quality, shelf life, and improving palatability. Physicochemical properties of the ghee are following:

i. **Reichert–Meissl (RM) value:** >23 (26–28) (cow ghee), >30 (buffalo ghee)
ii. **Polenske value (PV):** 1.5–3.0 (cow ghee), 1.5–2.0 (buffalo ghee)
iii. **Saponification value (SV):** >225 (225–230) (cow ghee), 226–234 (buffalo ghee)
iv. **Iodine value (IV):** (35–41) (cow ghee), (30–36) (buffalo ghee)

Apart from these, some other physiochemical properties of ghee are:

- Free fatty acid content (oleic acid),
- Moisture content or volatile content,
- Melting range,
- Bomer value,
- Peroxide value,
- Solidification temperature, etc.

### 7.7.2 Analysis of Adulteration of Ghee

Consumers judge the quality of ghee based on its flavor, color, and appearance (Kumar et al., 2016).

i. **Reichert–Meissl value:** This is the volume of N/10 sodium hydroxide needed to neutralize the water-soluble fatty acids that were distilled from 5 g of caproic acid during the steam distillation process. For cow ghee, the value has to be more than 23, and for buffalo ghee, it has to be more than 30.
ii. **Polenske value:** It is defined as the quantity of ml of N/10 sodium hydroxide needed, under the exact conditions outlined in the procedure, to neutralize the steam-volatile water-insoluble fatty acids distilled from 5 g of fat. To check the value of it, cow ghee and buffalo ghee should be 1.5–3 and 1.5–2, respectively.
iii. **Saponification value:** The amount of potassium needed to saponify one gram of fat is measured in milligrams. The saponification value of pure cow ghee is 225 or more, and for buffalo ghee, it is around 226–234.
iv. **Iodine method:** It is described as the quantity of iodine absorbed by 100 grams of fat under particular circumstances. In the case of pure cow ghee, the iodine value should be 35–41, for buffalo ghee, it should be 30–36.

## 7.8 FACTORS INFLUENCING THE YIELD OF GHEE

**Method of production:** The fat recovery ranges from 88 to 92% for the creamery butter method, from 80 to 85% for the indigenous approach, and from 90 to 95% for the straight cream method.

**The fat content of the raw material used:** A larger amount of fat will result in a higher yield, and vice versa.

**Quality of milk or cream:** If the acidity of the milk or cream that will be used to make ghee is higher, then there will be more losses in the ghee residue, which lowers the yield.

**Fat recovery from ghee residue:** Scientific reports suggest extracting as much fat as possible from ghee residue by dissolving ghee residue in hot water followed by filtration and centrifugation. By using this technique, the fat from the ghee residue can be removed, and the fat can then be added back to the cream or butter melter.

## 7.9 PACKAGING AND STORAGE OF GHEE

### 7.9.1 Packaging System

Ghee degrades when exposed to light, air, water vapor, and metals, as demonstrated in **Figure 7.8** (Kumar & Singhal, 1992).

Ghee is typically packaged in glass bottles, food-grade plastic containers such as high-density polyethylene pouches, laminates with metallic layer support (aluminum), and tin cans (Panjagari & Ganguly, 2020).

**Tin cans:** For bulk packs of 15 and 5 liters, lacquer-coated tin cans are used to block the entry of oxygen, which oxidizes the product during storage.

**Glass bottles:** Glass bottles offer exceptional product quality protection because they don't react with food. Glass bottles can be used for high-speed operation. Producers of ghee have begun storing the product in glass bottles with weights ranging from 100 g to 500 g for retailers.

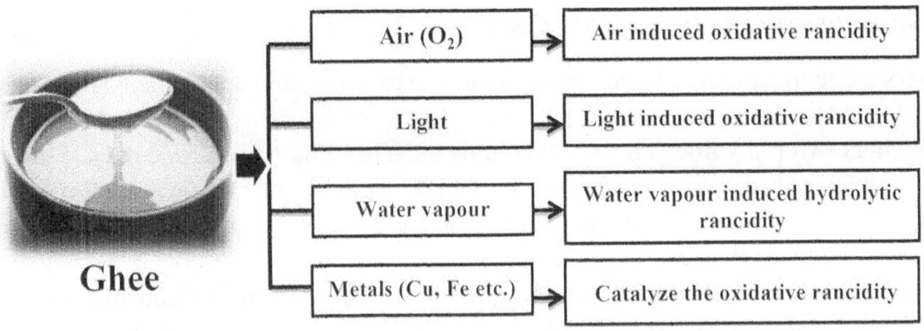


FIGURE 7.8 **Ghee degradation process.** It's becoming rancid. Ghee turns rancid when it is oxidized or exposed to air, heat, moisture, or light for an extended period. In addition to having a terrible smell and sour taste, rancid ghee might appear white rather than yellow.

**Semi-rigid containers:** Tinplate containers are being replaced with semi-rigid plastic containers. These containers have the benefits of being portable, affordable, and light. Ghee packaging options are ideal for semi-rigid containers.

**Flexible films/pouches/laminates:** Flexible pouches are the most appealing way to package ghee because they are the most affordable option among all other options. The compatibility of the contact layer, the capacity for heat sealing, the strength of the heat seal, and the desired shelf life are the main factors that determine whether to choose a laminate or multilayer film.

**The following qualities of packing materials for ghee are desired:** (i) Ghee and packaging materials shouldn't react, (ii) it should be easily accessible and inexpensive, (iii) it ought to be harmless, (iv) it must prevent printing ink from penetrating the product, (v) it must guard against tempering, (vi) it needs to have effective spoilage-preventing characteristics, and (vii) it must survive deterioration while being transported.

### 7.9.2 Storage System

Oxidized flavor, especially when ghee has a noticeable initial acidity, develops at a higher storage temperature. Lower-temperature storage gives ghee a fatty and pasty texture, even if it slows acid production and lengthens shelf life. Therefore, a storage temperature of 21°C is advised. Ghee can be kept at 21°C for up to 12 months (Singh & Ram, 1978).

## 7.10 QUALITY JUDGING OF GHEE

The quality of ghee depends on the following factors:

i. Method of preparation
ii. Quality of cream or butter used
iii. Boiling temperature
iv. Other ingredients and flavors, if added
v. Storage conditions of the finished product

The difference in quality between fresh-milk ghee and acid-milk ghee is shown in **Table 7.4**.

**TABLE 7.4**
**Quality Difference between Fresh-Milk Ghee and Acid-Milk Ghee**

| Parameter | Fresh-milk ghee | High acidity-milk ghee |
|---|---|---|
| Liquid portion | Less | More |
| Color units | Usually high (about 19) | Less (about 16) |

The Hedonic Type scale is used to assess ghee sensory qualities. Usually, sensory evaluation is performed using a 9-point hedonic scale (1: dislike extremely, 9: like extremely), where panelists evaluate the sensory attributes, i.e., texture, color, flavor, taste, and overall acceptability of ghee (Bajwa & Kaur, 1995). The Hedonic Type scale is illustrated in **Table 7.5**.

## 7.11 DEFECTS IN GHEE

Ghee can be stored at temperatures between 5 and 38°C depending on the time of year and location. Higher storage temperatures (over 30°C) hasten chemical degradation, especially oxidative deterioration, whereas lower temperatures (below 10°C) delay chemical spoilage and degrade the texture of ghee. Ghee hardens and becomes oily at low temperatures. Ghee and butter oil should be kept between 20 and 30°C for optimum storage results. The following table covers the numerous ghee defects that are typically found, as well as their causes (**Table 7.6**):

**TABLE 7.5**
**Score Card for the Sensory Evaluation of Ghee**

| Name: | | Sample no: | | | Date: |
|---|---|---|---|---|---|
| Sl. no | Color and appearance | Flavor | Body and texture | Overall acceptability | Total remarks |
| 1 | | | | | |
| 2 | | | | | |
| 3 | | | | | |
| 4 | | | | | |
| 5 | | | | | |

| Rate | Organoleptic score |
|---|---|
| Like extremely | 9 |
| Like very much | 8 |
| Like moderately | 7 |
| Like slightly | 6 |
| Neither like nor dislike | 5 |
| Dislike slightly | 4 |
| Dislike moderately | 3 |
| Dislike very much | 2 |
| Dislike extremely | 1 |

**TABLE 7.6**
**Defects in Ghee**

| Defects | Causes | Remedies |
|---|---|---|
| Acidic | i. Cooking butter with high acidity<br>ii. High initial moisture of ghee | Maintain optimum moisture content and acidity. |
| Curdy | i. Cream or butter undercooked<br>ii. All non-fat solid content is not properly removed | Remove all non-fat solid content properly and cook the cream perfectly. |
| Smoky | i. Use of smoky fire<br>ii. Storage of ghee in a smoky environment | Avoid smoky environments and fire. |
| Burnt | Heating of butterfat at a very high temperature at the last stage of preparation | Maintain optimum temperature for heating. |
| Flat | i. Using butter with an extremely low curd content<br>ii. Maintaining a low temperature of heating under vacuum | Use butter containing enough curd. |
| Hydrolytic rancidity | i. Low-quality raw materials<br>ii. High-heat treatment | Use premium quality raw materials. |
| Oxidative rancidity | i. Default packaging<br>ii. Improper storage facility | Ensure proper packaging and storage facility. |
| Greasy | i. Improper storage of ghee, particularly frequent thermal shocks<br>ii. Prolonged storage of ghee under refrigeration | Avoid long-term refrigeration and ensure proper storage facility. |

## 7.12 HEALTH BENEFITS OF GHEE

Ghee has the potential to provide health advantages. Ghee has been recognized as superior to other fats due to the presence of unique short-chain fatty acids and as a carrier of the four fat-soluble vitamins, A, D, E, and K, and essential fatty acids such as linolenic acid and arachidonic acid (Kumar et al., 2018). Because of its antidiabetic, anticancer, anti-stress, eye lubricant, hepatoprotective, cardioprotective, and wound-healing qualities, it is regarded as a healthy fat. Ayurveda also uses cow ghee for a variety of medical purposes. Ayurveda uses medicated ghee made with various botanical extracts to prescribe various treatment methods for various illnesses. Numerous health advantages and high popularity may be found in Ayurvedic ghee such as Amrutprash, Arjuna ghrita, Ashoka ghrita, Ashwagandha ghrita, Kalyan ghrita, and Vachadi ghrita. Currently, health centers, yoga studios, and fitness facilities advise using ghee as a nutritious food (Sindhuja et al., 2020; Pandey, 2021). **Figure 7.9** illustrates the key potential health benefits of ghee.

### 7.12.1 Association of Ghee Consumption with Providing Nourishment

Many studies suggest that ghee is suitable for ingestion by people of all ages and has a variety of health benefits due to its distinctive flavor and bio-functional components (Ray, 2019; Changhk & Kim, 2014). The fat-soluble vitamins A, D, E, and K are abundant in ghee. These nutrients are essential to many body functions, from the brain to the immune system. Ghee also facilitates the body's assimilation of fat-soluble nutrients, including vitamins and minerals from other diets. According to the spectral fingerprints of vitamins, cow ghee has a comparatively higher content of the vitamins $B_{12}$, D, and K than buffalo ghee. Similarly, cow ghee contains considerably more CLA and

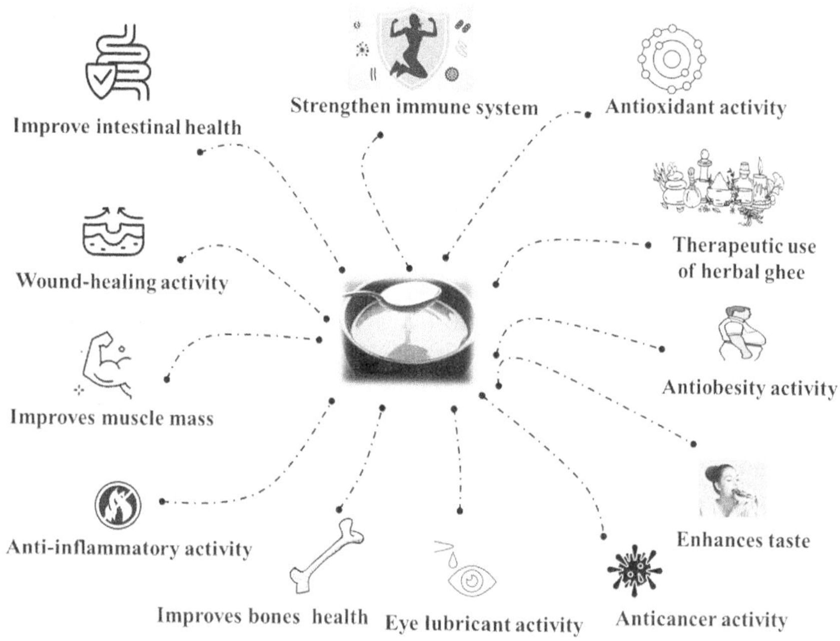


**FIGURE 7.9 Key potential health benefits of ghee.** Despite its high fat content, ghee includes a high concentration of monounsaturated omega-3 fatty acids. These beneficial fatty acids promote heart and cardiovascular health. According to research, eating ghee as part of a balanced diet can help lower harmful cholesterol levels.

vitamin A. Both forms of ghee were found to contain significant amounts of vitamin E. Therefore, beta-carotene, CLA, and vitamin A levels can be utilized as biomarkers to distinguish between cow and buffalo ghee. The successful detection of adulteration of blind samples has been proven using spectroscopic analysis and principal component analysis (PCA) (Ahmad & Saleem, 2020).

### 7.12.2 Association of Ghee Consumption with Digestive System/Intestinal Health

Ghee consumption is strongly related to a healthy gut. Before every meal, our ancestors used to eat a teaspoon of ghee in the past. It lined the gut and reduced the chances of ulcers and cancer (Benjamin & Spener, 2009). In contrast to other oils, ghee includes butyric acid, a short-chain fatty acid that imparts a distinctive flavor and aids in digestion (Kumar et al., 2015). Beneficial intestinal microorganisms that use butyric acid as a source of energy and to strengthen the intestinal wall transform fiber into butyric acid (Maurice, 1987). Studies have shown that butyric acid is not produced by those with compromised digestive systems. According to research, the production of butyric acid provides sufficient support for the gut's generation of killer T cells, leading to a strong immune system (Changhk & Kim, 2014). Ghee is a great choice to support the health of the intestinal walls because it is one of the highest-quality food sources of butyric acid (Park & Haenlein, 2013). The cells of the colon use butyric acid as their preferred source of energy (Evans et al., 2010).

### 7.12.3 Association of Ghee Consumption with Antioxidant and Antiatherogenic Activity

In a study, Chinnadurai et al. showed that ghee high in CLA enhances the activity of antioxidant enzymes like CAT, SOD, and GST, demonstrating the substance's antioxidant nature. While lipid-soluble antioxidants defend the cell membranes from lipid peroxidation, water-soluble antioxidants interact with oxidants (free radicals) in the blood plasma and cell cytoplasm (Chinnadurai et al., 2013). Feeding CLA-enriched ghee also resulted in lower triglycerides, high-density lipoproteins, and cholesterol. This resulted in lower levels of low-density lipoproteins, resulting in a lower atherogenic index, demonstrating the substance's antiatherogenic effect. The study shows that ghee (clarified butter) with a high CLA content possesses antioxidant and antiatherogenic properties, indicating that ghee may be an essential food component for lowering the risk of cardiovascular illnesses (Chinnadurai et al., 2013; Spiteller, 2007).

### 7.12.4 Association of Ghee Consumption with Wound-Healing Activity

By measuring collagen estimation, wound contraction, and skin breaking strength, Datta et al. examined the effects of five selected formulated variants of topical application materials (cow ghee, flax seed oil, amalaka fruit extract, shoreabusta resin, and yashadabhasma) on the functional status of skin and tissue regeneration capacity in wound-healing models. It had been selected based mostly on the findings from Ayurvedic literature, with the conclusion that it can be helpful in wound contraction, enhancement of tensile strength, and augmentation in hydroxyproline content or collagen content. This combination of qualities creates anti-aging effects that are especially beneficial for skin health (Datta et al., 2009).

### 7.12.5 Association of Ghee Consumption with Eye Lubricant Activity

The cure for computer vision syndrome (CVS) is cow ghee. The Goghrita has a lubricating quality that helps to lessen the symptoms of CVS and includes 98% glycerides and some fatty acids. It contains vitamin A 3500 IU/100 g. Vitamin A is responsible for keeping the surface of the eyeballs wet and preventing blindness. Beta-carotene and vitamin E, which have antioxidant properties, are also present. Therefore, aschyotan (Goghrita eye drops) may be a useful treatment for computer vision syndrome (Mulik & Bhusari, 2013).

### 7.12.6 Association of Ghee Consumption with Cancer Prevention

To test the anticancer potential of cow ghee, a recent study examined the effects of feeding a mixture of cow ghee and soybean oil on 7, 12-dimethylbenz (a)-anthracene (DMBA)-induced carcinogenesis and expression of cyclooxygenase-2 (*COX-2*) and peroxisome proliferator-activated receptor gamma (*PPAR-γ*) in rat mammary glands (Rani & Kansal, 2012). The animals fed soybean oil in the DMBA (a carcinogen)-treated groups had higher tumor incidence (65.4%), tumor weight (96.18 g), and tumor volume (6285 $mm^3$) than the rats who were only given cow ghee (26.6%, 1.67 g, and 1925 $mm^3$, respectively). The tumor latency period was 27 weeks in cow ghee group compared to 23 weeks in soybean oil group. They came to the conclusion that dietary cow ghee, as opposed to soybean oil, attenuates mammary carcinogens, which are caused by DMBA. The effect is mediated by decreased expression of *COX-2* and improved expression of *COX-2* and *PPAR-γ* in the former group (Rani & Kansal, 2012).

### 7.12.7 Association of Ghee Consumption with Obesity Prevention

According to study, the weight of the animals in the cow ghee group decreased (Karandikar et al., 2016). This weight loss may be attributed to the medical benefits of cow ghee, which promotes quick absorption and digestion of meals. While other fats and oils may slow down the body's digestion and make the stomach feel fuller, ghee encourages the production of stomach acids to aid in digestion.

### 7.12.8 Association of Ghee Consumption with Anti-Inflammatory Activity

Lauric acid, one of the medium- and short-chain fatty acids found in ghee, is a strong antibacterial and antifungal compound. Due to its anti-inflammatory properties, topical use of ghee aids in wound healing and reduces swelling.

### 7.12.9 Association of Ghee Consumption with Immune System Health

Ghee is rich in butyric acid, which helps the body produce T cells that fight diseases. Butyrate is beneficial to the immune system and the digestive system. Staying active requires a healthy stomach and a robust immune system. To reap the advantages of ghee for better immunity, drink 100% certified cow ghee produced using the conventional Bilona approach.

### 7.12.10 Association of Ghee Consumption with Healthy Bone Development

Vitamin K, which is abundant in ghee, aids in calcium absorption. Calcium is beneficial for bone health. Ghee contributes vitamin K to the diet and provides passive support for bone health.

### 7.12.11 Association of Ghee Consumption with Taste Enhancement

Ghee is an excellent taste enhancer for all foods. Its neutral taste and nutty scent complement the flavor of food and spices in a holistic way. However, adding or seasoning with ghee offers a different flavor, frequently feeling buttery but never with the buttery, creamy texture.

### 7.12.12 Association of Ghee Consumption with Thyroid Function

Ghee consumption is important in thyroid dysfunction since it helps to balance hormones (Hazra & Parmar, 2014). Selected examples of the therapeutic use of herbal ghee (Pandya & Kanawjia, 2002; Gandhi, 2015) are as follows:

- Amrutprash for anti-aging
- Arjuna ghrita for preventing heart disease
- Ashoka ghrita and kaghrita for preventing leucorrhea
- Kalyan ghrita for treatment of madness
- Treatment of various CNS disorders
- Samhit ghee is a good supplement for malnutrition and has positive effects on intelligence, memory, longevity, enhancing vision and complexion, cooling action, and detoxifying.
- Satavarighrita is an antispasmodic and diuretic that supports patients in overcoming the side effects of chemotherapy during cancer treatment. It boosts the immune system and is beneficial for AIDS as well as many other known health-stimulating qualities for women.
- It is also said to have antidiarrheal, antihepatotoxic, and immune-stimulant properties. Brahmi is utilized in Ayurvedic treatment in the form of herbal ghee.
- Anticonvulsant, antidepressant, antiepileptic, antipsychotic, anti-stress, hepato-protective, and many different therapeutic uses are still to be explored.

## 7.13 GHEE INNOVATIONS

Efforts have been made to increase the shelf life and functionality of ghee by adding many functional ingredients, flavors, and natural antioxidants from different sources (Kumbhare et al., 2023). **Figures 7.10, 7.11, and 7.12** illustrate ghee innovations from production to nutritional and health attributes (Kumbhare et al., 2023).

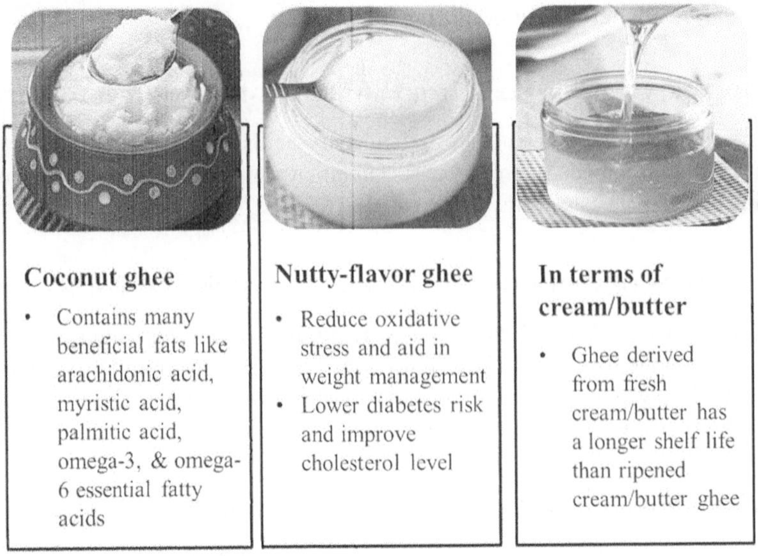


FIGURE 7.10 Ghee innovations in production attributes.

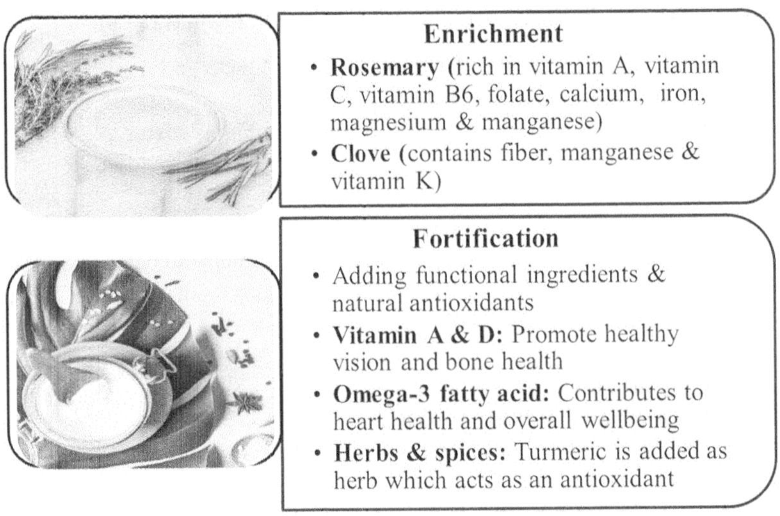


FIGURE 7.11 Ghee innovations in nutritional attributes.

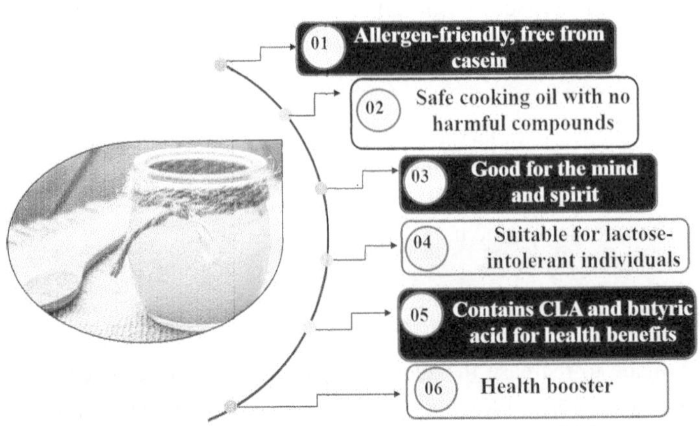


FIGURE 7.12 Ghee innovations in health attributes.

## 7.14 NEGATIVE PUBLICITY OF GHEE

Despite its many health advantages, ghee has received unfavorable publicity in recent years because of its high cholesterol and saturated fatty acid levels. Although these are necessary for health up to a point, over that point, they may potentially have negative consequences on well-being. To lessen the risk of cardiovascular disease, the American Coronary Heart Affiliation suggests keeping saturated fat intake to less than 7% of our total caloric intake (Lichtenstein et al., 2006). Therefore, it can be indicated that someone who has cardiac and renal issues should stay away from ghee (Shukla et al., 2012; Lordan et al., 2018).

## 7.15 GHEE YIELD

Ghee yield is calculated by the following formula:

$$\text{Percentage of ghee obtained} = (\text{Weight of ghee} \times 100)/\text{Weight of fat in butter}$$

$$\text{Weight of fat in butter} = \text{weight of butter} \times 80\%$$

## 7.16 CONCLUSIONS

Ghee is an anhydrous milk fat that is mostly made using conventional techniques in Asia, the Middle East, and Africa. Recently, it has gained considerable popularity in some areas outside of these regions. The qualities and manufacturing processes differ. Ghee is broadly prepared by two methods: a traditional method and industrial method, namely the creamery butter method, direct cream method, pre-stratification method, and continuous method. According to market dynamics, the traditional process of manufacturing makkhan before turning it into ghee accounts for more than 90% of the ghee produced. More research is required on novel manufacturing methods that are energy efficient, cost effective, and have maximum yield without compromising the quality of ghee or raising cholesterol levels, and on new bioactive components that are beneficial to human health.

## REFERENCES


Abichandani, H., Bector, B. S., & Sarma, S. C. (1995). Continuous ghee making system-design, operation and performance. *Indian Journal of Dairy Science, 48*(11), 646–650.

Ahmad, N., & Saleem, M. (2020). Characterisation of cow and buffalo ghee using fluorescence spectroscopy. *International Journal of Dairy Technology, 73*(1), 191–201.

Akalln, A. S., & Tokusoglu, Ö. (2003). A potential anticarcinogenic agent: Conjugated linoleic acid (CLA). *Pakistan Journal of Nutrition, 2*, 109–110.

Bajwa, U., & Kaur, A. (1995). Effect of ghee (butter oil) residue and additives on physical and sensory characteristics of cookies. *Chemie, Mikrobiologie, Technologie der Lebensmittel, 17*(5–6), 151–155.

Benjamin, S., & Spener, F. (2009). Conjugated linoleic acids as functional food: An insight into their health benefits. *Nutrition & Metabolism, 6*, 1–13.

Changhk, P. E., & Kim, M. (2014). Gut microbiota-derived short-chain fatty acids, T cells, and inflammation. *Immune Network, 14*(6), 277–288.

Chinnadurai, K., Kanwal, H. K., Tyagi, A. K., Stanton, C., & Ross, P. (2013). High conjugated linoleic acid enriched ghee (clarified butter) increases the antioxidant and antiatherogenic potency in female Wistar rats. *Lipids in Health and Disease, 12*, 121.

Datta, H. S., Mitra, S. K., & Patwardhan, B. (2009). Wound healing activity of topical application forms based on ayurveda. *Evidence-Based Complementary and Alternative Medicine, 2011*, 1–10.

Evans, N. P., Misyak, S. A., Schmelz, E. M., Guri, A. J., Hontecillas, R., & Bassaganya-Riera, J. (2010). Conjugated linoleic acid ameliorates inflammation-induced colorectal cancer in mice through activation of PPARγ. *The Journal of Nutrition, 140*(3), 515–521.

Gandhi, K. (2015). Potential of herbal nutraceuticals in ghee: A review. *Research and Reviews: Dairy Science and Technology, 4*(2), 1–5.

Hazra, T., & Parmar, P. (2014). Natural antioxidant use in ghee-A mini review. *Journal of Food Research and Technology, 2*(3), 101–105.

Karandikar, Y. S., Bansude, A. S., & Angadi, E. A. (2016). Comparison between the effect of cow ghee and butter on memory and lipid profile of wistar rats. *Journal of Clinical and Diagnostic Research: JCDR*, *10*(9), 11.

Kumar, A., Goyal, S. K., Munesh, K. V., & Kumar, L. (2016). Study on physico-chemical analysis of ghee. *South Asian Journal of Food Technology and Environment*, *2*(3&4), 448–451.

Kumar, A., Tripathi, S., Hans, N., Pattnaik, H. S. N., & Naik, S. N. (2018). Ghee: Its properties, importance and health benefits. *Lipid Universe*, *6*, 6–14.

Kumar, A., Upadhyay, N., Padghan, P. V., Gandhi, K., Lal, D., & Sharma, V. (2015). Detection of vegetable oil and animal depot fat adulteration in anhydrous milk fat (Ghee) using fatty acid composition. *MOJ Food Processing & Technology*, *1*(3), 13.

Kumar, M., Pandya, H. B., Dodiya, K. K., Bhatt, R., & Mangukiya, M. (2017). Advancement in industrial method of ghee making process at Sarvottam Dairy, Bhavnagar, Gujarat (India). *International Journal of Science, Environment and Technology*, *6*(3), 1727–1736.

Kumar, M., Sharma, V., Lal, D., Kumar, A., & Seth, R. (2010). A comparison of the physico-chemical properties of low-cholesterol ghee with standard ghee from cow and buffalo creams. *International Journal of Dairy Technology*, *63*(2), 252–255.

Kumar, N., & Singhal, O. P. (1992). Effect of processing conditions on the oxidation of cholesterol in ghee. *Journal of the Science of Food and Agriculture*, *58*(2), 267–273.

Kumbhare, S., Prasad, W., Khamrui, K., Wani, A. D., & Sahu, J. (2023). Recent innovations in functionality and shelf life enhancement of ghee, clarified butter fat. *Journal of Food Science and Technology*, *60*, 11–23.

Kwak, H. S., Ganesan, P., & Mijan, A. M. (2013). Butter, ghee, and cream products. *Milk and Dairy Products in Human Nutrition: Production, Composition and Health*, 390–411.

Lichtenstein, A. H., Appel, L. J., Brands, M., Carnethon, M., Daniels, S., Franch, H. A., Franklin, B., Kris-Etherton, P., Harris, W. S., Howard, B., Karanja, N., Lefevre, M., Rudel, L., Sacks, F., Van Horn, L., Winston, M., & Wylie-Rosett, J. (2006). Diet and lifestyle recommendations revision 2006: A scientific statement from the American heart association nutrition committee. *Circulation*, *114*(1), 82–96.

Lordan, R., Tsoupras, A., Mitra, B., & Zabetakis, I. (2018). Dairy fats and cardiovascular disease: Do we really need to be concerned? *Foods*, *7*(3), 29.

Mahakalkar, A., Kashyap, P., Bawankar, R., & Hatwar, B. (2014). The versatility of cow ghee-an ayurveda perspective. *American Journal of Drug Delivery and Therapeutics*, *1*(1), 28–34.

Maurice, B. (1987). Occurrence, absorption and metabolism of short chain fatty acids in the digestive tract of mammals. *Comparative Biochemistry and Physiology. B, Comparative Biochemistry*, *86*(3), 439–472.

Mulik, S. S., & Bhusari, D. P. (2013). Conceptual study of goghrita eye drops (aschyotana) in computer vision syndrome. *Asian Journal of Multidisciplinary Studies Oct*, *1*(3), 1–6.

Pandey, A. (2021). Therapeutic potential of vachadi ghrita (a medicated ghee) on CNS and other ailments—a review. *Journal of Ayurveda and Holistic Medicine (Jahm)*, *4*(3), 36–46.

Pandya, N. C., & Kanawjia, S. K. (2002). Ghee: A traditional nutraceutical. *Indian Dairyman*, *54*(10), 67–77.

Panjagari, N. R., & Ganguly, S. (2020). Packaging of dairy products. *Online Training for Master Trainers on Dairy Processing*, *131*.

Park, Y. W., & Haenlein, G. F. (Eds.). (2013). *Milk and dairy products in human nutrition: Production, composition and health*. John Wiley & Sons.

Patel, R. S., Mathur, R. S., Sheth, S. A., Patel, N. N., & Sharma, P. (2006). Industrial method of ghee making at panchmahal dairy, Godhra. *Indian Dairyman*, *58*(8), 49.

PFA. (2001). *Preventation of food adulteration Act, 1954 & Rules 1955*. Eastern BookCompany, 1267 Kashmir Gate.

Rajorhia, G. S. (1993). Ghee and anhydrous milk fat. In *Encyclopaedia of food science, food technology and nutrition* (Vol. –4, pp. 2186–2192). Pub. Academic Press.

Rani, R., & Kansal, V. K. (2012). Effects of cow ghee (clarified butter oil) & soybean oil on carcinogen-metabolizing enzymes in rats. *The Indian Journal of Medical Research*, *136*(3), 460–465.

Ray, P. R. (2019). Technological and biochemical aspects of ghee (butter oil). *Engineering Practices for Milk Products: Dairyceuticals, Novel Technologies, and Quality*, 83–109.

Shukla, D. J., Vyas, H. A., Vyas, M. K., Ashok, B. K., & Ravishankar, B. (2012). A comparative study on chronic administration of Go Ghrita (cow ghee) and Avika Ghrita (ewe ghee) in albino rats. *AYU*, *33*(3), 435–440.

Sindhuja, S., Prakruthi, M., Manasa, R., Shekhara Naik, R., & Shivananjappa, M. (2020). Health benefits of ghee (clarified butter)—A review from ayurvedic perspective. *IP Journal of Nutrition, Metabolism and Health Science*, *3*(3), 64–72.

Singh, S., & Ram, B. P. (1978). Effect of ripening of cream, manufacturing temperature and packaging materials on flavour and keeping quality of ghee. *Journal of Food Science and Technology*, *15*, 142–145.

Spiteller, G. (2007). Review the important role of lipid peroxidation processes in aging and age dependent diseases. *Molecular Biotechnology*, *37*(1), 5–12.

# 8 Long-Life Dairy Food—Powdered Milk

## 8.1 LEARNING OBJECTIVES

By the end of the chapter, the reader will be able to:

- Understand the composition and uses of various types of powdered milk
- Gain knowledge of the production and processing of powdered milk
- Learn about the functional advantages and applications of powdered milk
- Understand the detection of adulteration in powdered milk
- Learn how to judge and improve the quality of the powdered milk
- Make powdered milk enterprises profitable
- Know the key potential health benefits of powdered milk
- Discover powdered milk innovations from production to nutritional and health attributes

Powdered milk is a well-balanced combination of nutrients/good taste along with its new bioactive components beneficial to healthy aging. Supplemented milk powder improves glycemic control and insulin resistance in the elderly and improves bone mineral density in adolescents.

## 8.2 INTRODUCTION

Milk powder (also known as powdered milk, dried milk, or dry milk) is a suitable alternative for those who do not immediately have access to sufficient refrigeration and fresh dairy products (**Figure 8.1**). It is made by removing the water from milk. The main objective of milk powder manufacturing is to convert the liquid perishable raw material into a product that can be kept for a certain period without significantly losing quality due to low water activity that impedes microbial metabolism. It has numerous uses in bakeries, confectioneries, baby formula, nutritional foods, etc. (Caballero et al., 2015).

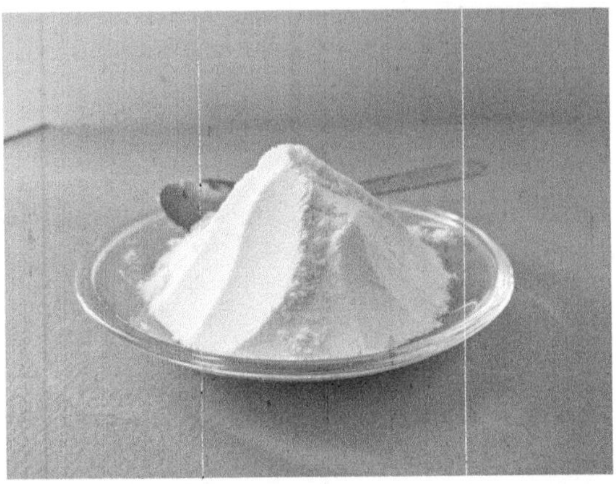

FIGURE 8.1 **Image of powdered milk.** Fresh instant full-cream milk powder is an easy-to-use product that may be reconstituted with water to make liquid milk. It is produced by extracting water from fresh milk and then spray drying the remaining milk solids to produce a powdered form.

The same dry milk product has gone by a number of names and is produced by leading companies (**Figure 8.2**). Some other names for non-fat dry milk are dried skim milk, non-fat dry milk solids, and skim milk powder (SMP).



DOI: 10.1201/9781003397786-8

**Key Players in Milk Powder**

Dairy farmers of America Inc.
Nestle
Nestle S.A
Danone
Friesland Campina
Arla Foods amba
Yili
Mengniu
Parmalate
Dean Foods company
Fonterra Co-operative Group
Burra Foods
Lactalis Group
Kraft Food Inc.
Ausino
Tarur

**FIGURE 8.2 Leading companies in the global powdered milk market.**

Dry whole milk, dry cream, dry buttermilk, and others are sometimes referred to as dried or powdered whole milk, despite their different identities (Caballero et al., 2015). Milk powders are used by consumers to make a range of processed food products and to substitute fresh milk. Milk powders need to be of a high standard if they are to be accepted by consumers and users of ingredients. Milk powders are made to meet a variety of specifications and compositional norms. These milk powders have been created by organizations including the American Dairy Products Institute, the International Dairy Federation, the Food and Agricultural Organization of the United Nations, and national food authorities in several countries. Milk powders vary in their functional properties while having a similar composition. Because dried milk and milk products have superior keeping qualities, need less storage space, and have reduced shipping costs, all of which are commercially desirable, there are strong signs that the manufacturing of these goods may increase in the future. Due to the superior keeping quality of non-fat dry milk, it is produced more often than whole-milk powder. The ultimate goal of the sector is to produce dry goods that, when mixed with water again, exhibit little to no change from the initial liquid product. While reconstituted non-fat dry milk is nearly comparable in flavor to the original skim milk, much improvement needs to be made with dry whole milk. The other aims are to ensure good keeping quality and a low manufacturing cost. During the flush season, dry milk gives a dairy plant a way to deal with the surplus milk supply, while during the lean season, milk intended for the manufacturing of dry milk may be switched to market milk. Consequently, dry milk might be referred to be the current dairy industry's balancing wheel.

### 8.2.1 Definition

The term "powdered milk" refers to milk products that are produced by partially removing the water from milk (Kalyankar et al., 2015). The only reason is the fat and/or protein content of the milk may be altered is to comply with the compositional requirements in Section 3 of the Codex Standard (Caballero et al., 2015) by adding or deleting milk components without affecting the milk's whey protein-to-casein ratio.

The product formed by removing water from milk by heat or other acceptable methods to produce a solid containing 5% or less moisture is known as dried milk or milk powder. Drying can be done using whole milk, defatted milk, or skim milk. The product made from skim milk is known as dried skim milk, skim milk powder, or non-fat dry milk (NFDM), whereas that made from whole milk is known as dried whole milk or whole-milk powder (WMP). There are distinct names assigned to the many dried milk products.

Milk powders are widely used as components in processed and produced dairy goods. Traditional recombined dairy products like evaporated milk, sweetened condensed milk, and UHT milk all include a sizable quantity of milk powder in nations where the availability of fresh milk is insufficient. A variety of culinary products, including ice cream, cultured milk and yogurts, chocolate, candies, baked goods, soups, and sauces, also use milk powder as an ingredient. In situations where increased dairy tastes are needed, buttermilk powders are utilized to substitute skim milk powder.

## 8.3 HISTORY AND DEVELOPMENT OF POWDERED MILK

**TABLE 8.1**
**Timeline Showing the Most Important Scientific Achievements Related to the Research on Powder Milk Production**

| Year | Achievements in powdered milk manufacturing |
|---|---|
| **13th century** | Marco Polo said that soldiers of Kublai Khan would bring dried milk with them during their trips. The common perception is that the milk underwent a fat removal process before it was dried through the application of solar heat. |
| **1832** | M. Dirchoff, a Russian scientist, developed the first usable commercial method for manufacturing dried milk. |
| **1850** | In order to create a solid, Birdseye condensed milk was made with more sugar. |
| **1855** | A modified dry product made by Grimwade utilizing sodium (or potassium) carbonate, sugar, and highly concentrated milk was granted a British patent. |
| **1855** | Despite William Newton having invented a vacuum drying method, T. S. Grimwade obtained a patent for a dried milk system. |
| **1898** | Patents and papers were published focused on methods for producing dry milk without the addition of additional products. |
| **1909** | Frenchman Nicholas Appert created dried milk tablets by air drying concentrated milk solids until they resembled "dough." |
| **1901** | Americans Campbell and Danish Wimmer dried condensed milk on trays. |
| **1902** | Hall received a patent for a novel method of producing dry condensed milk. |
| **1970** | Powdered milk was routinely created by spray drying non-fat skim milk, whole milk, buttermilk, or whey. Spray drying was invented in the 1920s and became well liked in powdered milk. |
| **1980** | Imported powdered milk had established itself as a key rival in developing nations for individuals who did not have access to refrigeration. |

## 8.4 TYPES OF POWDERED MILK

i. Full-fat milk powder
ii. Dry milk without fat
iii. Milk with malt
iv. Dried buttermilk
v. Dry whey
vi. Infant formula
vii. Special dried milk

These different types of dried milk are described along with their various uses.

### 8.4.1 Full-Fat Milk Powder

The end product of partially extracting the water from pasteurized milk is whole-milk powder (WMP). The powder can contain between 26% and 40% milk fat (by weight) on an "as-is" basis and offers all the nutritional qualities of milk in its dry form.

**Uses:** Used to improve food's dairy flavor, used in dairy reconstituted foods like yogurt, and used in making tea and coffee.

### 8.4.2 Non-Fat Dried Milk

Non-fat dried milk is white to light cream in color and has a definite dairy taste. It is obtained by removing the water from pasteurized skim milk. It has 1.5% or less milk fat and 5% or less moisture (by weight). It is sometimes referred to as skim milk powder.

**Uses:** Powdered milk can be used in lieu of fresh milk in baked items that call for milk.

### 8.4.3 Milk with Malt

A soluble powder created from a combination of malted barley, evaporated whole milk, and wheat flour.

**Uses:** Used to add its distinctive flavor to beverages and used in baking to aid with appropriate dough cooking.

### 8.4.4 Dried Buttermilk

A fermented dairy beverage is a buttermilk. It has a light cream hue and a smooth, gratifying, sweet dairy flavor. Dry buttermilk (DBM) is made by pasteurizing and drying liquid buttermilk that was created during the churning of butter. DBM contains no less than 30% protein.

**Uses:** Used in baking to aid with appropriate dough cooking and enrich the nutritive value of prepared foods, bread, and ice cream.

### 8.4.5 Dry Whey

Dry whey is the material that is produced when water is removed from whey while maintaining all other ingredients in their original relative proportions.

### 8.4.6 Infant Formula

Infant formula is often created from cow's milk that has undergone various treatments to make it better suited for infants.

### 8.4.7 Special Dried Milk

Special dried milk is manufactured depending on specific diseases, health status, age, etc.

**Other special dried milk:**

**Diabetic milk:** Unlike regular milk, it does not increase the blood sugar level.

**Milk for growing-age children:** Milk contains pro-bones, minerals, immune guards, energy boosters, and brain developers.

**Nutrients:** Vitamin A, B complex, D, E, K, calcium, magnesium, iodine.

**Milk for pregnant women:** This special type of milk for pregnant women contains probiotics, folic acid, iron, calcium, vitamins, and choline.

**Milk for old age (40+):** This kind of special milk is for those who need more calcium intake because as we grow, our calcium intake gets low. This type of milk contains more calcium than other conventional milk.

**Instant milk:** Instant milk powder has one major advantage over regular powdered milk. It mixes up much more easily. Regular non-fat milk is used to make instant milk powder. Phospholecithin is used as an emulsifier, which is why it can dissolve more quickly than normal powder milk.

## 8.5 NUTRITIONAL FACTS

The nutritional content of milk is largely retained by contemporary drying techniques. While it seems like lysine is only slightly destroyed during spray drying, more lysine is destroyed with roller drying's intense heat treatment. Large amounts of calcium, phosphorus, and vitamin A may be found in dry whole milk. Additionally, it is a good source of riboflavin. Unfortunately, it loses some vitamins like $B_1$, $B_6$, $B_{12}$, vitamin C, and some minerals. Different types of milk powder compositions are illustrated in **Table 8.2.**

**TABLE 8.2**
**Different Types of Powdered Milk Composition (%)**

| Type of dried milk | Type/brand | Moisture | Fat | Protein | Lactose | Ash | Lactic acid | Carbohydrate |
|---|---|---|---|---|---|---|---|---|
| Whole-milk powder | – | 2.0 | 27.4 | 26.5 | 38.2 | 5.9 | – | – |
| Non-fat dry milk | – | 3.0 | 0.8 | 35.9 | 52.3 | 8.0 | – | – |
| Malted milk | – | 3.22 | 7.55 | 13.19 | 72.40 | 3.66 | – | – |
| Buttermilk powder | Sweet | 2.8 | 5.3 | 34.3 | 50.0 | 7.6 | – | – |
| | Sour | 4.4 | 5.7 | 37.6 | 38.8 | 7.4 | 5.7 | – |
| Whey powder | Cheddar cheese whey | 4.5 | 0.9 | 12.9 | 73.5 | 8.0 | 2.3 | – |
| | Cottage cheese whey | 3.2 | 0.0 | 13.0 | 66.5 | 10.2 | 8.6 | – |
| Infant formula | Amul | 3.0 | 18.0 | 22.0 | – | 5.0 | – | 52.0 |
| | Glaxo | 2.9 | 26.5 | 24.9 | – | 5.6 | – | 38.5 |
| | Lactogen | 3.0 | 19.0 | 21.6 | – | 4.8 | – | 50.8 |

*Source:* Anandharamakrishnan, 2017

## 8.6 WORLDWIDE MILK POWDER PRODUCTION AND CONSUMPTION TRENDS

In 2020, the global total output of milk powder was 11.10 million metric tons, with a 20% increase projected between 2021 and 2026. Surprisingly, the top ten highest-generating countries produce nearly 90% of the global amount. New Zealand was the biggest producer of all sorts of milk powder, with 1.535 million metric tons produced yearly. China produced 1.2 million metric tons of milk powder, followed by Brazil (580 thousand metric tons), Argentina (250 thousand metric tons), and Mexico (129 thousand metric tons). Other notable manufacturers of milk powder worldwide were Indonesia, Chile, the United States of America, Russia, and Australia. **Table 8.3** describes the top powdered milk (dry whole powdered milk)-consuming countries in the world in 2021.

**TABLE 8.3**
**Top Powdered Milk-Consuming Countries in the World in 2021**

| Rank | Country | Production (1000 MT) |
|---|---|---|
| 1 | China | 1940 |
| 2 | New Zealand | 1555 |
| 3 | Brazil | 670 |
| 4 | Algeria | 270 |
| 5 | Argentina | 258 |
| 6 | Indonesia | 141 |

## 8.7 ROLE OF MILK CONSTITUENTS

Dried milk constituents play a specific role that determines the possibility of forming quality dried milk powder.

### 8.7.1 Milk Proteins

The behavior of the caseinate system and, in particular, the aggregation of casein particles by heat, salts, acid, etc., are at the heart of many of the issues with dairy technology. Milk proteins are easily altered by heat processing and to some extent by storage; these alterations have a negative impact on their solubility or dispersibility. As the heat treatment intensifies, it causes irreversible denaturation (coagulation), which further destabilizes the proteins by causing first-stage denaturation. It appears that some proteins, most likely lactoglobulin, are sources of the sulfhydryl chemicals responsible for the cooked and caramelized flavor.

### 8.7.2 Milk Fat

This may be present in dried milk or milk products either in the original globule, i.e., in de-emulsified form, in emulsion form, or as free fat. Free fat adds an oily finish to the reconstituted milk and makes the dry product greasy. The unsaturated fatty acids of milk fat, e.g., oleic acid, have a significant impact on oxidative degradation. Free fat promotes oxidation. The oxidized flavor of milk appears to be caused by its phospholipids. Butyric acid, which is generated when glycerides are digested by the action of the lipase enzyme, is primarily responsible for the sour flavor of milk.

### 8.7.3 Milk Sugar

This is crucial to the production and preservation of dried milk products. Lactose is still present in the amorphous or glass (non-crystalline) state in freshly dried milk. It rapidly collects moisture when exposed to the atmosphere in this state since it is very hygroscopic, which leads to crystallization. This absorbed humidity then causes the powder to become sticky and then to cake (this tendency toward stickiness and caking increases in the presence of lactic acid). The browning (color defect) of dried milk products can occur during production, primarily as a result of high temperatures and prolonged heat exposure. Browning discoloration may also occur during storage, especially under conditions of high moisture, high storage temperature, and packaging in air-packed containers—all of which hasten and intensify browning.

### 8.7.4 Milk Salts

These have a significant impact on the physical condition and stability of milk proteins, especially the caseinates. The optimum heat stability, according to Sommer and Hart's well-known "salt balance theory," requires the proper ratio of calcium and magnesium ions to citrate and phosphate ions (Webb et al., 1965). This equilibrium is easily broken by slight pH and salt balance changes, which also tend to destabilize and precipitate the casein particles. Low solubility will be seen in the resulting dry milk (dispersibility). Copper and iron exert a catalytic action in the oxidation of milk lipids, which produces undesirable flavors in dried milk products.

## 8.8 MANUFACTURING PROCESS

The technological steps of the production of milk powder are illustrated in **Figures 8.3 and 8.4.** There are two methods:

i. Cold treatment
ii. Heat treatment

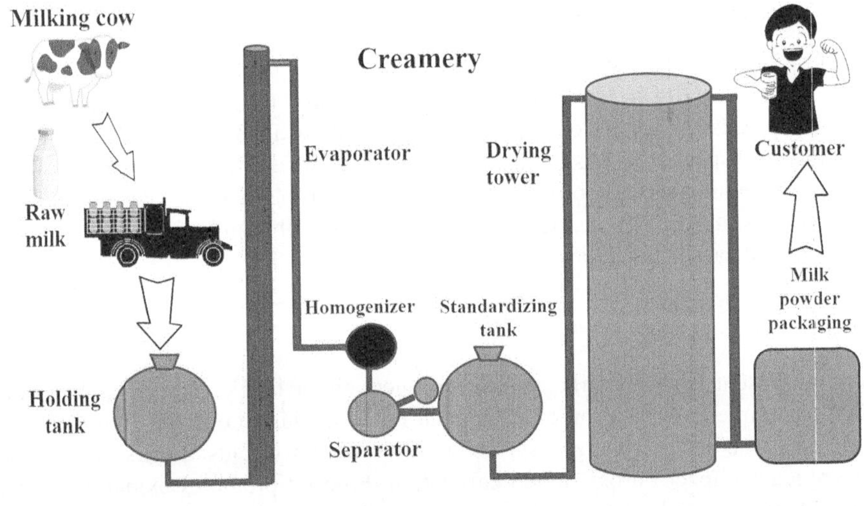


**FIGURE 8.3 Pictorial diagram of the milk powder production process.**

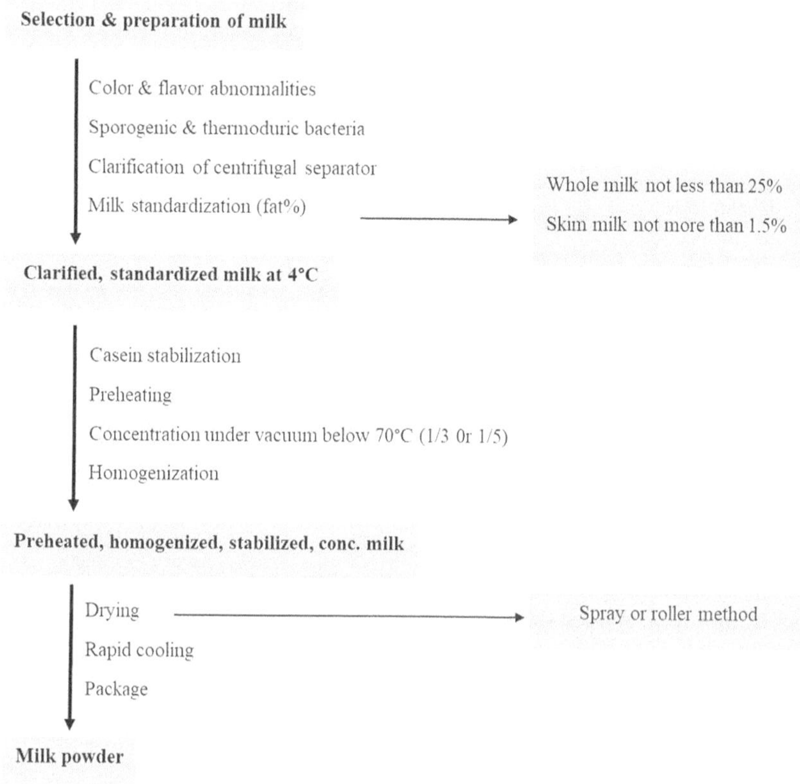


**FIGURE 8.4 Technological steps for the production of powdered milk.**

### 8.8.1 Cold Treatment (Freeze Drying)

- Cold treatment processes include concentration freezing, sublimation, cake formation, grinding, high vacuum belt drying, and screening.
- A thin layer of the liquid is frozen, where upon the ice is sublimated under a high vacuum.
- A voluminous cake is left (the space of the ice crystal is now occupied by holes) and is subsequently grounded.
- A batch processing or a continuous operation in a high-vacuum belt drier can be applied.

#### 8.8.1.1 Merits of Freeze Drying

- Can be designed for continuous operation.
- Almost complete absence of air.
- Moisture content of the final product remains very low.
- Heat damage to protein stability, flavor, solubility, and color of the final product is minimal.

#### 8.8.1.2 Demerits of Freeze Drying

- Fat globules undergo partial coalescence. It causes freeze-dried whole-milk powder to segregate after reconstitution.
- The plant is complicated.
- Very expensive and thus not suitable for commercial production.

#### 8.8.1.3 Technological Steps of Milk Powder Production

### 8.8.2 Heat Treatment

It includes three processes:

i. Drum drying process
ii. Spray drying process
iii. Foam spray drying process

#### 8.8.2.1 Drum Drying Process

The milk is applied in a thin coating to the smooth surface of a constantly spinning, steam-heated metal drum, roller, or cylinder. The milk is ideally concentrated. A sanitary knife, doctor blade, or scraper is continually scraping the dried milk film off in the opposite direction from where the milk is applied. For the powder to be produced, the milk film must be crushed. Drum drying includes two methods, the atmospheric process and the vacuum process.

**Atmospheric Process** Commonly used in the production of dry skim milk, dried sour cream, and dried buttermilk.

**Vacuum Process** In this process, milk is dried at a lower temperature; thus, the quality of the final product is improved. A vacuum is used in this process.

##### *8.8.2.1.1 Advantages of Drum Drying*

- Capital and operational costs are quite modest.
- Plant is portable, manageable, and takes up little floor space.
- Effective for producing tiny amounts of milk.
- Produces milk powder that is more suited for storage.

##### *8.8.2.1.2 Disadvantages of Drum Drying*

- Low-quality milk powder is produced.
- Provides reconstituted milk with a cooked/scorched taste.

#### 8.8.2.2 Spray Drying Process

This calls for a large drying chamber into which hot air is rapidly blasted (**Figure 8.5**). Usually, a suction pan is used to extract some of the milk's water first. In the heated chamber where the outgoing air is, the condensed milk is subsequently sprayed or atomized. Through free-meshed screens, which are frequently employed, the air is filtered. Dried milk that has landed on the drying chamber's flooring is removed mechanically or by suction (Schuck et al., 2009) (**Figure 8.6**).

##### *8.8.2.2.1 Advantages of Spray Drying*

- Superior quality in appearance, flavor, and solubility.
- Most economic when large quantities of milk are handled.
- Suitable for industrial production.

##### *8.8.2.2.2 Disadvantages of the Spray Drying Process*

- Large capital investment.
- Plant is complicated.

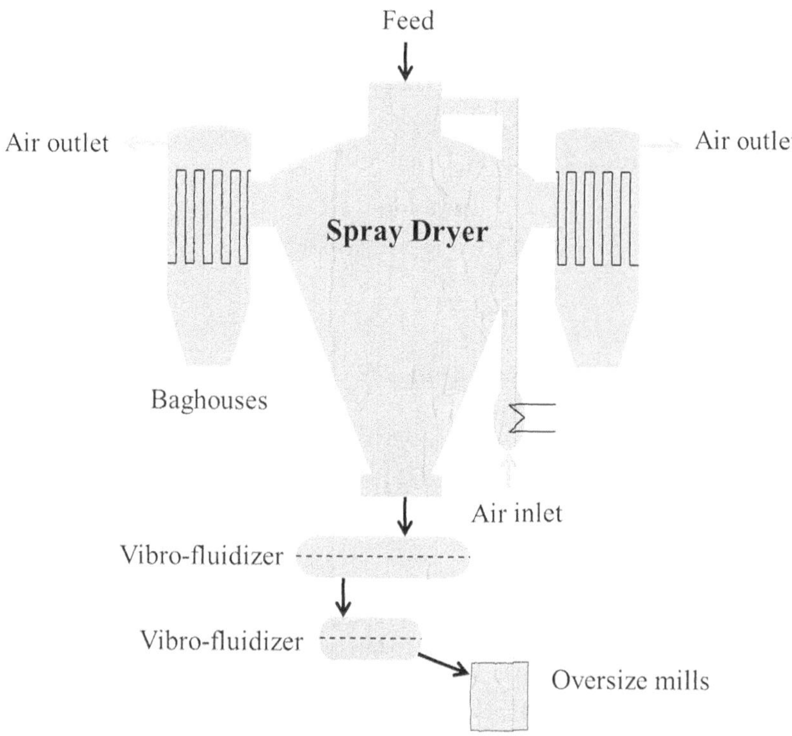


**FIGURE 8.5** Industrial powdered milk spray dryer with the internal fluid bed.

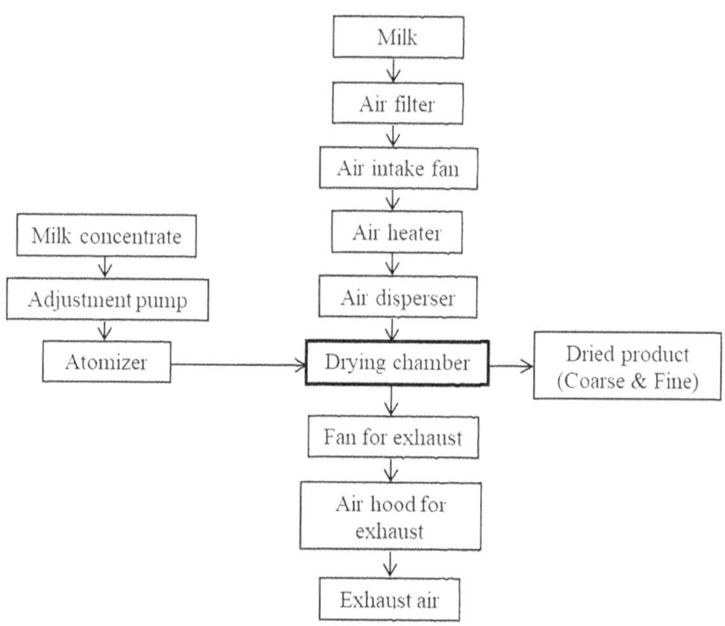


**FIGURE 8.6** General flow diagram of the procedure of spray drying.

The comparison between drum- and spray-dried milk is shown in **Table 8.4**.

**TABLE 8.4**
**Comparison between Drum- and Spray-Dried Milk**

| Properties | Drum dried | Spray dried |
|---|---|---|
| Color and appearance | Deep yellow or greenish white | Light yellow or creamy white |
| Flavor | Heated/cooled | Same as pasteurized milk |
| Surface | Wrinkled | Smooth |
| Particle size | 8–20 μm | 10–25 μm |
| Shape | Irregular/angular | Regular/spherical |
| Air cells | Absent | Present (one or more) |
| Bulk density | 0.3–0.5 g/ml | 0.5–0.6 g/ml |
| Solubility | 85% | 98% |

#### 8.8.2.3 Foam Spray Drying Process

This is done by forcing the "gas" into the liquid product after the pump but before the atomizer. Air is commonly used as the added gas for making foam-spray non-fat dry milk and nitrogen for foam-spray dried whole milk. Common dairy products such as skim milk, whole milk, buttermilk, sweet and sour cream, whey, and emulsified cheese slurry can be foam-spray dried.

##### *8.8.2.3.1 Advantages of Foam Spray Drying Process*

- Suitable for drying specialized goods such as whey, cottage cheese, and malted milk.
- The particles of the dried products are more uniform in size.

##### *8.8.2.3.2 Disadvantages of Foam Spray Drying Process*

- Low bulk density of non-fat dry milk (less than or equal to 0.35 g/ml).
- Higher packaging cost.

A process flow diagram for the spray-drying system used to produce whole-milk powder (WMP) and skim milk powder (SMP) is shown in **Figure 8.7**.

A process flow diagram for making whole-milk powder (WMP) and skim milk powder (SMP) using a drum dryer is shown in **Figure 8.8**.

## 8.9 HUMANIZED BABY MILK POWDER FROM COW'S MILK

Formula milk, often known as baby formula or infant formula, is typically prepared from processed cow's milk. Various procedures have been devised for producing adapted or "humanized" products from cow's milk, the content of which is as near to that of mother's milk as feasible. In one approach, "humanized" milk is made by partially demineralizing whey over ion-exchange resins and then adding milk enhanced in lactose, fat, minerals, and vitamins to it (**Figure 8.9**).

## 8.10 FUNCTIONAL PROPERTIES

As a food ingredient, milk powder offers a variety of functional advantages (**Table 8.5**). The three main milk powder ingredients—proteins, lactose, and milk—affect the way milk powder functions and whether it is suitable for a certain application (Attaie et al., 2003; Tamime, 2009).

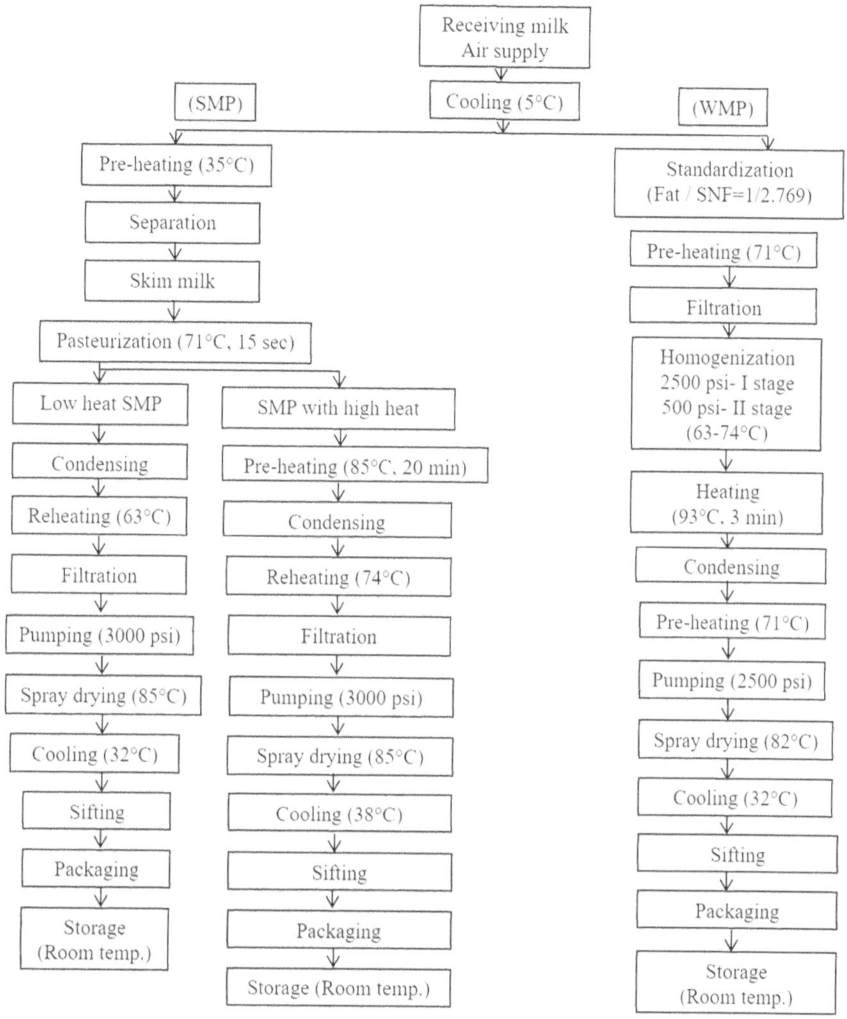


**FIGURE 8.7 General flow diagram for the manufacturing of WMP and SMP by spray drying.**

## 8.11 PACKAGING AND STORAGE OF POWDERED MILK

Dried milk powder packaging is significant because it affects marketing, quality, safety, and customer acceptance. Milk powder should be packed to avoid contact with moisture, light, and oxygen since milk powder is susceptible to lipid oxidation due to its hygroscopicity and fat content. Innovative technologies have recently been launched to increase the functionality of packaging materials and improve the quality of food, such as active packaging, intelligent packaging, and nanotechnology. This entails enhancing barrier qualities, using indicators to detect deterioration and freshness, and adding active substances to extend the shelf life of the packaged dairy product.

Dry milk is hygroscopic, and it must be protected from moisture during packaging and storage. Dry whole milk for export or use in infant formula is packed in tin containers in which the atmosphere has been replaced by an inert gas such as nitrogen or carbon dioxide to minimize the oxidative changes that may occur during storage. Non-fat dry milk is packed in barrels with moisture-proof double liners, containers, or corrugated paper.

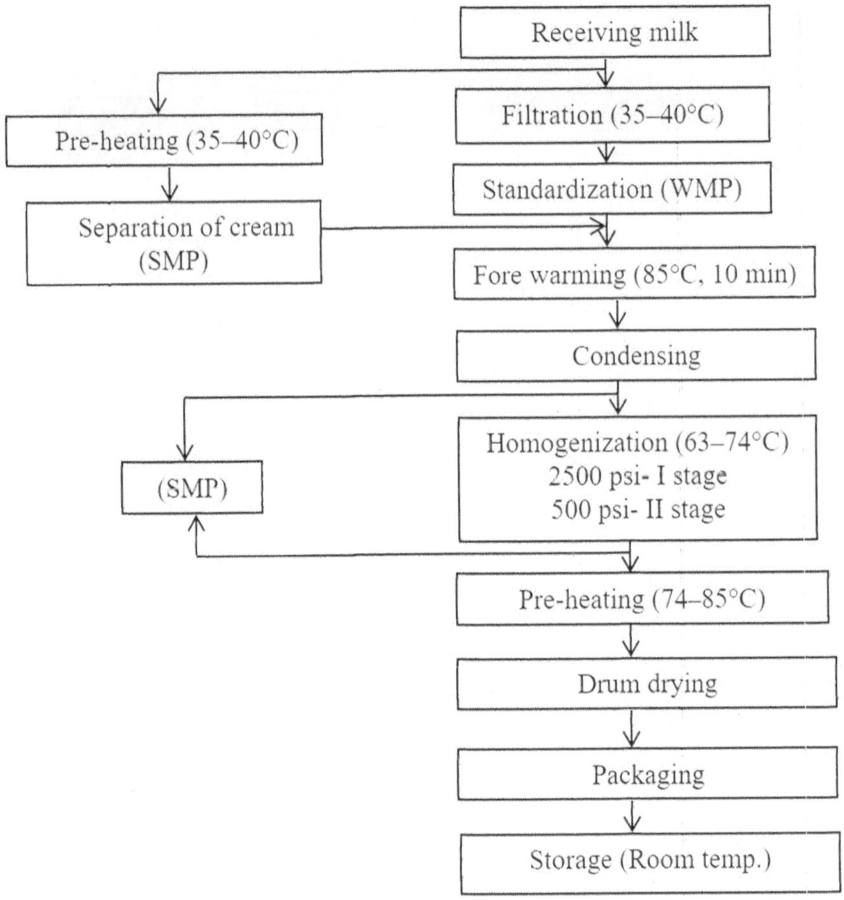


**FIGURE 8.8 The general manufacturing procedure for WMP and SMP by drum drying.**

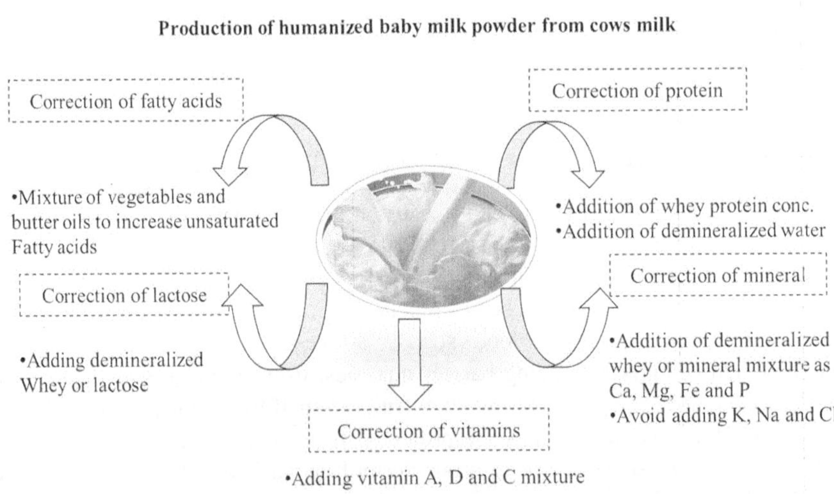


**FIGURE 8.9 General flow diagram for the manufacturing of humanized baby powdered milk from cow's milk.**

**TABLE 8.5**
**Functional Advantages and Applications of Powdered Milk**

| Function | Benefits | Applications |
|---|---|---|
| Browning/color | Highlights the development of color when heating and baking. Helps to improve the color of viscous foods like sauces and soups. | Baked goods, confections, mixed dairy and milk, dietary beverages, finished goods, soups and sauces |
| Flavor enhancement | Baking and heating may give a baked taste. This can offer notes of creamy dairy and ensures a uniform dispersion of taste. | Baked goods, confections, dairy/recombined milk, meat, beverages |
| Emulsification | Prevents fat globules from forming one large mass, improving product appearance. All-natural emulsifying ingredient. | Baked goods, confections, dairy/recombined milk, beverages, prepared foods |
| Gelling and heat setting | Enhances the mouthfeel. Helps create the smooth, creamy feel of fat, increasing the attractiveness of lower-fat goods to consumers. | Confections, dairy/recombined milk, meat, prepared foods |
| Solubility | Some milk powders mix easily with meals. Prevents settling in drinks, soups, and sauces. | Bakery, beverages, confections, frozen desserts, infant formula, soups and sauces |
| Water binding and viscosity building | Allows for a decrease in the amount of fat by giving items qualities similar to those of fat. | Baked goods, confections, dairy/recombined milk, nutritional beverages, prepared foods |
| Whipping, foaming, and aeration | Maintains foam characteristics, improving the end product's flavor and texture as well as its aesthetic attractiveness. | Baked products, confections, dairy/recombined milk, beverages |

Powdered milk has a long shelf life. Most manufacturers advise consuming powdered milk within 18 months of purchase; however, this is only a "best by" date. Powdered milk, according to the USDA, may be kept forever. An unopened product is likely to be usable for 2 to 10 years beyond the indicated "best by" date.

## 8.12 HYGIENIC ASPECTS

The specifications for the bacteriological purity of milk powder partially rely on the application for which it is intended, as well as the production procedure. For instance, it matters if the powder is intended for immediate consumption or if it undergoes a heat treatment following reconstitution (for example, in recombined milk). Many germs may survive the production process as the low-heat treatment used to produce (skim) milk powder, is often not more intensive than the low heat (72°C for 20 s) heat treatment used to pasteurize milk.

There are three possible reasons why milk powder could be unsafe (Walstra et al., 2006):

i. Fresh milk contains microorganisms that are not destroyed by the heat treatments are applied to it before and during drying.
ii. Conditions can support the growth of some bacterial species during the various manufacturing phases until the product is dry.
iii. Incidental contamination may happen during manufacturing. The degree of contamination is often modest and stays low if the contaminated bacteria are prevented from growing.

### 8.12.1 Bacteria in the Original Milk

Psychotropic Gram-negative rods can form in deep-cooled milk after extended storage (e.g., *Pseudomonas* spp.). These bacteria, as is widely known, cannot endure even a low-heat treatment.

These rods' produced proteinases and lipases could endure and end up absorbed into the powder. It is important to prevent contamination and growth while storing thermalized milk.

### 8.12.2 Growth during Manufacture

Some thermophilic bacteria can easily develop during the various manufacturing phases because of the temperature and water activity levels, and drying does not completely or effectively destroy them. The kind of bacteria is frequently indicative of the source of the infection.

### 8.12.3 Incidental Contamination

A distinction can be found between contamination during or after drying (dry part) and contamination before drying (wet portion). These sorts of contamination-related bacteria often do not develop during the procedure and add little to the powder's bacterial count.

## 8.13 INSTANTIZATION

Compared to other milk powders, instant milk powder has greater reconstitution abilities. The instantization method, which Peebles developed, greatly enhanced the drying technology's efficiency and quality. The main goal of instantiating is to increase the speed and thoroughness of milk powder reconstitutability. Producing particles with a high surface-to-mass ratio is the goal of the spray-drying process. Small powder particles are difficult to reconstitute in water, and their dispersion requires vigorous mixing. Instant powder production by agglomeration is one of the main goals of advances in the spray- and fluid bed-drying fields. Agglomeration creates the structure of porous aggregates that disperse easily and quickly to generate stable reconstituted milk without the need for intense agitation. The instantizing process enhances the wettability, penetrability, sinkability, dispensability, and dissolvability of dry materials (Millqvist-Fureby & Smith, 2007). The procedure enables a better balance between these factors. Either the rewetting process, where the instantization is completed after the powder is received in dry form, or the straight-through technique, where the instantization is completed while drying, can produce a successful agglomeration. The raw material for the rewetting process is dry MP. Powder particle agglomeration results from the powder being disseminated in the wetting chamber and gaining a water content of 5–10%. The agglomerated product is moved to the vibrating fluid bed dryer and cooler, where it is instantly chilled to around 10°C after being re-dried in a hot airstream at 90–120°C. The fluid bed dryer produces a finished product with a water concentration of 4% (2–4%). Hot air, forced upward via the fluid bed dryer's, fluidizes the powder and carries the smallest powder particles or fines to the cyclone, where separation occurs. After the heat and solids have been recovered and the fines have been returned to the process' beginning, the air is released into the atmosphere. WMP has a milk fat film covering the surface of the particles, complicating the instantization process. Free fat coats the particle surfaces with a hydrophobic coating, impregnating them and reducing their capacity to bind water. Powder particles are lecithinated by adding lecithin combined with butter oil before instantization to avoid this and enhance the recombination characteristics. The particles are cycled back to the wet zone when the powder is dried in two phases throughout this operation. To prevent the agglomerates from disintegrating, the lecithinated powder needs to be chilled and packaged in an appropriate material.

## 8.14 ADULTERATION OF POWDERED MILK

Adulteration is the process of adding substances to gain profit through an unfair process. In dried milk, the most common adulterants are melamine, caustic soda, bleaching powder, vegetable fat, expired milk powder, synthetic powdered milk etc.

### 8.14.1 Melamine

A chemical compound that contains high nitrogen is mainly used to increase the percentage of protein in proximate analysis, even though the dried milk doesn't possess that amount of protein. If melamine is used, a false reading of protein may be found.

### 8.14.2 Caustic Soda and Bleaching Powder

Recently, in the dried milk of a few companies, some dangerous chemicals like bleaching powder and caustic soda have been found to be used for attractive color and texture. These chemicals are very harmful to human health.

### 8.14.3 Vegetable Fat

Vegetable fat is mixed with skim milk powder and marketed as full cream milk powder. People in developing countries continue to drive the demand for affordable milk powder, so they can turn to vegetable fat-filled milk powders to meet their needs.

### 8.14.4 Expired Milk Powder

Expired milk powder can be mixed with fresh milk powder and marketed as fresh powdered milk. It is most common in developing countries, including Bangladesh.

### 8.14.5 Synthetic Powdered Milk

Maize powder, calcium carbonate, dried milk flavor, expired milk powder, and some unknown chemical substances are used to make synthetic powdered milk. This product is marketed as fresh milk powder by some miscreant businessmen. This is an inhumane practice that is very dangerous for our health.

## 8.15 DEFECTS IN POWDERED MILK

A defect is defined as a lack of something that results in its incompleteness, inadequacy, or imperfection. There are three types of defects in powdered milk.

i. Flavor defects (**Table 8.6**)
ii. Body and texture defects (**Table 8.7**)
iii. Color and appearance defects (**Table 8.8**)

### 8.15.1 Flavor Defects

**TABLE 8.6**
**Flavor Defects, Causes, and Possible Remedies**

| Name of defect | Causes | Remedies |
|---|---|---|
| Stale or aged | i. High-temperature extended storage<br>ii. Excessively high preheating temperature<br>iii. Removing the dried product from the drying chamber and delaying cooling<br>iv. High moisture content during storage | i. Short storage and storage at low temperatures (24°C or 75°F or below)<br>ii. Optimum preheating temperature<br>iii. Removal of the dried product from the drying chamber as soon as it has cooled<br>iv. Ideal moisture level for storage |

*(Continued)*

**TABLE 8.6 *(Continued)***
**Flavor Defects, Causes, and Possible Remedies**

| Name of defect | Causes | Remedies |
|---|---|---|
| Oxidized | i. High-temperature storage<br>ii. Action of sunlight (because of transparent packaging material)<br>iii. High acidity in milk<br>iv. Metallic (copper and iron) contamination due to direct contact with milk<br>v. Excessively high preheating temperature<br>vi. Delayed cooling and product removal from the drying chamber<br>vii. Higher oxygen content in the headspace of the container | i. Storage at low temperature<br>ii. Avoid the action of sunlight by using opaque packaging material<br>iii. Using fresh, sweet milk<br>iv. Using stainless steel/aluminum alloy milk contact surface only<br>v. Optimum preheating temperature<br>vi. Removal of the dried product from the drying chamber as soon as it has finished cooling<br>vii. Vacuuming or gas packaging |
| Rancid | Low preheating temperature (lipase not inactivated) | Optimum preheating temperature (50°C to inactivate lipase) |
| Scorched/burnt | i. Excessively high temperature of drying (in drum process)<br>ii. If the surface of the drum is pitted<br>iii. Sharpening scraper knives (in drum process) | i. Optimum drying temperature (in drum process)<br>ii. Maintaining the drum's surface smooth.<br>iii. Scraper knives kept sharp |
| Cooked flavor | Any stage of milk processing that involves overheating | Recommended timing and temperature settings for processing |

### 8.15.2 Body and Texture Defects

**TABLE 8.7**
**Body and Texture Defects, Causes, and Possible Remedies**

| Name of defect | Causes | Remedies |
|---|---|---|
| Lumpy body | i. Inadequate drying<br>ii. Taking up moisture (due to exposure to a humid atmosphere)<br>iii. Drippage from a pressure spray nozzle | i. Adequate drying<br>ii. Employing packaging that is moisture-impervious to stop moisture from being absorbed<br>iii. Using a centrifugal disc atomizer |
| Gummy body | Caused by the large proportion of high-melting triglycerides (solid fat) | Elimination of feeds containing high-melting-points fats |
| Leaky body | Caused by the presence of high temperature of churning and wash water | At various phases of processing, the control methods include appropriate working, optimal churning, and utilization of the right temperature. |

### 8.15.3 Color and Appearance Defects

**TABLE 8.8**
**Color and Appearance Defects, Causes, and Possible Remedies**

| Name of defect | Causes | Remedies |
|---|---|---|
| Browning/darkening of color | i. Long storage<br>ii. High-temperature storage<br>iii. Removing the dried product from the drying chamber and delaying cooling<br>iv. High moisture content during storage | i. Short storage<br>ii. Low-temperature storage<br>iii. Removal of the dried product from the drying chamber as soon as it has finished cooling<br>iv. Optimum moisture content during storage |
| Charred or burned look | i. Very high drying temperature<br>ii. The drum's surface is pitted | i. Optimum drying temperature<br>ii. Drum surface kept smooth |
| Lack of uniformity in appearance | i. Partial scorching during manufacture<br>ii. Partial discoloration after packaging | i. Careful control of operators<br>ii. Careful control of storage conditions influencing discoloration |

## 8.16 HEALTH BENEFITS OF POWDERED MILK

Powdered milk has the same nutritional value as fresh milk. It offers minerals that help develop bones, including protein, calcium, and vitamins A, D, E, and K. Protein-rich powdered milk can be used in recipes to boost their protein and energy levels (especially for people with health conditions that need extra protein) (Davoodi et al., 2016). Whole-milk powder is also one of the best proteins and amino acid sources, including immunoglobulins, protease-peptones, alpha-lactoglobulin, etc. Additionally, it contains lactose, which does not increase blood glucose and is digested more slowly than glucose and fructose. **Figure 8.10** summarizes the health claims considered here that are related to it.

### 8.16.1 Association of Powdered Milk Consumption with Cardiovascular Health

A smart way to supplement a diet with the micronutrients it lacks is through milk powder. Research has revealed that the use of milk powder supplemented with potassium and phytosterols, together with other preventive treatments, provides an efficient way to slow the sharp rise in cardiovascular problems across a number of nations (Gandola et al., 2019). The risk of cardiovascular disease may be decreased by this fortified milk powder, which results in lowering blood pressure and low-density lipoprotein levels. Overall, the intake of dairy products, excluding butter, has been linked to reduced arterial stiffness and a decreased risk of stroke (Diez-Fernăndez et al., 2019). Despite the high levels of saturated fat in whole milk and whole powdered milk, evidence suggests that dairy consumption has a favorable or indifferent impact on people's cardiovascular health (Thorning et al., 2016).

### 8.16.2 Association of Powdered Milk Consumption with Diabetes Prevention

Researchers have investigated the effects of milk powder supplemented with insulin and resistant dextrin on glycemic management, insulin resistance, and blood pressure in older individuals with type 2 diabetes mellitus (Cai et al., 2018). A unique set of substances, including oxylipins and endocannabinoids, were discovered in research to be present in the blood plasma of diet-induced obese rats that were fed a diet high in non-fat milk powder and calcium. These animals had much less fat accumulation, less adiposity, less inflammation in the fat tissues, and better glucose homeostasis (Cai et al., 2018). Consuming modest amounts of dairy products, especially powdered milk, has

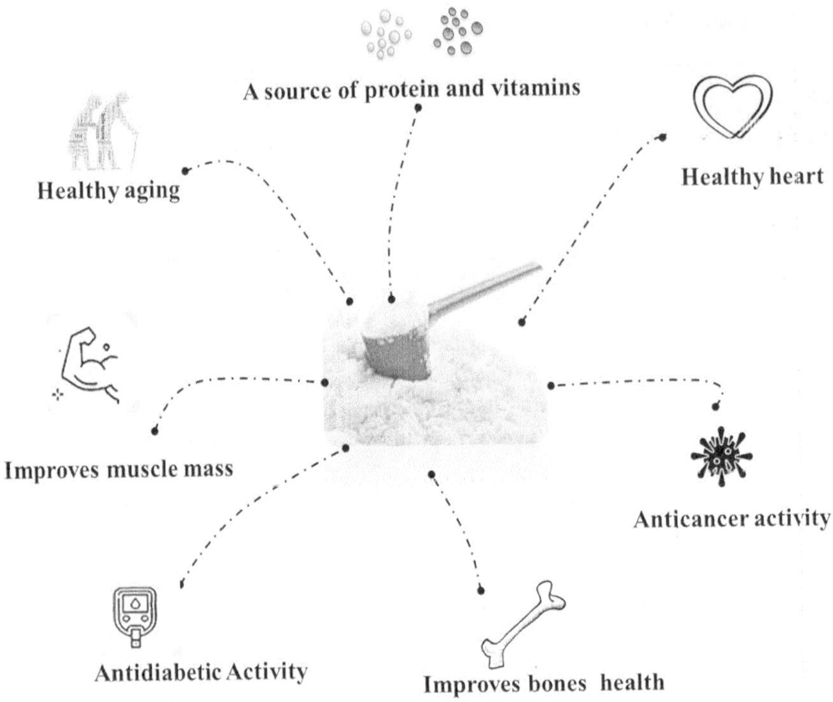


FIGURE 8.10 **Key potential health benefits of powdered milk.** Powdered milk is high in amino acids, calcium, potassium, phosphorus, and protein, all of which are beneficial to bone health. Many kinds are additionally supplemented with vitamin D, which aids in calcium absorption.

been linked to a lower incidence of type 2 diabetes mellitus as well as positive changes in waist circumference, body mass index, and blood pressure (Cai et al., 2018). Additionally, research has been done on camel milk powder as a possible functional food to help prevent type 2 diabetes mellitus (Mirmiran et al., 2017).

### 8.16.3 Association of Powdered Milk Consumption with Bone Health

Dairy products are crucial for strong bones due to their high calcium content. High dairy intake can support oral health maintenance and osteoporosis prevention. Hormonal changes put postmenopausal women at an increased risk of getting osteoporosis. Healthy postmenopausal women who consume high-calcium milk powder significantly decrease bone loss at the lumbar spine. The added benefit of supplementing with high-calcium milk powder was that it prevented height reduction (Chen et al., 2015). Children's bone development can also be accelerated by using milk powder supplements (Chen et al., 2015). Milk powder supplementation, however, may not have a substantial impact on bone mineralization and turnover in healthy pubescent teenagers (Lu et al., 2019).

### 8.16.4 Association of Powdered Milk Consumption with Cancer Prevention

The link between dairy consumption and cancer risk has not been conclusively shown by studies. According to research, drinking milk reduces the incidence of bladder and colorectal cancer (Barrubés et al., 2019). The main protein in milk powder, casein, has an anticarcinogenic effect. Additionally, whey-containing diets have been demonstrated to lower breast and colon malignancies in experimental animals (Davoodi et al., 2016).

### 8.16.5 Association of Fat-Free Powdered Milk Consumption with Health Benefits

i. Supplies a good source of protein
ii. Offers a source of calcium
iii. Takes care of the body from diseases
iv. Maintains a healthy heart and slim body
v. Provides all nutritional constituents of calcium, proteins, vitamins, and carbohydrates

## 8.17 POWDERED MILK INNOVATIONS

The benefits of powdered milk to human health have recently been recognized globally, and usage is likely to rise significantly in the next years, particularly in developing nations. This is especially due to the progress that has been made in the past decade in all areas of research related to powdered milk, from production to nutritional and health attributes. Recent research on the role of spray drying, along with other processes, in the development of dairy ingredients for applications in chocolate and the preparation of microencapsulated powders, lactose-free skimmed milk powder, milk powder for immune booster, etc., has been done. Low-heat treatment (spray drying) makes the powder easier to reconstitute and keeps the biological availability of the bioactive compounds. **Figures 8.11 and 8.12** illustrate powdered milk innovations from production to nutritional and health attributes (Patel, 2015; Sunartaty, 2019).

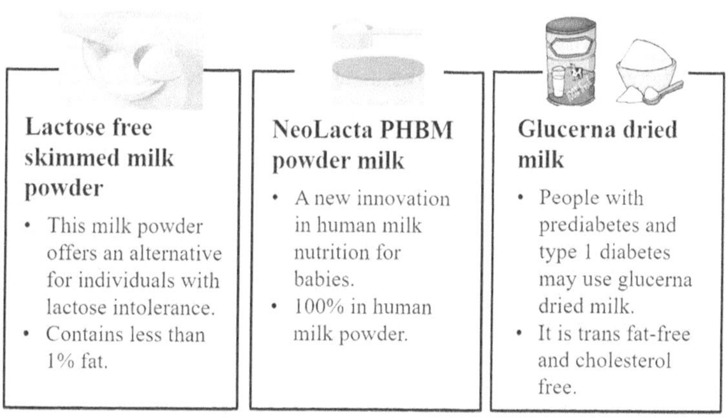


**FIGURE 8.11 Powdered milk innovations in production attributes.** Powdered milk has changed a lot, such as chocolate, the preparation of microencapsulated powders, and so on.

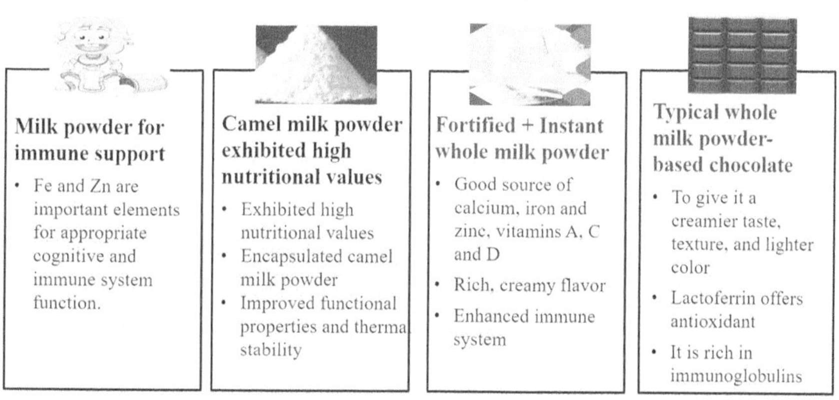


**FIGURE 8.12 Powdered milk innovations in nutritional and health attributes.** To meet the increased demand for health and nutritional products, manufacturers are developing powdered milk including changes in the fat quantity and source, protein boosts, etc.

## 8.18 POWDERED MILK YIELD

**Skim milk:** Considering the skim milk of 9% SNF, then quantity required for 1 kg powdered milk will be (1.0/9) × 100 =11.11 liter

**Whole milk**: Considering the whole milk of 12% total solids, then quantity required for 1 kg of powdered milk will be (1.0/12) × 100 = 8.33 liter. Thus, theoretically 8.5 liters fresh milk will produce 1 kg of powdered milk.

## 8.19 CONCLUSIONS

Powdered milk is an acceptable substitute for people who do not have rapid access to sufficient refrigeration systems and dairy products. It is made by removing the water from milk. Consumers use milk powders to replace fresh milk and as a component in the creation of a variety of processed food products. The separation, heat treatment, pasteurization, evaporation, concentration, dehydration (drying process), agglomeration, packaging, and storage of milk powder are all steps in the manufacturing of powdered milk. New technologies have emerged as a result of recent advancements and innovations in the processing of powdered milk. Spray-drying processes/methods have also been optimized, including downstream fluidized bed granulation operations. In this regard, understanding the relationship between process, formulation, and final powder product properties has become an important scientific challenge for food scientists. Technological aspects of nutritional mineral (calcium) and vitamin D fortification and much more remain to be exposed. However, more research is needed in the advanced investigation of powdered milk processing covering all processing steps from separation to evaporation, drying, and agglomeration, and a well-balanced combination of nutrients/good taste in milk powder and their new bioactive components to benefit healthy human aging and overall well-being.

## REFERENCES

Anandharamakrishnan, C. (Ed.). (2017). *Handbook of drying for dairy products*. John Wiley & Sons.

Attaie, H., Breitschuh, B., Braun, P., & Windhab, E. J. (2003). The functionality of milk powder and its relationship to chocolate mass processing, in particular the effect of milk powder manufacturing and composition on the physical properties of chocolate masses. *International Journal of Food Science & Technology*, *38*(3), 325–335.

Barrubés, L., Babio, N., Becerra-Tomás, N., Rosique-Esteban, N., & Salas-Salvadó, J. (2019). Association between dairy product consumption and colorectal cancer risk in adults: A systematic review and meta-analysis of epidemiologic studies. *Advances in Nutrition*, *10*(Suppl. 2), S190–S211.

Caballero, B., Finglas, P., & Toldrá, F. (2015). *Encyclopedia of food and health*. Elsevier Science.

Cai, X., Yu, H., Liu, L., Lu, T., Li, J., Ji, Y., Le, Z., Bao, L., Ma, W., Xiao, R., & Yang, Y. (2018). Milk powder co-supplemented with inulin and resistant dextrin improves glycemic control and insulin resistance in elderly type 2 diabetes mellitus: A 12-week randomized, double-blind, placebo-controlled trial. *Molecular Nutrition & Food Research*, *62*(24), 1800865.

Chen, Y., Zhang, Q., Wang, Y., Xiao, Y., Fu, R., Bao, H., & Liu, M. (2015). Estimating the causal effect of milk powder supplementation on bone mineral density: A randomized controlled trial with both non-compliance and loss to follow-up. *European Journal of Clinical Nutrition*, *69*(7), 824–830.

Davoodi, S. H., Shahbazi, R., Esmaeili, S., Sohrabvandi, S., Mortazavian, A., Jazayeri, S., & Taslimi, A. (2016). Health-related aspects of milk proteins. *Iranian Journal of Pharmaceutical Research*, *15*(3), 573.

Diez-Fernández, A., Álvarez-Bueno, C., Martínez-Vizcaíno, V., Sotos-Prieto, M., Recio-Rodríguez, J. I., & Cavero-Redondo, I. (2019). Total dairy, cheese and milk intake and arterial stiffness: A systematic review and meta-analysis of cross-sectional studies. *Nutrients*, *11*(4), 741.

Gandola, A. E., Dainelli, L., Zimmermann, D., Dahlui, M., & Detzel, P. (2019). Milk powder fortified with potassium and phytosterols to decrease the risk of cardiovascular events among the adult population in Malaysia: A cost-effectiveness analysis. *Nutrients*, *11*(6), 1235.

Kalyankar, S. D., Deshmukh, M. A., Chopde, S. S., Khedkar, C. D., Lule, V. K., & Deosarkar, S. S. (2016). Milk powder. In B, Finglas, P and Toldra (Eds.), *The encyclopedia of food and health* (Vol. 3, pp. 724–728). Academic Press.

Lu, J. X., Pan, H., Hu, X. Q., Huang, Z. W., & Zhang, Q. (2019). Effects of milk powder intervention on bone mineral density and indicators related to bone metabolism in Chinese adolescents. *Osteoporosis International*, *30*, 2231–2239.

Millqvist-Fureby, A., & Smith, P. (2007). In-situ lecithination of dairy powders in spray-drying for confectionery applications. *Food Hydrocolloids*, *21*(5–6), 920–927.

Mirmiran, P., Ejtahed, H. S., Angoorani, P., Eslami, F., & Azizi, F. (2017). Camel milk has beneficial effects on diabetes mellitus: A systematic review. *International Journal of Endocrinology and Metabolism*, *15*(2).

Patel, S. (2015). Emerging trends in nutraceutical applications of whey protein and its derivatives. *Journal of Food Science and Technology*, *52*, 6847–6858.

Schuck, P., Doli vet, A., Méjean, S., Zhu, P., Blanchard, E., & Jeantet, R. (2009). Drying by desorption: A tool to determine spray drying parameters. *Journal of Food Engineering*, *94*, 199–204.

Sunartaty, R. (2019). The innovation of making powder milk from jackfruit waste (Artocarpus Heterophllus) with Maltodextrin Addition. *Journal of Physics Conference Series*, *1232*(1), 012047.

Tamime, A. Y. (Ed.). (2009). *Dairy powders and concentrated products*. John Wiley & Sons, Ltd.

Thorning, T. K., Raben, A., Tholstrup, T., Soedamah-Muthu, S. S., Givens, I., & Astrup, A. (2016). Milk and dairy products: Good or bad for human health? An assessment of the totality of scientific evidence. *Food & Nutrition Research*, *60*(1), 32527.

Walstra, P., Wouters, J. T., & Geurts, T. J. (2006). *Dairy science and technology* (2nd ed.). CRC Taylor & Francis Group (*Food Science and Technology 147)*.

Webb, B. H., Johnson, A. H., & J. A. Alford (Ed.). (1965). *Fundamentals of dairy chemistry*. AVI Publishing Company Inc.

# 9 Concentrated Dairy Food—Condensed Milk

## 9.1 LEARNING OBJECTIVES

By the end of the chapter, the reader will be able to:

- Understand the classification and composition of condensed milk
- Gain knowledge of condensed milk production and processing
- Learn how to judge and improve the quality of the condensed milk
- Make condensed milk enterprises profitable
- Learn about the key potential health benefits of condensed milk
- Discover condensed milk innovations from production to nutritional and health attributes

New flavored functional condensed milk has developed to meet consumer demand by adding cinnamon extract and replacing sugar used in the formulation of SCM, which may boost consumers' healthy aging.

## 9.2 INTRODUCTION

People have known since the beginning of time that milk could only be kept fresh for a short period. According to Marco Polo, the Tatars were able to condense milk in the thirteenth century. He claimed that each man carried 10 pounds (4.5 kg) of milk paste, which they afterward combined with water. However, this statement most likely relates to a fermented milk concentrate rather than fresh milk, as the soft Tatar curd katyk may be turned into a drink (ayran) by diluting it. Condensed milk (**Figure 9.1**) was developed by Nicolas Appert in France in 1820 and by Gail Borden Jr. in the United States in 1853 as a result of the difficulty of keeping fresh milk for more than a few hours. After returning from a trip to England in 1851, Borden was heartbroken to learn that some of his kids had died, reportedly from consuming milk from shipboard cows that were of low quality. Borden was finally successful in reducing milk without scorching or curdling it due to the vacuum pan that shakers used to condense fruit juice. Even then, only the third factory he created in New York with his new partner Jeremiah Milbank produced milk that could be used as a derivative that

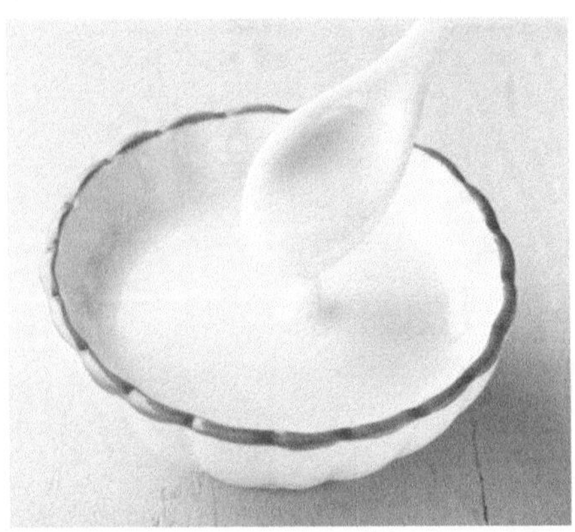

**FIGURE 9.1 Image of condensed milk.**


DOI: 10.1201/9781003397786-9

was durable and did not require refrigeration. His first two factories had failed even then. Products made from condensed milk have a number of advantages over fresh milk, including the need for reduced storage space, retaining supreme quality, preserving beneficial additional nutrients in milk, and reducing transport expenses. These goods can be employed in vulnerable situations like wars, epidemics, earthquakes, or other natural disasters when there are no fresh milk supplies. They are also appropriate for specialty foods made for persons like athletes, the elderly, or those recovering from illness.

### 9.2.1 Definition

Sweetened condensed milk (SCM) is defined by the US Department of Agriculture as the end product obtained after the removal of a significant amount of water from the milk that has been sweetened with sugar or dextrose. This product can be taken as a dessert and is produced by heating it and adding sweeteners like sucrose (Silva et al., 2020). According to Nieuwenhuijse (Nieuwenhuijse & van Boekel, 2003a, 2003b; Nieuwenhuijse, 2011), SCM is concentrated milk with sugar added as a preservative that is then sterilized at a high temperature after manufacturing to maintain freshness. In general, SCM contains 20% non-fat solid, 45% sugar, and 8% fat. It has at least 28% milk total solids (TS) and at least 8.5% milk fat (Siddique et al., 2017). However, SCM contains added sugars, while evaporated milk does not. Condensed dairy goods are value-added milk products with a longer shelf life.

## 9.3 HISTORY OF CONDENSED MILK

The first person to concentrate milk for preservation was Nicolas Appert. He did this in the early nineteenth century by boiling milk in a water bath over a fire, cooling it, and then pouring it into glass bottles. He then sterilized the finished product by heating the bottles for two hours in a boiling water bath. The procedure that is still in use today was primarily created by two inventions that were made in the second part of the nineteenth century. The method of evaporating milk under low pressure to create sweetened condensed milk was invented by Gail Borden in 1856. A method for sterilizing condensed milk in tin cans that rotated under pressurized steam and permitted a short sterilization time was patented by John B. Meyenberg in 1884. **Table 9.1** gives a summary of the historical advancements in condensed milk production.

**TABLE 9.1**
**Timeline Showing the Most Important Scientific Achievements Related to Research on Condensed Milk Production**

| Year | Achievements in condensed milk manufacturing |
|---|---|
| **Before the common era** | Compared to butter and cheese, which were popular, condensed milk is of earlier origin. |
| **1357** | The procedure for making pasty milk concentrate, which was combined with water, was documented by Marco Polo (Mongolia). |
| **1820** | Condensed milk was first developed in France by Nicolas Appert, a confectioner and inventor of airtight food preservation. |
| **1853** | The process of making condensed milk was invented by Gail Borden Jr., who is referred to as "the Father of the Process of Milk Condensing." |

*(Continued)*

**TABLE 9.1 (*Continued*)**
**Timeline Showing the Most Important Scientific Achievements Related to Research on Condensed Milk Production**

| Year | Achievements in condensed milk manufacturing |
|---|---|
| **1858** | Borden's milk, marketed under the Eagle brand, became well known for its excellence, shelf life, and affordability. |
| **1864** | The largest and most modern condensery, the New York Milk Condensery, was built in Brewster, New York, by Borden's New York Condensed Milk Company. |
| **1883** | Scientific developments in the realm of sterilizing led to a significant improvement in the vacuum pan. |
| **1884** | John B. Meyenbarg (Switzerland) conducted experiments to develop the method for sterilizing condensed milk by applying steam under high pressure. He came up with the concept of manufacturing condensed milk without the use of sugar or other preservatives and without refrigeration. |
| **1906** | The term "evaporated cream" was changed to "evaporated milk" by the Federal Food and Drug Act of 1906. |
| **1911** | In Dennington, Victoria, Australia, Nestle constructed the biggest condensed milk plant in the world. |
| **1914** | "Condensed Milk and Milk Powder" was written by Professor Otto F. Hunziker, head of the dairy division at Purdue University. Condensery operations in the US and other countries were standardized and improved by Professor Hunziker and other members of the American Dairy Science Association |
| **1958** | A plate-type evaporator was invented. |
| **1961** | India's Anand Milk Producer's Union Ltd. (AMUL) began producing sweetened condensed milk commercially for the first time ever. |
| **2017** | HOCHDORF reintroduced its own blue tube brand to Swiss supermarket shelves. |

## 9.4 TYPES OF CONDENSED MILK

i. **Sweetened condensed milk:** One of the earliest industrial dairy products is SCM. Fresh cow's milk is processed to remove the majority of the water, and sugar is then added to preserve it. Sterilization is not used in the production of this product.
ii. **Unsweetened condensed milk (evaporated milk):** Unsweetened condensed milk that has been sterilized is known as "evaporated milk" (EM). It is made from fresh milk that has had a significant amount of water drained (nearly half) from it (**Figure 9.2**). After homogenizing the product, it is canned, and the cans are subjected to thermal sterilization.
iii. **Recombined evaporated milk:** When fresh milk isn't readily available, milk powder may be used in place of any or all of the non-fat solids. Similarly, the fat portion can be obtained from anhydrous milk fat (AMF). The product made exclusively by the homogenization of skim milk powder and anhydrous milk fat is known as recombined evaporated milk (REM). Some milk solids are frequently obtained from sources other than milk, skim milk, and cream, such as sweet cream buttermilk. Sweet cream buttermilk enhances the flavor and heat stability of items, particularly REM, by containing a significant amount of the fat globule membrane lipids found in milk. The properties of REM are similar to those of EM.

## 9.5 NUTRITIONAL FACTS

Condensed milk has a lot of protein, vitamins, and minerals like calcium, potassium, and phosphorus. The nutritional composition of various types of condensed milk is shown in **Tables 9.2 and. 9.3.**

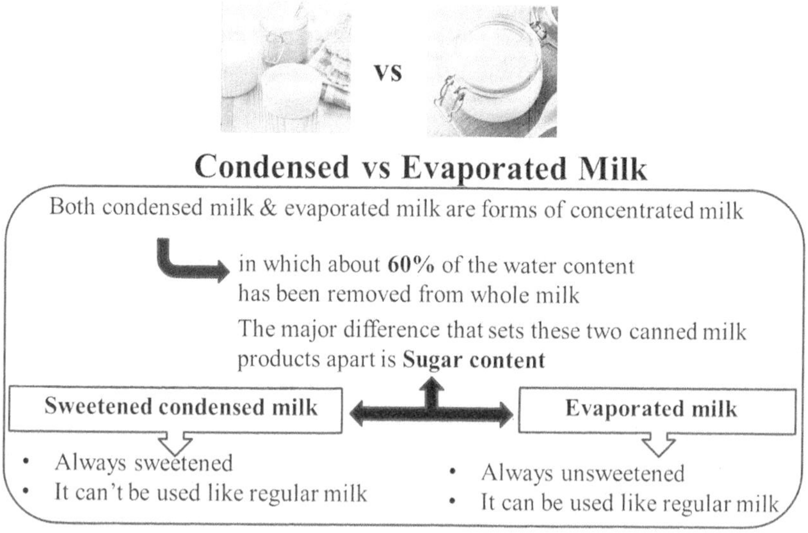


**FIGURE 9.2** **Sweetened condensed milk vs. evaporated milk.** Evaporated milk is milk that is heated and loses about 60% of its water. Then, it is put into cans and can be used like half-and-half because it is extra creamy. Condensed milk is made similarly, but sugar is added to it so about 45% of it is sugar.

**TABLE 9.2**
**Nutritional Composition of Various Types of Condensed Milk (%)**

| Type of condensed milk | Water | Total solids | Fat | Milk non-fat solids | Protein | Lactose | Ash | Total milk solids | Sucrose |
|---|---|---|---|---|---|---|---|---|---|
| Sweetened condensed milk | 26 | 74 | 9 | 22 | 8.3 | 12.2 | 1.5 | 31 | 43 |
| Unsweetened condensed milk | 31 | 69 | 9 | 22 | 8.3 | 12.2 | 1.5 | 31 | – |
| Skim sweetened | 29 | 71 | 0.5 | 25.5 | 9.3 | 14 | 2.2 | 26 | 45 |

*Source:* Asaduzzaman et al., 2007; Dydenkov, 1996; Newstead, 1999

**TABLE 9.3**
**Nutritional Composition of Condensed Milk**

| Components | Values (per 100 g) |
|---|---|
| Water | 27.2 g |
| Energy | 321 kcal |
| Carbohydrates | 54.4 g |
| Total fat | 8.7 g |
| Protein | 7.91 g |
| Total sugar | 54.4 g |
| Potassium | 371 mg |
| Calcium | 284 mg |
| Phosphorous | 253 mg |
| Sodium | 127 mg |
| Magnesium | 26 mg |
| Iron | 0.19 mg |

The majority of the nutrients in milk are still there in the condensed form because condensed milk is essentially produced from milk. Let's explore condensed milk's nutritional worth (per 100 g) according to the US Food and Drug Administration (**Table 9.3**).

## 9.6 WORLDWIDE CONDENSED MILK PRODUCTION AND CONSUMPTION TRENDS

The worldwide sweetened condensed milk market was about $6118.41 million in 2021 and is predicted to grow at a CAGR of 0.78% through 2027, reaching $6412.04 million. Top sweetened condensed milk production countries are shown in **Table 9.4.**

The United States, Peru, and Malaysia had the greatest levels of consumption in 2021, accounting for 33% of the worldwide consumption.

**TABLE 9.4**
**Top Sweetened Condensed Milk Production Countries in the World in 2021**

| Rank | Country | Production (Metric tons) |
|---|---|---|
| 1 | Malaysia | 274,718 |
| 2 | Saudi Arabia | 151,000 |
| 3 | USA | 97,326 |
| 4 | Moldova | 74,540 |
| 5 | Brazil | 66,884 |
| 6 | Mexico | 62,077 |

## 9.7 MANUFACTURING PROCESS

Milk is subjected to the first main treatment (filter, cream separation/standardization). The surplus water content is then removed by evaporation, and sugar is added. Following that, the mixture is homogenized. **Figure 9.3** illustrates the process of manufacturing sterilized and UHT-sterilized EM (Carić, 1994). The following sections explain the main processing steps.

### 9.7.1 Preheating

Before being concentrated, fresh milk is heated. The primary goal of this treatment is to improve the concentrated milk's heat stability. If the milk is not preheated, the homogenized full-cream EM cannot be sterilized. To produce EM with the highest heat stability, milk is often warmed at 110–130°C for around 1–3 min in a continuous flow. As preheating inactivate microbial spores, it also serves as a significant barrier to microbial growth. The manufacturer of the powder undergoes preheating for REM before concentration and drying. This makes it possible to reconstitute the powder at the precise concentration needed for REM.

### 9.7.2 Concentration of Milk

For milk concentration, energy-efficient multi-stage falling film evaporators are generally utilized. To reduce the chance of reducing the milk's heat stability, overconcentration should be avoided.

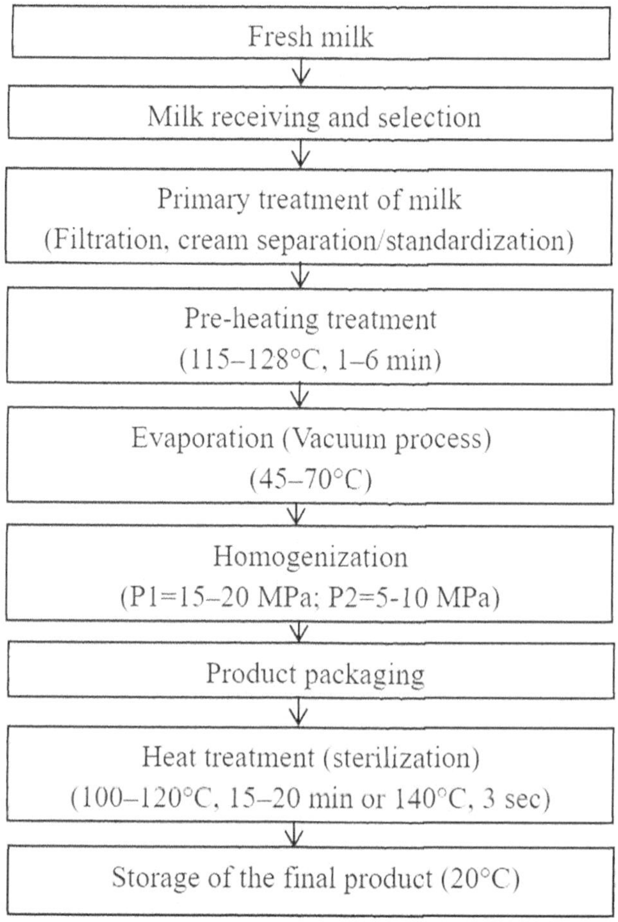


**FIGURE 9.3** General flow diagram of the manufacturing process of condensed milk.

Likewise, excessive concentration reduces output capacity and necessitates more energy use. At the point where the product leaves the evaporator, the total solid (TS) content is adjusted based on the continuous measurement of the refractive index or density of the concentrate. Between the concentrating and sterilizing operations, the final standardization of fat and TS is often completed. Reverse osmosis (RO) concentrates the milk, which can also be used to make unsweetened condensed milk. Although the composition and characteristics of EM produced by RO and those formed by evaporation are nearly identical, RO's industrial use for this purpose seems to be relatively limited.

### 9.7.3 Homogenization

The homogenization of milk slows the frequency of creaming while the product is being stored and inhibits the coalescence of fat globules. Higher pressures cause a significant decrease in heat stability, while homogenization pressures up to about 5 MPa often have little impact on or only slightly increase heat stability. As soon as the concentrated milk exits the evaporator, it is homogenized. At the same pressure, smaller fat globules with superior heat stability are produced by a higher homogenization temperature.

### 9.7.4 Heat Stability Test

It is clear that the product's heat stability varies from batch to batch during the preparation of EM. Stabilizers are added to regulate heat stability. The quantity of stabilizer required differs widely as well. A series of cans holding the product is combined with various amounts of stabilizers to determine the appropriate amount to be added. Following sterilization, the inside of the cans is examined for thermal stability. The batch as a whole is stabilized with the amount that yields the best properties (Singh et al., 1995).

### 9.7.5 Cooling and Cold Storage

A predetermined amount of stabilizer (dissolved in water) is added after EM has been homogenized, cooled, and stored. This amount is decided by the stability test results. To reduce microbial growth at this stage, long storage should be avoided. At this point, the final standardization of the fat and TS can be done while taking into account the amount of water added along with the stabilizer. The risk of the sterilized product's age gelation is significantly increased when unsterilized EM is kept in the freezer for longer than 24 hours.

Since it is anticipated that EM will be kept for a longer time, special storage conditions are needed to prevent the product's quality from degrading. The product's shelf life is mostly influenced by the storage temperature. EM and condensed milk are kept in storage at 10–15°C. The storage of condensed milk at low temperatures, such as 0°C or lower, may cause sugar separation, resulting in sandiness; this sugar separation is caused by the formation of very large lactose crystals. An extremely low storage temperature also makes the product more viscous, which may be advantageous up to a point but has an impact on the product's body and texture. Commercial EM has been demonstrated to remain acceptable while stored below 15°C for 2 years, but it degrades quickly when stored at 21°C or higher. To prevent the spoiling of cans and labels, the humidity level of the storage area should be kept low (below 50%). Fat separation in EM is minimized during storage by inverting the cans.

### 9.7.6 Packaging

One of EM's distinguishing characteristics is its prolonged shelf life at room temperature, which places high demands on the packaging materials. The materials used for packaging must be mechanically durable and permeable to water, light, gases, and hydrophobic substances. Those parts that are in direct contact with the product must be made of food-grade materials. The can is the most common EM container and typically contains 170 or 411 g of EM (6 or 14.5 oz, respectively). Concentrated milk products are frequently packaged in cans with mechanical seals. In order to stop the tin and iron from dissolving into the product, current tinned plates are covered in a polymer layer. Glass bottles with twist-off tops are sometimes used to package EM used as coffee creamer in Western European nations. Single-portion cups made of aluminum or polystyrene and milk cartons lined with aluminum foil are also frequently used. Due to this material's permeability to air and light, EM delivered in translucent (white) polystyrene single-portion cups typically gets an oxidized flavor.

### 9.7.7 Sterilization

In addition to eliminating all germs, sterilization also renders dormant any microbial spores that could potentially grow when EM is stored. During preheating, the native milk enzymes are turned inactive. It is important to take note of the milk's high microbiological quality when choosing it to manufacture concentrated milk. Due to their thermostability and inability to be rendered inactive by sterilization, the enzymes generated by microbes (particularly psychrotrophic microbes) should be absent. Cans of condensed milk can be filled with a variety of techniques. Concentrated milk pours into cans through a tiny hole (3 mm or 1/8 in diameter) in a technique that is frequently employed. The cans are securely sealed after filling because the seal needs to resist the heat of sterilization. To prevent contaminating the milk, it is also crucial that the cans be filled as soon as possible. Typically, a mechanical finger is used to solder the aperture in the cans. The filled and sealed cans are then submerged in a hot water tank to check for leaks. Any cans that lift or release air bubbles are eliminated as unsuitable for sterilizing. Modern sealing techniques are so quick that many cans can be sealed in a single minute. Open or sanitary-type cans are employed in this operation. The open can is filled with concentrated milk, and after filling it to the top, an automatic seaming machine seals the can's opposite end. Cans are sterilized in a horizontal rotating system with rotary airlocks, while the bottles are sterilized in hydrostatic sterilizers. These systems feature a significant amount of heat regeneration, making them very energy efficient.

## 9.8 PACKAGING AND STORAGE OF CONDENSED MILK

Bulk packaging is done in barrels of various sizes, drums with polythene liners, or tin containers. For retail packs, cans are mostly used.

| | | Safe storage time | |
|---|---|---|---|
| **Dairy food** | **How to store** | **In refrigerator or pantry 35–40°F (2–4°C)** | **In freezer 0°F or below** |
| Condensed milk (opened) | Keep covered | 2 weeks | Do not freeze. |

When kept in the can, condensed milk can last for approximately 1 year. Once opened, the shelf life is reduced (around 2–3 weeks for SCM and about 2 weeks for unsweetened condensed milk).

## 9.9 USES OF CONDENSED MILK

Condensed milk has good storage capabilities, making it a handy product for domestic use. It is especially helpful onboard ships and in tropical climates. It is frequently used in the house to prepare baked goods, tea, coffee, and puddings. Additionally, SCM is utilized as a bulk product in the ice cream and frozen dessert sectors as well as in the chocolate and confectionery industries as a retail-packed product. It can be quickly reformed by diluting it with water to the consistency of raw milk. The chocolate and confectionery industries also utilize a lot of this type of milk (Ahmed et al., 2019).

Milk is transformed into EM to maintain its nutrients, which shouldn't degrade over the course of weeks, months, or even years in storage without refrigeration. EM is also easily transportable over large distances. For countries with insufficient milk supply, especially in the tropics, EM is a general-purpose milk product. In some markets, EM is used for various functions like preparing food, tea, or coffee. After being diluted 1:1 with boiling water, EM is consumed like fluid milk. This results in a product that has a slightly greater non-fat solid concentration and fat:non-fat solid ratio than conventional full-cream milk with 3.5% fat. Compared to pasteurized or UHT-sterilized milk, some people prefer the taste of sterilized milk. To give coffee, cocoa, or tea a milky flavor and a white look, only a small amount of EM is needed. The yellowish color that the Maillard reaction's byproducts give coffee, chocolate, or tea in EM is preferable to the grayish hue that results from adding pasteurized or UHT milk. Because EM is made from homogenized milk, it is suggested for infant feeding due to the stomach's tendency to develop a soft curd. Since EM has a smooth consistency, it is a crucial component in many different kinds of puddings, sauces, and gravies. It is used to make ice cream due to its high TMS content. Additionally, it is used to make bread and confectionery goods, as well as chocolate. SCM milk is used in a variety of dessert recipes around the world.

## 9.10 QUALITY EVALUATION OF CONDENSED MILK

High-quality condensed milk needs to smell fresh and pleasant, taste very sweet, have a smooth, consistent body and texture, and be a uniformly light in color. Cow milk should be yellow, and buffalo milk should be a light greenish white color. A moderate, pleasing flavor, a somewhat thick body, a typically smooth texture, and a consistent color are all characteristics of high-quality evaporated milk. The Hedonic Type scale is used to assess condensed and evaporated milk sensory qualities (Asaduzzaman et al., 2007). The Hedonic Type scale is illustrated in **Tables 9.5** and **Tables 9.6.**

**TABLE 9.5**
**Score Card for Sensory Evaluation of Condensed Milk**

| Name: | Sample no: | Date: |
|---|---|---|
| **Traits** | | **Score** |
| Flavor and odor | | 30 |
| Body and texture | | 25 |
| Color | | 5 |
| Fat content | | 10 |
| Milk solids | | 10 |
| Bacteria | | 10 |
| Sugar | | 10 |
| Adulterants and preservatives are not permitted | | |
| | | Total score: 100 |

**TABLE 9.6**
**Score Card for Sensory Evaluation of Evaporated Condensed Milk**

| Name: | Sample no: | Date: |
|---|---|---|
| **Traits** | | **Score** |
| Flavor and odor | | 40 |
| Body and texture | | 35 |
| Color | | 5 |
| Fat content | | 10 |
| Total solids | | 10 |
| Adulterants and preservatives are not permitted | | |
| | | Total score: 100 |

**TABLE 9.7**
**Defects in Condensed Milk with Their Causes and Possible Remedies**

| Name of defect | Causes | Remedies |
|---|---|---|
| **Microbial defects** | | |
| Gassy fermentation/ bloating | Gas-producing yeasts Source: Raw milk, low-quality sugar, or unhygienic conditions such as inadequately cleaned and sterilized equipment and filling machines | It is recommended to utilize high-quality raw milk and a suitable preheating temperature. The only sugar to be used is premium grade, free of yeast contamination. The production and packaging of condensed milk should be done in a sanitary manner. The containers should be completely filled, with minimal area left for air. |
| Bacterial thickening | Microorganisms that produce enzymes similar to rennet | In the course of the preheating process, these organisms are simply eliminated. The growth of bacteria is also inhibited by an ideal sugar ratio. Low-temperature storage also contributes to lowering bacterial thickening. |
| Mold buttons | Mold (*Aspergillus repeno*) makes an enzyme similar to rennet that induces localized coagulation. Storage at a high temperature encourages the organism's growth. | Careful cleaning and maintenance of dairy equipment are necessary to prevent this problem. This defect can be avoided by storing condensed milk at a lower temperature. |
| **Non-microbial defects** | | |
| Sandiness | The milk could be grainy and packed with large lactose crystals. Due to using an excessive amount of sugar during manufacture, the sugar may crystallize out and cause sandiness. | Condensed milk should be cooled to facilitate the formation of numerous minute sugar crystals, which gives the product its smooth texture. To prevent this problem, the ideal storage temperature is also crucial. |
| Age thickening | Storage (at room temperature or above), high packaging and heating temperatures and increased concentration of milk solids | An optimum preheating temperature and addition of the proper type of stabilizers and only sugar at the very end of the milk condensing process should be used, and the finished product should be stored below 15°C. |
| Brown color | Associated with age thickening, both of which intensify with storage. The rate of this change is determined by the acidity and storage temperature. | This defect can be avoided by storing condensed milk at a lower temperature. |
| **Flavor defects** | | |
| Rancid, tallowy, and metallic flavor | Raw milk, or unhygienic conditions such as inadequately cleaned and sterilized equipment and filling machines | These defects can be avoided by good manufacturing practices; using good-quality raw materials, fresh milk, and well packaging; and storing at a low temperature. |

## 9.11 DEFECTS IN CONDENSED MILK

Condensed milk contains about 40–45% sugar to protect condensed milk against bacterial defects and against causing sugar crystallization. In **Table 9.7**, a few common defects of sweetened condensed milk are described.

## 9.12 HEALTH BENEFITS OF CONDENSED MILK

Sweetened condensed milk contains essential nutrients for human growth. It is a very thick, sweet product with a high calorie content that may cause people who are calorie concerned to rethink using it frequently. When used moderately, some of its potential advantages are still there. **Figure 9.4** gives a summary of the health benefits of condensed milk.

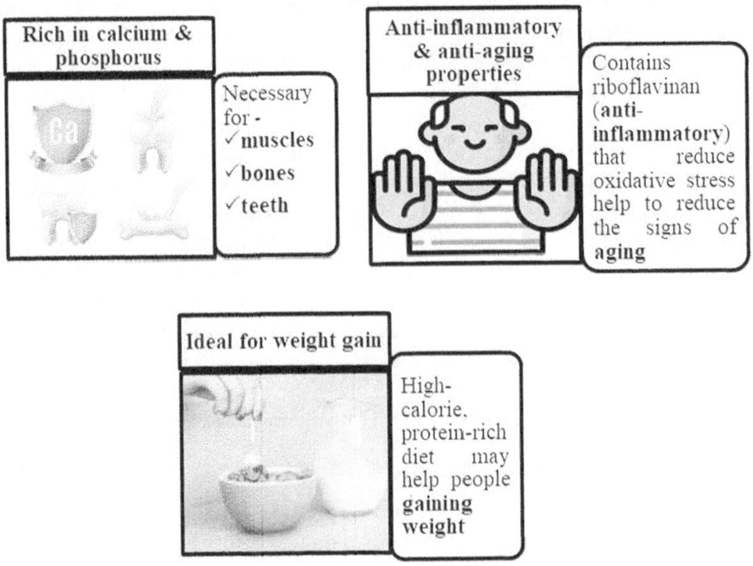


FIGURE 9.4 **Key potential health benefits of condensed milk.** Condensed milk has the concentrated advantages of ordinary milk but with a greater sugar level. Condensed milk, like milk, is an excellent source of calcium, vitamin D, vitamin $B_{12}$, vitamin A, riboflavin, phosphorus, and protein. These nutrients are required for strong teeth and bones, as well as a healthy immune system and cardiovascular system.

### 9.12.1 Association of Condensed Milk Consumption with Bone Health

Sweetened condensed milk contains calcium. Calcium is necessary to properly function muscles, bones, and teeth. In addition to improving bone health, calcium has been shown in studies to help with hypertension during pregnancy and osteoporosis. It also helps in the re-establishment of calcium levels in postpartum women.

### 9.12.2 Association of Condensed Milk Consumption with Weight Gain

Underweight people can put on weight by eating a high-calorie, protein-rich diet. This type of diet may aid in the improvement of overall body mass index. Compared to condensed milk, sugar only contains empty calories, whereas condensed milk contains other nutrients such as protein, calcium, and phosphorus.

### 9.12.3 Association of Condensed Milk Consumption with Cholesterol Reduction

Milk and other dairy products include cholesterol and saturated fats, which might have the risk of heart disease. However, research on Maasais, a tribe of Africans who consume a lot of milk, showed that they have a low level of cholesterol in their systems. Scientists think that dairy

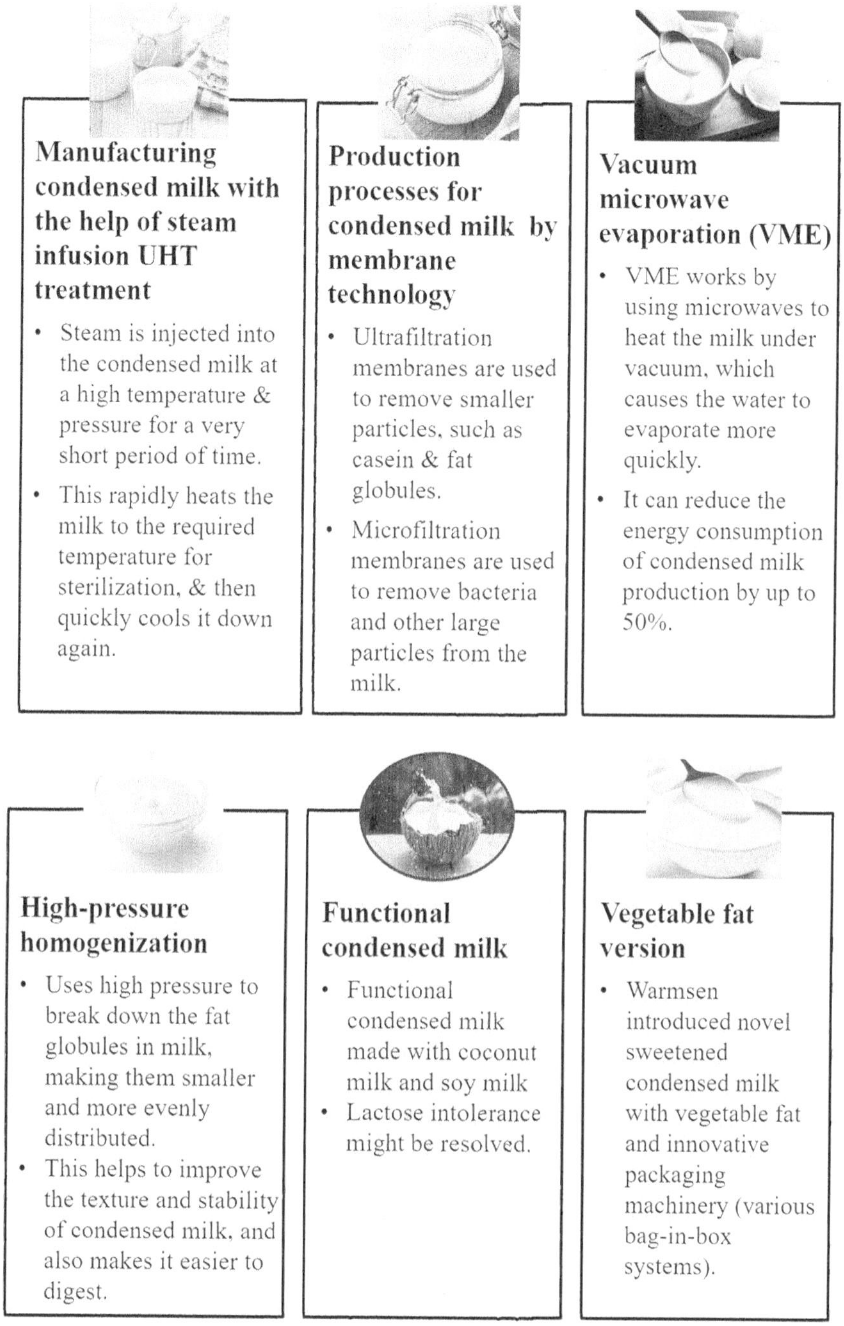


**FIGURE 9.5** **Condensed milk innovations from production to nutritional and health attributes.**

products contain carbohydrates (sugars) that cannot be completely broken down during digestion (Gibney & Burstyn, 1980). The activity of gut bacteria allows for the breakdown of these carbohydrates. It alters the mechanism of cholesterol production in the body and reduces the amount of cholesterol in the circulation.

### 9.12.4 Association of Condensed Milk Consumption with Anti-Inflammatory and Anti-Aging Effects

In addition to having a lot of protein, sweetened condensed milk also has a small amount of riboflavin, an anti-inflammatory vitamin. By reducing oxidative stress caused by free radicals, riboflavin may also help to reduce the signs of aging.

### 9.12.5 Association of Condensed Milk Consumption with Boosting Energy Levels

Condensed milk has both added sugars and natural sugars, which gives a quick boost of energy.

**Other benefits of condensed milk:**

- Helps muscle development
- May help prevent osteoporosis
- Great for hair well-being
- Prevents gum diseases
- Might reduce blood pressure
- Might move forward metabolic health

## 9.13 CONDENSED MILK INNOVATIONS

Product innovation in sweetened condensed milk is a crucial component contributing to the industry's growth. Furthermore, due to its thick texture and sweet flavor, sweetened condensed milk is a common component in sweets such as cakes and ice cream. **Figure 9.5** illustrates condensed milk innovations from production to nutritional and health attributes (Ahmed et al., 2019; Behera et al., 2013).

## 9.14 CONCLUSIONS

Condensed milk has good storage properties, making it a practical product for household uses, and the global condensed milk market demand is huge ($9.9 billion in 2021, projected to reach $15.2 billion by 2031, growing at a CAGR of 4.4% from 2022 to 2031). However, the condensed milk industry did not develop in the same way as did the other dairy food industry, that is, by successive, accidental, or incidental practices. Finally, considering the present situation, there is a need for more research to be undertaken, especially to boil milk and add sugar to it in order to enhance the milk's ability to keep; however, from a practical perspective, these attempts proved more or less futile with added ingredients that may boost consumer's healthy life/aging (Asaduzzaman et al., 2007).

## REFERENCES

Ahmed, E., Rita, R. P., Huq, S., Kabir, E., Rana, M. S., & Mazumder, M. A. R. (2019). Development of functional condensed milk from coconut milk and soy milk. *Asian Food Science Journal*, *6*(4), 1–7.

Asaduzzaman, M., Miah, K. Y., Mannan, A. K. M. A., Haque, M. E., Ara, A., Khan, M. M. H., Dawlatana, M., & Rahim, M. (2007). A study on the quality of sweetened condensed milk available in the local market of Bangladesh. *Bangladesh Journal of Scientific and Industrial Research*, *42*(2), 147–156.

Behera, B. K., Dash, S. S., & Swain, S. K. (2013). Steam infusion UHT treatment of condensed milk. *Journal of Food Engineering*, *119*(3), 473–479.

Carić, M. (1994). *Concentrated and dried dairy products*. VCH Publishers Inc.

Dydenkov, A. A. (1996). Modification of kofranyi method for determination of quality of protein substances in milk and sweetened condensed milk. *Dairy Science. Abstracts*, *28*(11), 596.

Gibney, M. J., & Burstyn, P. G. (1980). Milk, serum cholesterol, and the Maasai. A hypothesis. *Atherosclerosis*, *35*(3), 339–343.

Newstead, D. F. (1999). Sweet-cream buttermilk powders: Key functional ingredients for recombined milk products. *3rd international symposium on recombined milk & milk products (Penang, 23–26 May 1999)* (pp. 55–60).

Nieuwenhuijse, J. A. (2011). Concentrated dairy products I sweetened condensed milk. *Encyclopedia of dairy sciences* (2nd ed., pp. 869–873). Academic Press.

Nieuwenhuijse, J. A., & van Boekel, M. A. (2003a). Protein stability in sterilised milk and milk products. *Advanced dairy chemistry-1 proteins: Part A/Part B* (pp. 947–974). Springer US.

Nieuwenhuijse, J. A., & van Boekel, M. A. (2003b). Concentrated milk products-evaporated milk. *Encyclopedia of dairy science* (pp. 493–499). Elsevier Science.

Siddique, N. A., Islam, N., Habib, R., Ur-Rashid, H., Islam, A., & Afrin, S. (2017). Evaluation of the quality of sweetened condensed milk of different brands available in local markets of Bangladesh. *International Journal of Natural and Social Sciences*, *4*(1), 64–70.

Silva, R., Rocha, R. S., Guimarães, J. T., Balthazar, C. F., Pimentel, T. C., Neto, R. P. C., Tavares, M. I. B., Esmerino, E. A., Duarte, M. C. K. H., Freitas, M. Q., Silva, P. H. F., Cappato, L. P., Raices, R. S. L., Silva, M. C., & Cruz, A. G. (2020). Advantages of using ohmic heating in Dulce de Leche manufacturing. *Innovative Food Science & Emerging Technologies*, *65*, 102475.

Singh, H., Creamer, L. K., & Newstead, D. F. (1995). Heat stability of concentrated milk. *Heat-induced changes in milk* (2nd ed., pp. 256–278). International Dairy Federation.

# 10 Frozen Dairy Food—Ice Cream

## 10.1 LEARNING OBJECTIVES

By the end of the chapter, the reader will be able to:

- Understand the classification and composition of ice cream
- Know the role of different ingredients in making the body, texture, and taste of ice cream
- Gain knowledge of ice cream production and processing
- Understand how to improve the quality of the ice cream/be able to judge the ice cream
- Make ice cream enterprises profitable
- Learn about the key potential health benefits of ice cream
- Discover ice cream innovations from production to nutritional and health attributes

Ice cream is often referred to as the glamorous girl of the dairy industry. Although ice cream is typically consumed for refreshing experience, it now offers various health advantages. According to a recent study, functional ice cream is an excellent carrier of bioactive compounds that promote a healthy lifestyle. Furthermore, adding fruit fiber to the mixture before freezing results in the slow melting of ice cream for several hours, and low-sugar ice cream also is available for the health-conscious.

## 10.2 INTRODUCTION

Ice cream is a frozen dairy product manufactured by freezing a pasteurized mixture of sugar and other ingredients (**Figure 10.1**). Ice cream is often referred to as the "glamorous girl of the dairy industry" (Hossain & Kober, 2008). Agitation is used to add air to ensure uniform consistency. It is made up of a mix of food items such as milk products, sugar, corn syrup (dry or liquid), dextrose, water, and possibly flavorings, eggs or egg products, and a stabilizer or emulsifier—all of which are wholesome edible ingredients (Goff, 2013). Ice cream has distinct characteristics such

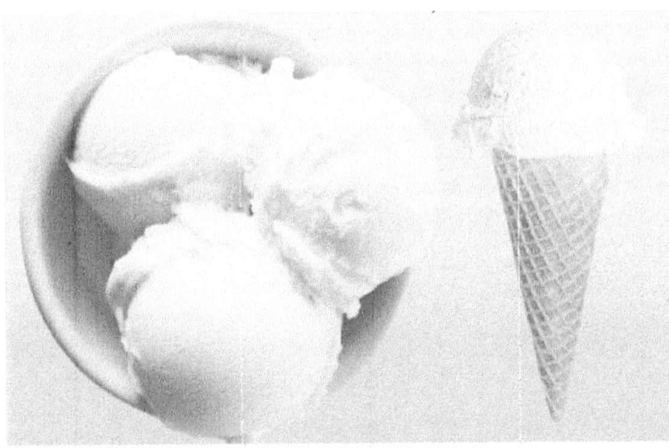

**FIGURE 10.1 Image of ice cream.** "Glamorous girl" of the dairy industry term can also be used for ice cream.



DOI: 10.1201/9781003397786-10

as being normally white in color (if no coloring agent is added), soft, firm, and malleable (the freezing point is approximately –2.5°C), glossy in appearance (density approximately 1.0554–1.1232 g/ml), with acidity of approximately 0.1–0.2% and a pH of approximately 6.3.

### 10.2.1 Definition

The definition of ice cream varies globally due to different regulations and methods used in various countries. Consequently, a variety of ice cream can be found, each containing distinct formulations.

i. Ice cream is a frozen dessert made up of ice crystals and solidified fat, which are mixed together with proteins, carbohydrates, salts, and gums that are liquid in phase. It needs to have at least 5% fat and 2.5% milk protein. If it is dairy ice cream, the fat content should exclusively derive from milk (Kilara & Chandan, 2008).
ii. Regular ice cream often includes a particular amount of fat, which may originate from either milk or alternative non-dairy sources. It also needs to have a certain amount of dietary solids or milk proteins or milk solids, either singly or together (Goff & Hartel, 2013; Arun & Ramesh, 2013).
iii. A frozen mixture containing milk/cream or fruit juice and sugar, emulsifiers and stabilizers, optionally flavorings or fruit, and usually air, whipped into the mixture during freezing and containing at least 10% milk fat (Arun & Ramesh, 2013).

## 10.3 HISTORY OF ICE CREAM

The origins of ice cream are unknown, but many accounts exist about their history. Between the years 618 and 697 AD, ice cream emerged as a delectable cuisine in China. King Tang of Shang was assisted by ice men, who aided him in creating a unique meal using buffalo milk, flour, and camphor. A type of ice cream was created in China around 200 BC. It was made by combining milk and rice together and then freezing it using snow. Some historians believe that ice cream was first brought to Italy by Marco Polo after he visited China. Some described ice cream-like desserts originating in ancient Persia approximately 550 BC, while others claim that Roman Emperor Nero would send his slaves to mountains in order to collect snow. He would then mix the snow with nectar, fruit pulp, and honey. Others said ice cream originated in the Mongol Empire and was first introduced to China during its reign (Stephens, 2007). Ice cream became more accessible to people from lower socioeconomic backgrounds as a result of the development of hand-cranked freezers and the improved availability of ice. Finally, by the end of the nineteenth century, it had made its way to urban areas and was being peddled on city streets.

**How ice cream became popular:** Ice cream became popular and affordable in England in the mid-nineteenth century, with a man named Carlo Gatti in 1851. For one cent, he sold scoops in shells. Agnes Marshall, known as the "queen of ices" in England, popularized an ice cream formula and made its consumption into a chic middle-class pastime. She is the one who proposed using liquid nitrogen to produce ice cream. After cheap refrigeration became common, ice cream became popular all over the world in the second half of the twentieth century.

**Häagen-Dazs:** In 1960, Reuben Mattus created Häagen-Dazs. This name appealed to him because it sounded Danish. He started with only three flavors: vanilla, chocolate, and coffee. It's an American brand that now has franchises throughout the UK, India, US, Japan, China, Brazil, Lebanon, Peru, and New Zealand.

**Dove Bar:** The Dove Bar is an American ice cream product founded by Leo Stefanos in 1956 at Dove Candies and Ice Cream on 60th Street and Pulaski Avenue in Chicago and launched nationally in 1984. The brand, which includes Dove chocolate and ice cream, was acquired by Mars Inc. in 1986, and Dove Bars are now manufactured by Mars.

**Good Humor:** The Good Humor Ice Cream Bar was invented by Harry Burt in 1920 and patented in 1923.

This ice cream has been known by different names and is made by top companies (**Figure 10.2**).

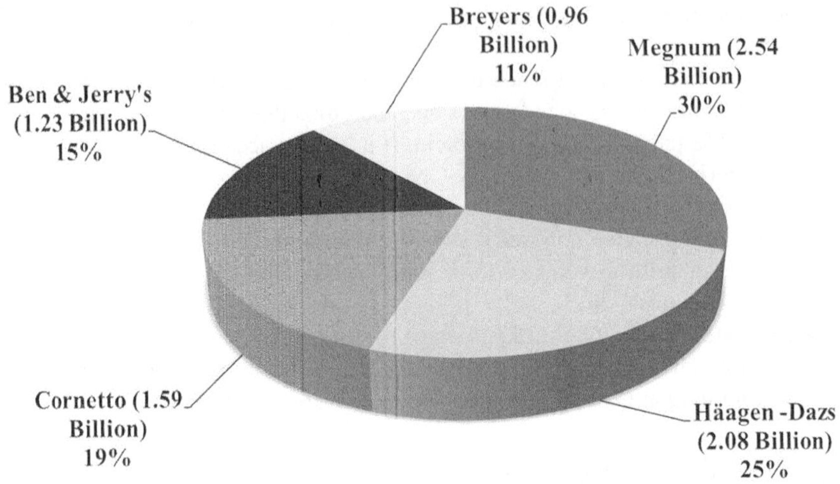


FIGURE 10.2 **Leading companies in the global ice cream market.**

## 10.4 TYPES OF ICE CREAM

In general, ice cream can be roughly categorized as super premium, premium, standard, or economy (**Table 10.1**). These ice creams usually vary by fat content, total solids, overrun, flavors, and cost (Tharp & Young, 2013) as shown in **Table 10.1**.

Moreover, ice cream can also be divided into four types according to the ingredients:

i. Ice cream is made exclusively from milk products (dairy ice cream).
ii. Ice cream containing vegetable fat.
iii. Sherbet ice cream is made of fruit juice with added milk fat and milk non-fat solids.
iv. Water ice is made of water, sugar, and fruit concentrate.

TABLE 10.1
Ice Cream Classifications

| Points | Economy | Standard | Premium | Super premium |
|---|---|---|---|---|
| Fat (%) | 10 (depending on legal requirements) | 10–12 | 12–15 | 15–18 |
| Total solids (%) | 30 (depending on legal requirements) | 36–38 | 38–40 | >40 |
| Overrun (%) | Legal maximum | 100–120 | 60–90 | 25–50 |
| Cost | Low | average | Higher than average | High |

## 10.5 NUTRITIONAL FACTS

Ice creams contain a lot of fat, carbohydrates, and protein, which means it gives you a lot of energy. The energy content of regular ice cream is about 200 calories per 100 grams. The ingredients in ice cream vary depending on the demand and place. Nutritional facts of ice cream are illustrated in **Figure 10.3** and **Table 10.2**. One serving of good average composition of vanilla ice cream (1/6 qt) contains 200 calories, 3.9 grams of protein, 0.31 grams of calcium, 0.104 grams of phosphorus, 0.14 milligrams of iron, 548 IU of vitamin A, 0.038 milligrams of thiamine, and 0.236 milligrams of riboflavin (Arbuckle, 1986).

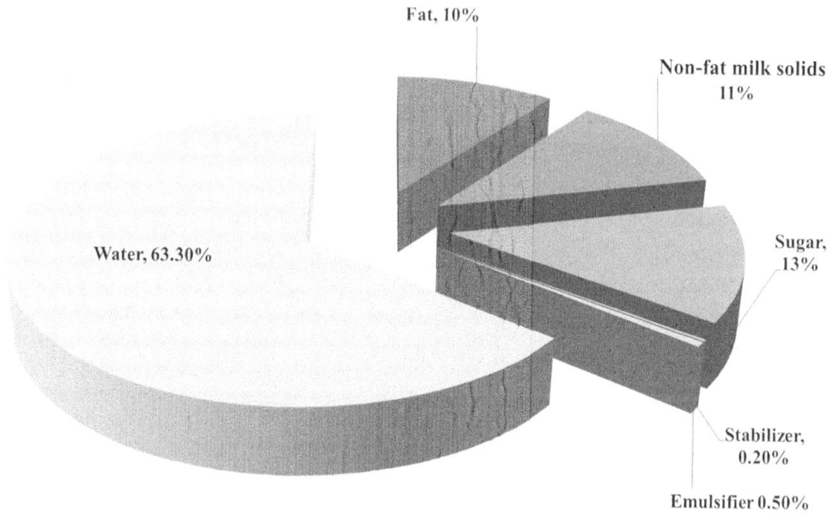


**FIGURE 10.3** Chemical composition of ice cream.

## TABLE 10.2
## Nutritional and Chemical Composition (% by wt.) of Commercially Available Ice Cream Varieties by Formulation Type

| Types | Milk fat | Milk non-fat solids | Sweeteners[a] | Stabilizers[b] | Total solids |
|---|---|---|---|---|---|
| Non-fat ice cream | <0.5 | 12–14 | 18–22 | 1.0 | 28–32 |
| Low-fat ice cream | 2–5 | 12–14 | 18–21 | 0.8 | 28–32 |
| Light ice cream | 5–7 | 11–12 | 18–20 | 0.5 | 30–35 |
| Reduced-fat ice cream | 7–9 | 10–12 | 18–19 | 0.4 | 32–36 |
| Economy ice cream | 10 | 10–11 | 15–17 | 0.4 | 35–36 |
| Standard ice cream | 10–12 | 9–10 | 14–17 | 0.2–0.4 | 36–38 |
| Premium ice cream | 12–14 | 8–10 | 13–16 | 0.2–0.4 | 38–40 |
| Super premium ice cream | 14–18 | 5–8 | 14–17 | 0–0.2 | 40–42 |
| Frozen yogurt: regular | 3–6 | 9–13 | 15–17 | 0.5 | 30–36 |
| Frozen yogurt: non-fat | <0.5 | 9–14 | 15–17 | 0.6 | 28–32 |
| Sherbet | 1–2 | 1–3 | 22–28 | 0.4–0.5 | 28–34 |

*Source:* Goff & Hartel, 2013; Akbari et al., 2019

[a] Includes sucrose, glucose, corn syrup solids, maltodextrins, polydextrose, and other bulking agents, some of which contribute little sweetness.

[b] Includes ingredients such as locust bean gum, guar gum, carrageenan, cellulose gum, and cellulose gel as stabilizers, and also mono- and diglycerides and polysorbate 80 as emulsifiers.

## 10.6 WORLDWIDE ICE CREAM CONSUMPTION TRENDS

The International Dairy Federation estimates that New Zealand holds the title for the most ice cream consumed per year per capita, but Finland is a close second. The information in **Table 10.3** shows how much ice cream people ate in different countries in 2021.

**TABLE 10.3**
**Per Capita Consumption of Ice Cream Worldwide in 2021**

| Country | Consumption (liters per capita/per year) |
|---|---|
| New Zealand | 28.4 |
| United States | 20.8 |
| Finland | 14.2 |
| Sweden | 12.0 |
| Canada | 10.6 |
| Denmark | 9.8 |
| Ireland | 8.4 |
| Italy | 8.0 |
| United Kingdom | 7.0 |
| Finland | 14.2 |
| Sweden | 12.0 |
| Canada | 10.6 |
| Denmark | 9.8 |
| Ireland | 8.4 |
| Italy | 8.0 |
| United Kingdom | 7.0 |

### 10.6.1 Economic Significance of Ice Cream

There are approximately 100 ice cream companies dispersed throughout several countries within the European Union. These small and medium-sized companies typically have a workforce of around 15,000 individuals. The projected growth of the global ice cream market is estimated to increase from $71.52 billion in 2021 to $97.85 billion by 2027, as per fortune business insights (The Content Bar, 2022). The significant surge of 37% in under a decade can be attributed primarily to the growing global demand for ice cream. In Europe, individuals typically consume around 620 liters of ice cream per year, according to the Ice Cream Association.

## 10.7 STRUCTURE OF ICE CREAM

In order to achieve a smooth texture, ice cream must contain small ice crystals. During freezing, most of the water freezes into ice. Whipping and aeration occur simultaneously with freezing to form small air bubbles, which are stabilized by the demulsified fat. The air takes up 30 to 50% of the final volume of the ice cream. The sugar sweetens the ice cream and lowers the freezing point of the water, thereby reducing the amount of ice cream. Soft-serve ice cream contains less ice. Usually, ice cream contains 30% ice crystals, 50% air bubbles, 5% fat droplets, and 15% liquid syrup (Kurt, 2018).

## 10.8 MANUFACTURING PROCESS

Ice cream is made by mixing the components and then pasteurizing them. The basic steps in the manufacturing of ice cream are generally as follows (**Figure 10.4**) (Goff, 2013).

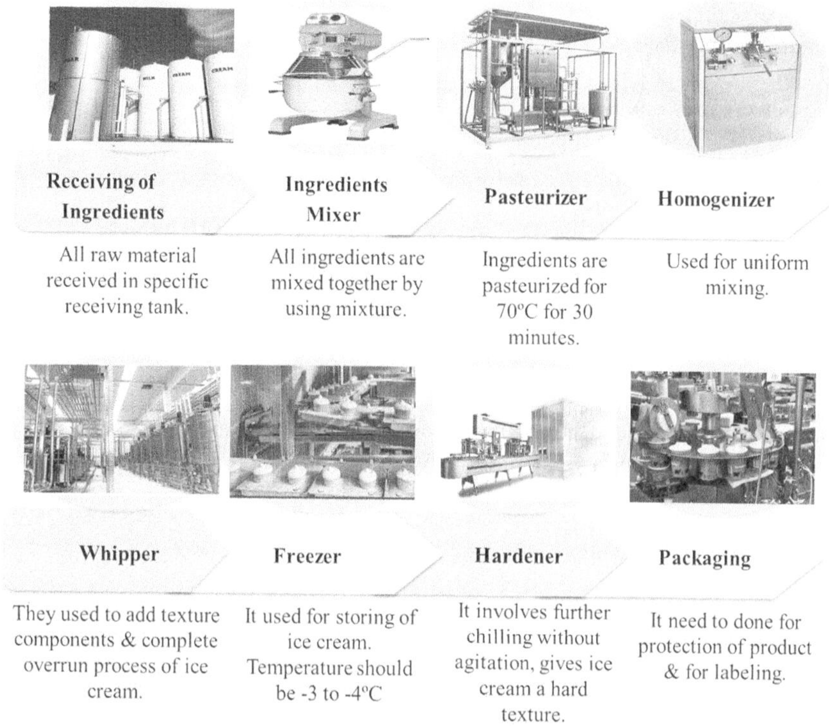


FIGURE 10.4 **Flow diagram of the ice cream manufacturing process.**

### 10.8.1 Blending/Ingredient Mixing

The "ice cream mix" is formed by combining and mixing ingredients according to desired proportions and the calculations derived from the selected ingredients and recipe. Powders must be quickly agitated during blending in order to be incorporated; thus, powerful blenders are often used.

### 10.8.2 Mix Pasteurization

In mix pasteurization, not only batch pasteurizers but also continuous (HTST) methods are applied. The proper ingredient amounts are blended in large jacketed vats fitted with some kind of heating, typically steam or hot water, in a batch pasteurization method. The product is then heated in the vat to at least 69°C (155°F) and kept for 30 minutes to meet legal pasteurization standards, which are required for the destruction of pathogenic bacteria. Following the blending of ingredients in a large, insulated feed tank, continuous pasteurization is typically done in a high-temperature short-time (HTST) heat exchanger.

### 10.8.3 Mix Homogenization

Through homogenization, the mixture is processed to break down the fat particles in milk or cream, resulting in a size smaller than 1 μm.

The following functions are given by homogenization in ice cream manufacture:

- Decreases the size of fat globules
- Increases surface area
- Forms membrane
- Allows the use of butter, frozen cream, etc.

By assisting in forming the fat structure, it also has the following indirect impacts:

- Makes ice cream smoother
- Increases palatability and apparent richness
- Improves air stability
- Increases melting resistance

In most conditions, a pressure of 2000–2500 psi on the first stage and 500–1000 psi on the second stage should suffice when using a two-stage homogenizer.

### 10.8.4 Mix Aging

The mixture is then aged for a minimum of 4 hours and usually overnight. As a result, the proteins and polysaccharides can fully hydrate and the fat can cool and crystallize. Aging provides the following functions:

- Enhances whipping qualities of the blend and body and texture of ice cream

### 10.8.5 Freezing

**Freezing with whipping (overrun):** The mix is first frozen in a continuous freezer concurrently with whipping (overrun). The word "overrun" is used to describe the amount of air incorporated into ice cream. The usual overrun is one of approximately 80–100% i.e., admixture of 0.6–1 liter of air per liter of ice cream mix. There are two basic ways to calculate percentage overrun, viz, by volume and by weight:

$$\%\text{ overrun} = \frac{(\text{volume of ice cream}) - (\text{volume of mix})}{\text{volume of mix}} \times 100$$

$$\%\text{ overrun} = \frac{(\text{Weight of unit volume of mix}) - (\text{Weight of unit volume of ice cream})}{\text{Weight of unit volume of ice cream}} \times 100$$

The freezing must take place quickly so that the ice crystals will be as small as possible. The frozen mix leaves the continuous freezer at a temperature of –3 to –4°C. Its texture will be similar to that of soft ice cream, and some 40–50% of the water content of the mix will be frozen. After the continuous freezing, fruits and nuts can be added before the mix is filled into molds or other packaging. The quantity of air infused into the ice cream varies depending on the composition of the mixture. Air being trapped during freezing is primarily responsible for the increased volume.

Factors that decrease overrun are (i) fat content, (ii) milk non-fat solid content, (iii) amount of mix in the batch freezer, (iv) poor homogenization, and (v) insufficient refrigeration (Sofjan & Hartel, 2004; Syed et al., 2018).

Factors that enhance overrun are (i) sodium caseinate, (ii) whey solids, (iii) emulsifiers, and (iv) pasteurization of the mix at higher temperatures (Sofjan & Hartel, 2004; Syed et al., 2018).

#### 10.8.5.1 Advantages of Overrun

- Improve texture to be light, creamy, less cold.
- Enhance the ease of chewing and taste quality of the food.
- Without overrun, ice cream turns into a frozen block, like an ice cube (Syed et al., 2018).
- Become convenient to scoop.

### 10.8.6 Hardening

The partly frozen mix is filled into molds in an ice cream bar freezer into other types of packaging material (cartons, cups, cones, containers) and then the temperature must be lowered to –15 to –18°C as quickly as possible, which is done by means a brine bath in the ice cream bar freezer or in a hardening tunnel in which air is circulated at high velocity at a temperature of –40 to –45°C. At the end of this stage, approximately 80% of the water is frozen. Ice cream bars are made by employing a unique machine equipped with freezing pockets (molds) to give them their distinctive shape. The pockets are immersed in a frigid brine, extremely cold at around –40 to –45°C. When placed inside the pockets, final crystallization takes place and the frozen ice cream transforms into a solid state. When it is hard, a wooden stick of considerable length is inserted into every pocket. In order to remove the hardened bars, the pockets are immersed in a liquid that melts the outer layer of ice cream. The bars are usually covered in chocolate or some other thick coating before being wrapped in paper.

### 10.8.7 Storage

After hardening, the ice cream is kept in a cold store at a temperature of –25°C. At this temperature, 90% of the water is frozen. It is important to maintain this temperature; if the ice cream is subjected to an increase in temperature and slow subsequent decreases in temperature, the result may be that large ice crystals form.

### 10.8.8 Packaging

Ice cream can be packaged in either paperboard or plastic cartons. Cartons are made from a special type of paper called wet-strength paperboard that is coated with polyethylene plastic to prevent it from collapsing in extreme freezer temperatures. Ice cream is carefully measured and placed into the cartons at a rate of 70 to 90 cartons per hour. Afterward, the cartons are fitted with a lid by a machine. An inkjet printer puts an expiration date and manufacturing code on every carton. Following that, the cartons go through a bundler, which is a hot tunnel that wraps a layer of plastic shrink wrapping around each cup.

The benefits and drawbacks of the different ingredients in ice cream have been summarized in **Table 10.4.**

## 10.9 STORAGE AND DISTRIBUTION OF ICE CREAM

Ice cream quality depends on many factors, including storage temperature. If kept at the correct temperature, ice cream is thoroughly frozen and can feel hard to the touch. If the final product is stored at a temperature between –20 and –25°C, it can be used for a duration of 12 to 18 months. It is recommended to keep the distribution temperature between –25 and –30°C. This range is safer because smaller changes in temperature are less risky.

### 10.9.1 Storage at Home

- Do not repeatedly soften and refreeze ice cream.
- The temperature of the freezer should be set between –5 and 0°F (–18°C). Ice cream is best to eat when it's between 6 and 10°F.

**TABLE 10.4**
**Advantages and Limitations of Various Components/Constituents of Ice Cream**

| Constituent | Advantages | Limitations |
|---|---|---|
| Milk fat | i. Enhances the flavor and makes the texture smoother<br>ii. Lubricates and insulates the mouth<br>iii. Important for the creaminess of ice cream | i. Comparatively high price<br>ii. Difficult to whip<br>iii. May limit consumption due to high calories and satiating effect |
| Non-fat milk solids (NMS) | i. Improves body and texture<br>ii. Promotes development of overrun | i. High amount may cause cooked or salty flavor<br>ii. Potential for sandiness at high concentrations |
| Whey solids | i. Less expensive than conventional sources of NMS | i. Large quantities lead to an excessive freezing point depression<br>ii. The possibility of having a sandy texture is more likely in NMS compared to other traditional sources |
| Sugar | i. Reduces freezing point<br>ii. Imparts sweetness to the ice cream<br>iii. Improves flavor/texture | i. Excess sweetness possible<br>ii. Lower hardening temperature needed<br>iii. Ice cream is softer, affecting scooping and the potential for greater recrystallization |
| Corn syrup solids | i. Lower cost than sugar<br>ii. Improve body and texture<br>iii. Increase stability of the ice cream | i. Impart off flavor and chewy texture when overused |
| Stabilizers | i. Enhance smooth texture<br>ii. Provide body | i. Excess chewiness may occur<br>ii. Increase melt resistance |
| Egg yolk solids | i. Improve whipping ability<br>ii. Impart custard flavor | i. Foamy melted product<br>ii. Egg flavor may be undesirable |
| Emulsifiers | i. Promote fat destabilization, leading to dryness, smoothness, and good melting properties | i. Increase potential for churning of fat |
| Total solids (TS) | i. Smoother texture<br>ii. Firmer body<br>iii. Higher nutrient content<br>iv. Less excess coldness | i. Heavy, soggy, or sticky body<br>ii. Reduce coldness |
| Flavoring | i. Increases acceptability | i. Intensities and harshness may be unacceptable |
| Coloring | i. Improves attractiveness<br>ii. Aids flavor identification | i. Artificial shades<br>ii. Allergic reactions of some people to yellow no. 5 or no. 6<br>iii. Some consumers dislike added colors |

*Source:* Marshall et al., 2003

- Storing ice cream in a gallon freezer bag for extended periods of time will reduce the formation of ice crystals.
- Ice cream should not be kept near uncovered food to prevent odors from affecting its taste.

### 10.9.2 Storage at the Store

- The optimal temperature is 0°F (–18°C) or below.
- To avoid excessive freezing, it is necessary to ensure that the freezer in the supermarket is set at a temperature below 10°F (–12°C).
- Place the ice cream products in a distinct area of the shopping cart, or alternatively, position them on the uppermost part of the other groceries.

- Keep the ice cream cold on the way home by wrapping it in a freezer bag or using an extra paper bag.
- Maintain the coldness of ice cream during transportation by placing it inside a freezer bag or an additional brown paper bag.

### 10.9.3 Transportation (Cold Chain)

Transporting ice cream in a cold chain might involve several steps:

**Supply:** The ice cream is made, packaged in a plant, and sent for transportation.
**Transport:** Refrigerated trucks are commonly used to transport ice cream, and they go through regular inspections to make sure they are in excellent condition.
**Storage:** Before being distributed, ice cream may be kept in a cold storage facility. The product could enter again into the cold chain for distribution after it has been bought.
**Market:** Delivery to the grocery store where customers buy ice cream is typically the last step in the cold chain. Before being placed in the frozen display for customers to purchase, the ice cream may be kept in a walk-in freezer here for a short while.

## 10.10 QUALITY JUDGING OF ICE CREAM

The sensory characteristics of the ice cream are measured by the following (**Table 10.5**) method described by Manoharan and Ramasamy (2013).

TABLE 10.5
Score Card for Sensory Evaluation of Ice Cream

Name: ________ Sample no: ________ Date: ________

| Sample. No | Color (5) | Flavor (45) | Body and texture (30) | Melting quality (5) | Bacterial count (15) | Total (100) |
|---|---|---|---|---|---|---|
| 1 | | | | | | |
| 2 | | | | | | |
| 3 | | | | | | |
| 4 | | | | | | |
| 5 | | | | | | |

## 10.11 DEFECTS IN ICE CREAM

### 10.11.1 Flavor Defects

These are classified according to the flavoring system (low flavor or very high flavor, unnatural flavor), the sweetening system (low sweetness or very sweet), processing-linked flavor defects (cooked), dairy component flavor defects (acidic, salty, old ingredient, oxidized, offensive, or whey flavors), and others (storage/absorbed, stabilizer/emulsifier, foreign).

### 10.11.2 Body and Texture Defects

**Coarse/icy texture:** It is noticeable when the ice cream is eaten. The causes are as follows:

(i) Inadequate total solids (high water content), (ii) inadequate protein, (iii) inadequate stabilizer, (iv) inadequate homogenizing force, (v) re-hardening soft ice cream, (vi) delayed hardening, and (vii) delayed freezing (Pon et al., 2015).

**Crumbly body:** The flaking or snowing feature is caused by: (i) low stabilizer, (ii) high overrun along with large air cells, (iii) low protein, and (iv) low total solids.

**Fluffy texture:** A porous characteristic caused by: (i) low total solids, (ii) incorporation of an enormous amount of air, and (iii) low stabilizer

**Gummy body:** This defect is the opposite of crumbly because it makes the substance feel like paste or putty. It occurs due to: (i) excess stabilizer, (ii) very low overrun, and (iii) poor stabilizer.

**Sandy texture:** Although it is the most annoying issue, it is also the simplest to identify. This happens because of lactose crystals, which are difficult to dissolve and provide a rough or gritty mouthfeel. This can be kept apart from "iciness" because the lactose crystals don't melt in your mouth when you have them. This problem can be solved by employing the following methods that prevent iciness: (i) maintaining low storage room temperature, (ii) hardening the ice cream immediately, and (iii) preventing temperature fluctuations from producer to customer.

**Weak body:** Ice cream lacks "chewiness" and melts quickly into a watery liquid. Gives the impression of lacking richness. May be caused by: (i) high overrun, (ii) low total solids, and (iii) insufficient stabilizer.

### 10.11.3 Melting Quality Characteristics

**Curdy melt-down:** It might be due to visible fat particles or milk protein coagulation, and it is influenced by variables that impact fat destabilization or protein stability, such as (i) high homogenizing pressure (fat coagulation), (ii) salt balance (protein coagulation), and (iii) over-freezing in the freezer (fat coagulation).

**Does not melt:** May be caused by: (i) over-emulsification, (ii) wrong emulsifier, (iii) high fat, (iv) excessive fat clumping in the mix due to homogenization at very low temperature or single-stage homogenizer, and (v) freezing to a very low temperature in the freezer.

**Wheying off:** The salt balance, protein composition, carrageenan addition, etc., are the factors.

### 10.11.4 Color Defects

**Color uneven:** It usually applies to ice cream where color has been used but can be seen in vanilla ice cream under certain circumstances.

**Color unnatural:** This may be caused by: (i) excess yellow coloring is used in vanilla ice cream, (ii) grayish color due to neutralization, and (iii) wrong shade of color used for flavored ice cream.

### 10.11.5 Shrinkage

It is caused by the loss of spherical air bubbles and the formation of continuous air channels. Some factors believed associated with the defect are: (i) freezing and hardening at very low temperatures, (ii) too much overrun, and (iii) both low and high temperature effects.

## 10.12 HEALTH BENEFITS OF ICE CREAM

Ice cream retains the nutritional qualities of milk due to its main ingredient being milk. It is found from many studies that ice cream is a good carrier of probiotic bacteria (Pankiewicz et al., 2019; Dos Santos Cruxen et al., 2017; Ayar et al., 2017; Vardar & Öksüz, 2007; Balthazar et al., 2018; Maurotti et al., 2023). Ice cream/functional ice cream (using various bioactive peptides, dietary fiber, vitamins, minerals, prebiotics, and probiotics) may provide potential health benefits (**Figures 10.5 and 10.6**).

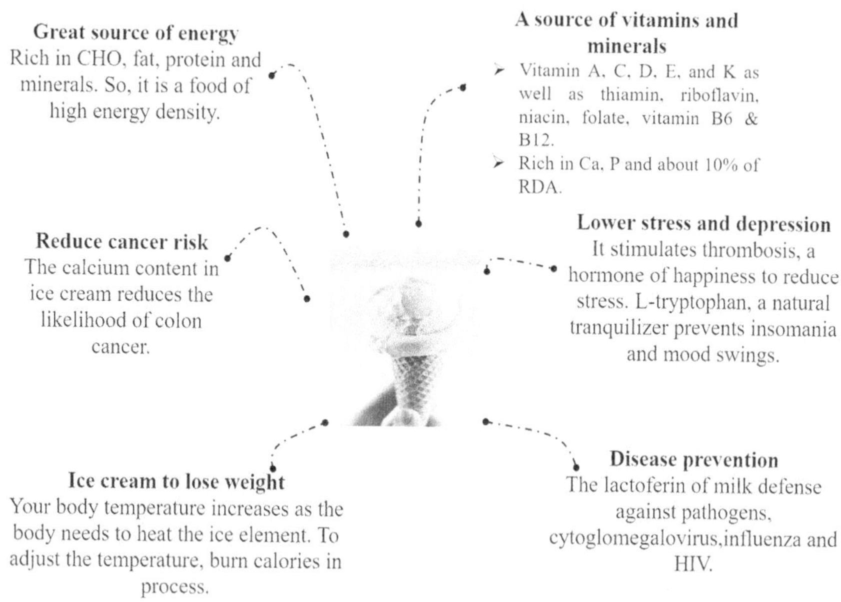


**FIGURE 10.5 Key potential health benefits of ice cream.** Ice cream is a calcium-rich meal, and calcium strengthens the body and increases metabolism.

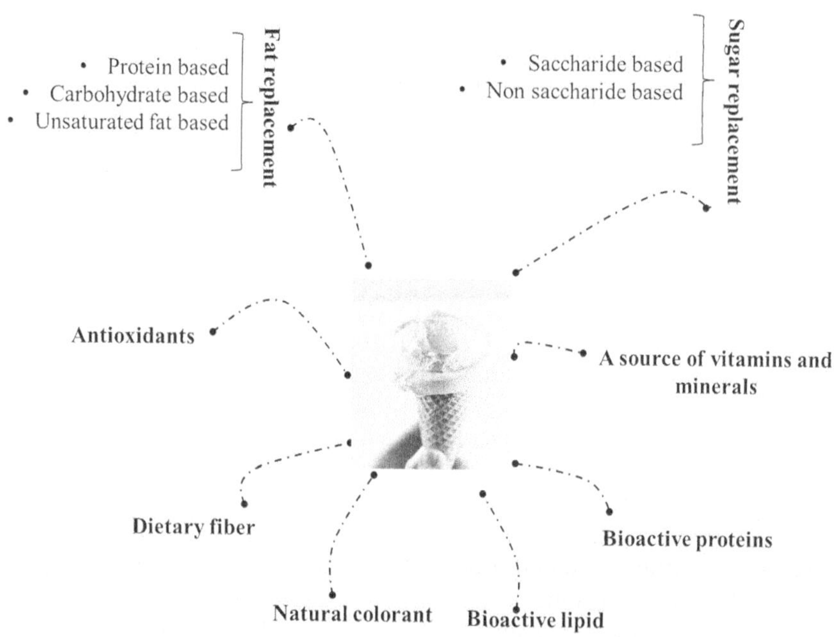


**FIGURE 10.6 Key potential health benefits of functional ice cream.** Functional ice cream is nutritious and helps to lower the risk of disease.

### 10.12.1 Association of Ice Cream Consumption with Bone Health

Calcium and phosphorus contents of ice cream are 0.132 g/100 g and 0.105 g/100 g, respectively. Ice cream helps in strengthening the bones because it is loaded with calcium and can be included in the diet to meet the calcium requirements. As a result, ice cream also contributes to fight osteoporosis. Ice cream is packed with minerals like calcium and phosphorus, which are essential for adequate nutrition.

### 10.12.2 Association of Ice Cream Consumption with Vitamin Intake

Ice cream is loaded with important vitamins including A, D, E, thiamin, riboflavin, pyridoxine, cyanocobalamin, niacin, folate, and ascorbic acid.

### 10.12.3 Association of Ice Cream Consumption with Energy Boosting

One of the most important health benefits of cream is an energy boost. Ice cream provides energy due to its high carbohydrate content, with about 15 g in a 1/2 cup serving. A serving contains about 7 g of fat and 2 g of protein, making it a high-energy food. For example, 1/2 cup of vanilla ice cream provides 137 kilocalories of energy, which is about twice than the quantity of 1/2 cup of whole milk (Spence et al., 2019).

### 10.12.4 Association of Ice Cream Consumption with Tissue Growth

Ice cream contains proteins that are highly significant for the body as they contain essential amino acids (tryptophan, lysine, etc.). These are very important for the development of infants and children and for building up tissues in adults.

### 10.12.5 Association of Ice Cream Consumption with Immuno-Boosting

Ice cream helps support immunity. As ice cream is loaded with lactoferrin and cytokines, it improved immunity against various diseases, including influenza.

### 10.12.6 Association of Ice Cream Consumption with Reproductive Health

High-fat dairy desserts like ice cream enhance the chances of ovulating. Therefore, ice cream improves the fertility of women.

### 10.12.7 Association of Ice Cream Consumption with Probiotics

Ice creams are food items showing the ability to be used as probiotic carriers, with the added benefit of being appreciated by people belonging to any or all age groups and social classes (Cruz et al., 2009). Lactic fermentation is a known alternative and natural method for creating novel ice cream formulations with improved nutritional, textural, physical, and rheological features (Aboulfazli et al., 2015). Cow milk can be enhanced by bioactive substances and postbiotics during fermentation, and these substances, together with microorganisms, can help the finished product's functional qualities (Peyer et al., 2016; Hossain & Kober, 2008). Additionally, fermentation by LAB has the ability to modify the sensory qualities of food without the use of additives by introducing welcoming flavors and enhancing their palatability (Mathur et al., 2020). Because different strains have varying tolerances for the relatively high sugar content that defines the composition of ice cream, the freezing processes, and the presence of oxygen in the cream, choosing starters is an important step (Alamprese et al., 2002). Dietary fiber additions can also improve the rheological, textural, and melting resistance of ice creams while keeping sensory qualities and probiotics (Akalın et al., 2018). The National Academies of Science (Washington, DC, USA) reports that the average daily intake of dietary fiber is far lower than the recommended intakes of 38 and 25 g for men and women, respectively (Sah et al., 2016). So, dietary fiber might be added to new ice cream formulations to enhance health benefits (such prebiotic activity, lowering cholesterol, and reducing blood glucose reactions) and providing laxative effects. Furthermore, due to the functional characteristics of these biopolymers, the production of exopolysaccharides (EPS) by lactic acid bacteria has attracted particular attention over the past 10 years (Duboc & Mollet, 2001). Despite this, there are just a few studies (Dertli et al., 2016; Zhang et al., 2017) that address the use of in situ EPS synthesis to functionalize ice cream. Another functional characteristic that can be enhanced in novel formulations through various techniques is antioxidant activity. Novel probiotic ice cream formulations have improved antiradical and anti-inflammatory features, according to a recent study (Polo et al., 2023).

### 10.12.8 Association of Ice Cream Consumption with Digestive Health

Many studies have shown that homogenized milk is more digestible than milk that has not been homogenized. This is because the homogenizer has broken down the fat globules into tiny particles, which are easier for the digestive juices to digest than the larger fat globules. When fat in ice cream mix is put into a homogenizer, as is now done in industrial ice cream plants, the same thing happens. Furthermore, the high palatability of ice cream quickens the flow of digestive juices. These two characteristics, combined with its sweet taste, velvety smooth texture, and glistening coolness, make it the perfect food (Arbuckle, 1986). These characteristics, along with its value as a morale booster, have led hospitals to include ice cream on their menus in large quantities. No other food commodity adds as much nutritional value in such an enticing and appealing shape or is as widely liked and sold as ice cream (Vardar & Öksüz, 2007).

## 10.13 ICE CREAM INNOVATIONS

Recently, the benefits of ice cream for public health have been recognized worldwide, and the sustainable food industry and consumption are expected to grow steadily over the coming years, especially in developed countries. This is especially due to the tremendous progress that has been made in the past decade in all areas of research related to ice cream, from production to nutritional and health attributes. Due to several health concerns and consumer demands, there have been innovations giving rise to a variety of health-friendly ice creams with ingredients that improve the overall nutrient content of the ice cream. Due to advances in ice cream from production to nutritional and health attributes ice cream offers a new perspective, combining the pleasure of a frozen dessert with health-enhancing ingredients and benefits. **Figures 10.7, 10.8, and 10.9** illustrate ice cream innovations from production to nutritional and health attributes (Arslaner & Salık, 2020; Shaunak, 2020).

## 10.14 ADVERSE HEALTH EFFECTS OF ICE CREAM

According to experts, it is advisable to consume foods containing additional sugar and saturated fat, such as ice cream, in a moderate, mindful manner. Excessive consumption of these foods can displace nutritious choices in the diet and increase the risk of enduring prolonged health issues such as cardiovascular disease, elevated cholesterol levels, excessive weight, diabetes, gastrointestinal complications, abdominal fat accumulation, renal disorders, cancer, eye irritation, sore throat, and allergic reaction (Goff, 2013).

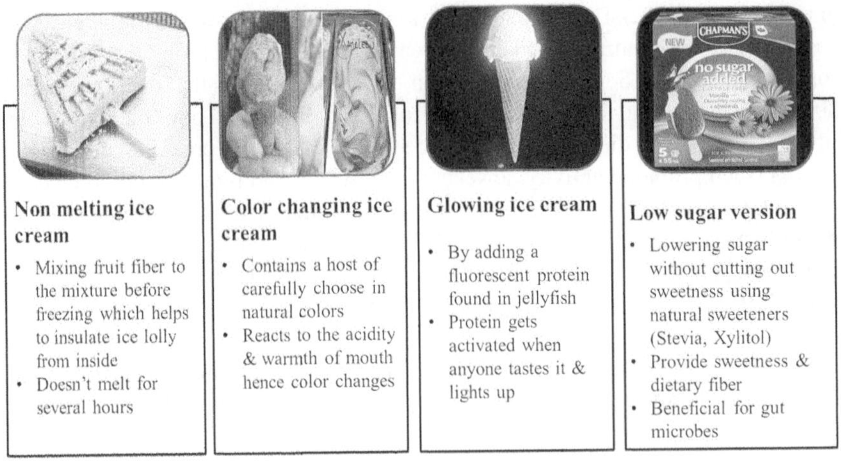


**FIGURE 10.7 Ice cream innovations in production attributes.** Modern-day ice cream has changed a lot such as non-melting ice cream, color-changing ice cream, and so on.

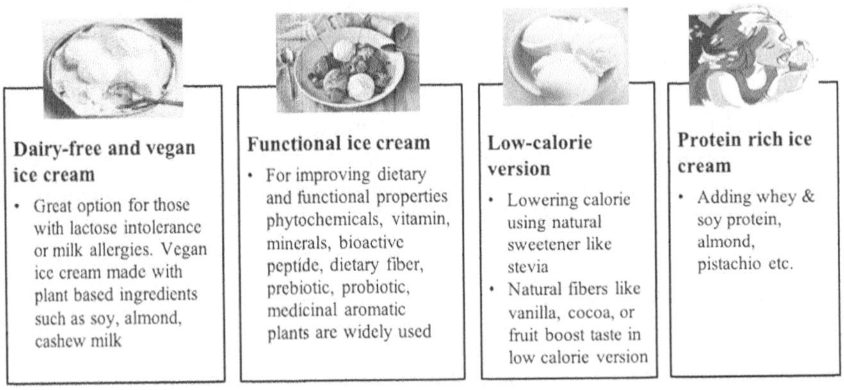


**FIGURE 10.8 Ice cream innovations in nutritional attributes.** Modern ice cream has evolved significantly, including changes to the fat quantity and source, reduced sugar varieties, protein boosts, and so on.

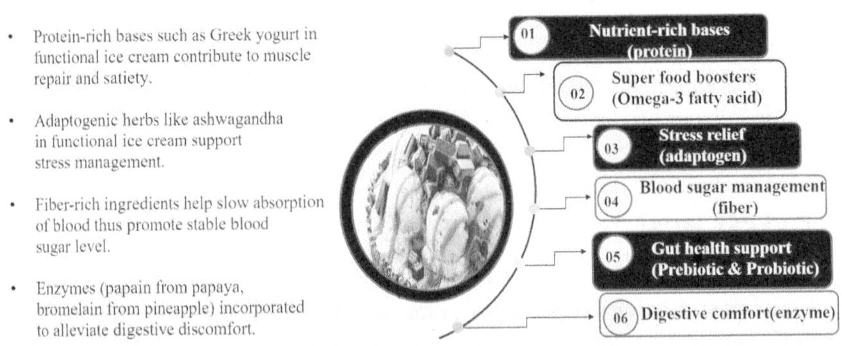


**FIGURE 10.9 Ice cream innovations in health attributes.** To meet the increased demand for health and wellness products, manufacturers are developing ice cream varieties that include probiotics, protein, and plant-based components.

## 10.15 CONCLUSIONS

Ice cream is a frozen dessert cherished by people across the globe. Adding milk and non-milk ingredients helps create the characteristics of structure, taste, body, and flavors in a product. Moreover, apart from incorporating new technologies, it is important to establish enhanced analytical methods to precisely assess the characteristics and manufacturing steps of ice cream (Kamińska-Dwórznicka et al., 2019). Nutraceutical substances that do not break down under freezing temperatures can be introduced with ice cream. Since ice cream is one of the most well-liked products, this type of fortification can be a great way to provide the elderly with the energy and nutrients they need, while also reducing their chances of being ill (Guo et al., 2018; Pintor et al., 2017).

## REFERENCES


Aboulfazli, F., Baba, A. S., & Misran, M. (2015). Effects of fermentation by Bifidobacterium bifidum on the rheology and physical properties of ice cream mixes made with cow and vegetable milks. *International Journal of Food Science & Technology*, *50*(4), 942–949.

Akalın, A. S., Kesenkas, H., Dinkci, N., Unal, G., Ozer, E., & Kınık, O. (2018). Enrichment of probiotic ice cream with different dietary fibers: Structural characteristics and culture viability. *Journal of Dairy Science*, *101*(1), 37–46.

Akbari, M., Eskandari, M. H., & Davoudi, Z. (2019). Application and functions of fat replacers in low-fat ice cream: A review. *Trends in Food Science & Technology*, *86*, 34–40.

Alamprese, C., Foschino, R., Rossi, M., Pompei, C., & Savani, L. (2002). Survival of Lactobacillus Johnsonii La1 and influence of its addition in retail-manufactured ice cream produced with different sugar and fat concentrations. *International Dairy Journal*, *12*, 201–208.

Arbuckle, W. S. (1986). *Ice cream* (4th ed.). Van Nostrand Reinhold Company Book of Firsts. RW Press.

Arslaner, A., & Salık, M. A. (2020). Functional ice cream technology. *Akademik Gıda*, *18*(2), 180–189.

Arun, K., & Ramesh, C. C. (2013). Frozen dairy food. *Milk and Dairy Products in Human Nutrition: Production, Composition and Health*, 390–411.

Ayar, A., Siçramaz, H., Öztürk, S., & Yilmaz, S. Ö. (2017). Probiotics properties of ice creams produced with dietary fibres from by-products of the industry. *International Journal of Dairy Technology*, *71*, 174–182.

Balthazar, C. F., Silva, H. L., Esmerino, E. A., Rocha, R. S., Moraes, J., Carmo, M. A., Azevedo, L., Camps, I., Abud, Y. K. D., Sant'Anna, C., Franco, R., Freitas, M. Q., Silva, M. C., Raices, R., Escher, G. B., Granato, D., Senaka Ranadheera, C., Nazarro, F., & Cruz, A. G. (2018). The addition of inulin and Lactobacillus casei 01 in sheep milk ice cream. *Food Chemistry*, *246*, 464–472.

Cruz, A. G., Antunes, A. E., Sousa, A. L. O., Faria, J. A., & Saad, S. M. (2009). Ice-cream as a probiotic food carrier. *Food Research International*, *42*(9), 1233–1239.

Dertli, E., Toker, O. S., Durak, M. Z., Yilmaz, M. T., Tatlisu, N. B., Sagdic, O., & Cankurt, H. (2016). Development of a fermented ice-cream as influenced by in situ exopolysaccharide production: Rheological, molecular, microstructural and sensory characterization. *Carbohydrate Polymers*, *136*, 427–440.

Dos Santos Cruxen, C. E., Hoffmann, J. F., Zandoná, G. P., Fiorentini, Â. M., Rombaldi, C. V., & Chaves, F. C. (2017). Probiotic butiá (Butia odorata) ice cream: Development, characterization, stability of bioactive compounds, and viability of Bifidobacterium lactis during storage. *LWT Food Science Technology*, *75*, 379–385.

Duboc, P., & Mollet, B. (2001). Applications of exopolysaccharides in the dairy industry. *International Dairy Journal*, *11*(9), 759–768.

Goff, H. D. (2013). *The ice cream ebook*. The dairy education series. The University of Guelph, Canada.

Goff, H. D., & Hartel, R. W. (2013). *Ice cream* (7th ed.). Springer.

Guo, Y., Zhang, X., Hao, W., Xie, Y., Chen, L., Li, Z., Zhu, B., & Feng, X. (2018). Nano-bacterial cellulose/soy protein isolate complex gel as fat substitutes in ice cream model. *Carbohydrate Polymers*, *198*, 620–630.

Hossain, M. T., & Kober, A. K. M. H. (2008). Microbiological quality of ice cream available in Chittagong. *Bangladesh Journal of Microbiology*, *25*, 135–136.

Kamińska-Dwórznicka, A., Gondek, E., Łaba, S., Jakubczyk, E., & Samborska, K. (2019). Characteristics of instrumental methods to describe and assess the recrystallization process in ice cream systems. *Foods (Basel, Switzerland)*, *8*(4), 117.

Kilara, A., & Chandan, R. C. (2008). Ice cream and frozen desserts. Chapter 16. In R. C. Chandan, A. Kilara, & N. P. Shah (Eds.), *Dairy processing and quality assurance* (pp. 357–386). Wiley-Blackwell.

Kurt, A., & Atalar, I. (2018). Effects of quince seed on the rheological, structural and sensory characteristics of ice cream. *Food Hydrocolloids*, *82*, 186–195.

Manoharan, A. P., & Ramasamy, D. (2013). Studies on sensory evaluation of aloe vera ice cream with artificial sweeteners and natural caramel colour. *International Journal of Food, Agriculture and Veterinary Sciences*, *3*(1), 109–116.

Marshall, R. T., Goff, H. D., & Hartel, R. W. (2003). *Ice cream* (6th ed.). Kluwer/Plenum Publishing.

Mathur, H., Beresford, T. P., & Cotter, P. D. (2020). Health benefits of lactic acid bacteria (LAB) fermentates. *Nutrients*, *12*(6), 1679.

Maurotti, S., Ferro, Y., Pujia, R., Frosina, M., Sciacqua, A., Mare, R., Mazza, E., Geirola, N., Romeo, S., Pujia, A., & Montalcini, T. (2023). Effects of a functional ice cream enriched with milk proteins on bone metabolism: A feasibility clinical study and in vitro investigation. *Nutrients*, *15*(2), 344.

Pankiewicz, U., Góral, M., Kozłowicz, K., & Góral, D. (2019). Novel method of zinc ions supplementing with fermented and unfermented ice cream with using PEF. *International Journal of Food Science & Technology*, *54*(6), 2035–2044.

Peyer, L. C., Zannini, E., & Arendt, E. K. (2016). Lactic acid bacteria as sensory biomodulators for fermented cereal-based beverages. *Trends in Food Science & Technology*, *54*, 17–25.

Pintor, A., Escalona-Buendía, H. B., & Totosaus, A. J. I. F. R. J. (2017). Effect of inulin on melting and textural properties of low-fat and sugar-reduced ice cream: Optimization via a response surface methodology. *International Food Research Journal*, *24*(4), 1728.

Polo, A., Tlais, A. Z. A., Filannino, P., Da Ros, A., Arora, K., Cantatore, V., Vincentini, O., Nicolodi, A., Nicolodi, R., Gobbetti, M., & Di Cagno, R. (2023). Novel fermented ice cream formulations with improved antiradical and anti-inflammatory features. *Fermentation*, *9*(2), 117.

Pon, S. Y., Lee, W. J., & Chong, G. H. (2015). Textural and rheological properties of stevia ice cream. *International Food Research Journal (Malaysia)*, *22*, 1544–1549.

Sah, B. N. P., Vasiljevic, T., McKechnie, S., & Donkor, O. N. (2016). Physicochemical, textural and rheological properties of probiotic yogurt fortified with fibre-rich pineapple peel powder during refrigerated storage. *LWT Food Science Technology*, *65*, 978–986.

Shaunak, A. (2020). *Ice cream of the future | 6 new ice cream innovations*. www.foodunfolded.com/article/ice-cream-of-the-future-6-new-ice-cream-innovations.

Sofjan, R. P., & Hartel, R. W. (2004). Effects of overrun on structural and physical characteristics of ice cream. *International Dairy Journal*, *14*(3), 255–262.

Spence, C., Navarra, J., & Youssef, J. (2019). Using ice-cream as an effective vehicle for energy/nutrient delivery in the elderly. *International Journal of Gastronomy and Food Science*, *16*, 100140.

Stephens, N. (2007). *Wine flavored ice cream*. Bordeaux-Undiscovered. Archived from the original on 27 July 2011.

Syed, Q. A., Anwar, S., Shukat, R., & Zahoor, T. (2018). Effects of different ingredients on texture of ice cream. *Journal of Nutritional Health and Food Engineering*, *8*(6), 422–435.

Tharp, B. W., & Young, L. S. (2013). *Tharp & Young on ice cream: An encyclopedic guide to ice cream science and technology* (pp. 181–182). DEStech Publications Inc.

The Content Bar. (2022). *Contentworks*. https://contentworks.agency/our-scoop-of-the-coolest-ice-cream-marketing.

Vardar, N. B., & Öksüz, Ö. (2007). Artisan strawberry ice cream made with supplementation of Lactococci or Lactobacillus acidophilus. *Italian Journal of Food Science*, *19*(4), 403–412.

Zhang, J., Zhao, W., Guo, X., Guo, T., Zheng, Y., Wang, Y., Hao, Y., & Yang, Z. (2017). Survival and effect of exopolysaccharide-producing lactobacillus plantarum yw11 on the physicochemical properties of ice cream. *Polish Journal of Food and Nutrition Sciences*, *67*, 191–200.

# 11 Traditional/Indigenous Dairy Foods

## 11.1 LEARNING OBJECTIVES

By the end of the chapter, the reader will be able to:

- Understand about different types of traditional dairy foods in various regions
- Know the methods of manufacture and nutritional facts of common traditional sweetmeats/traditional dairy foods
- Understand how to improve the quality of traditional dairy foods
- Make selected traditional dairy food enterprises profitable
- Gather information about the health benefits of traditional dairy foods
- Learn about selected traditional dairy food innovations from production to nutritional and health attributes

Traditional cuisines such as milk and dairy foods are popular and have been consumed all over the world since ancient times due to their social, economic, religious, and cultural significance. Dairy technologists have recently focused on the potential of these products due to their characterization of quality attributes, standardization of the manufacturing processes, and improvement of shelf life, which have led to their export and acceptance on a global scale.

## 11.2 INTRODUCTION

Dairy can be termed as "nature's gift," crafted with tradition and savored with delight. Traditional or indigenous dairy products are milk products that are indigenous to a region or nation and that have developed over time using readily available resources, such as local fuels and cooking utensils. Different types of nutritious and delicious traditional dairy foods are available around the globe (**Figures 11.1 and 11.2**). It is challenging to assess the market for locally produced dairy-based foods because the majority of these goods are produced in homes or in small cottage companies that serve small communities. A broad variety of South Asian milk sweets manufactured in various sections of the nation are popular with both men and women, young and old (**Figure 11.2**). Traditional dairy foods are broadly divided into four categories: fat-rich items, yogurt-based products (fermented), cheese/chhana (coagulum), and khoa-based products (**Figure 11.3**).

## 11.3 CLASSIFICATION OF TRADITIONAL DAIRY FOODS

Due to regional differences in the ingredients added and manufacturing processes, traditional dairy products are known by different names in different parts of the world. Traditional milk products might easily be divided into nine main groups for a better understanding of the products' nature.

DOI: 10.1201/9781003397786-11

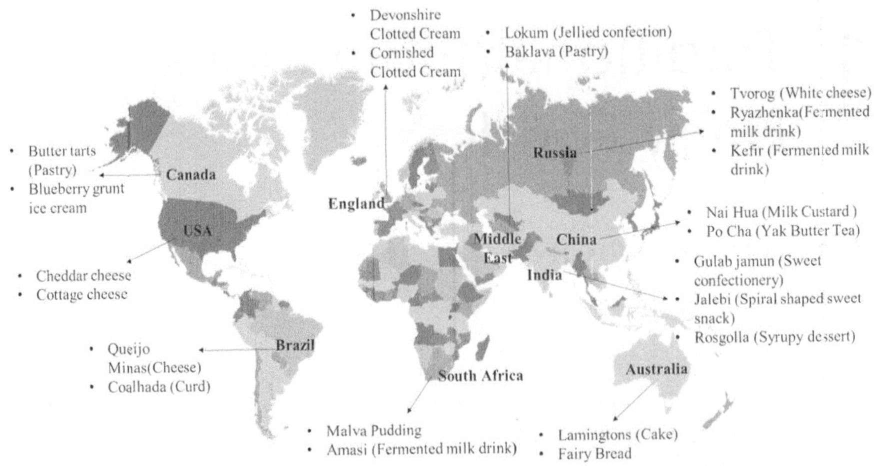


**FIGURE 11.1 Several varieties of nutritious and tasty traditional dairy foods are available around the world.** World's most popular traditional dairy foods, including laban (fermented milk), lassi (yogurt drink), rasgulla (syrup cheese ball), chomchom (sweetmeats), kheer (rice pudding), gulabjamun (rose berries dipped in sugar syrup), kachagolla (ricotta cheese sweets), peda (sweet made with full-fat milk and sugar), barfi (sweet confectionery), sandesh (sweet), rasmalai (cottage cheese balls), buttermilk, tvorog, ryazhenka, kefir, and so on.

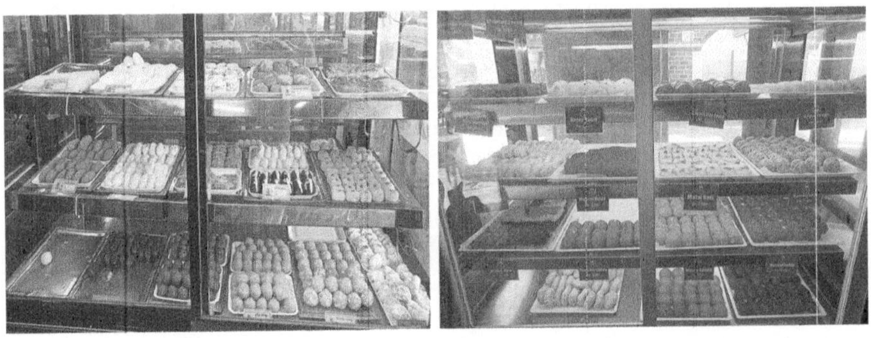

**FIGURE 11.2 Traditional South Asian milk sweets include common grocery store staples.** Milk is used to make a variety of sweetmeats such as rasgulla, rasmalai, malaikari, chomchom, kalojam, peda, chhanapolao, rajvog, kachagolla, rosokadam, gursandesh and so on. Indigenous sweetmeats are tasty, healthy, appealing, and widely consumed in South Asian countries such as India, Bangladesh, Pakistan, and Sri Lanka.

i. **Concentrated/partially desiccated products:** In this category of products, thermal energy is used to concentrate the milk. Milk's moisture content decreases as a result of product vapors evaporating.
ii. Based on the degree of heat treatment, which affects the items smell, color, aroma, and texture. Example: Khoa, Barfi, Rabri.
iii. **Heat and acid-coagulated products:** These are the products that coagulate when acidulants are added to warm milk. The amount of moisture removed determines the texture. Example—paneer, chhana (coagulum).
iv. **Cultured/fermented products:** Milk is fermented using lactic bacteria at a specified temperature and for a specific period of time. Sweet dahi is a well-known product in the eastern region since ancient times. Example—laban, lassi, buttermilk.

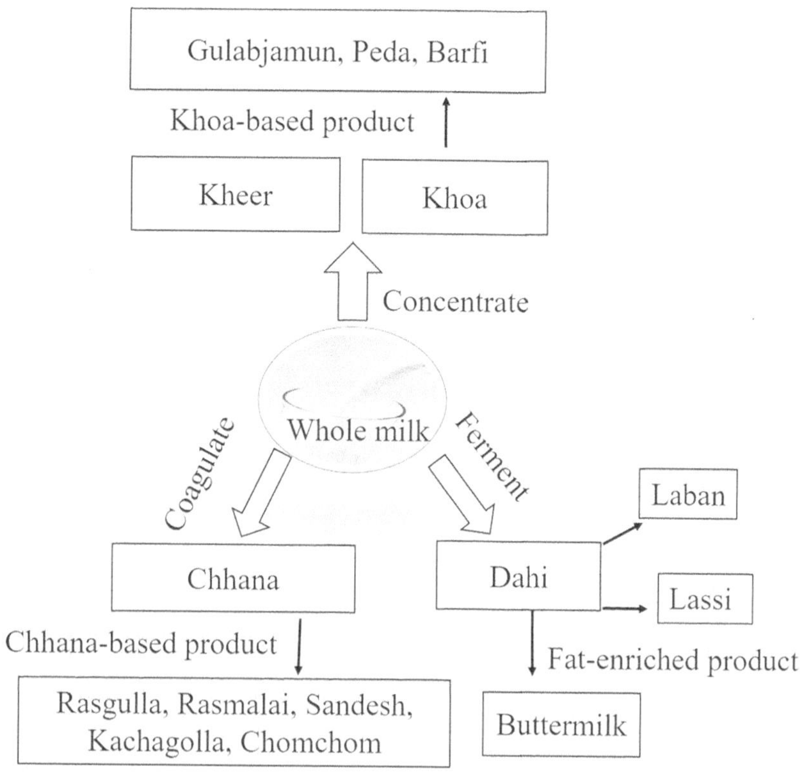


FIGURE 11.3 **Chart of major traditional dairy foods.** Traditional dairy foods are widely classified into four groups, notably the fat-rich products, yogurt-based products (fermented), cheese/chhana (coagulum), and khoa-based products.

v. **Frozen products:** Kulfi, malai-ka-baraf, milk ice
vi. **Cereal-based puddings:** Kheer, payasam
vii. **Milk confections:**
   a. **Khoa-based sweets:** Gulabjamun, barfi, kalak, milk cake, etc.
   b. **Chhana-based sweets:** Rasgulla, sandesh, rasmalai, etc.
   c. **Chhana and khoa-based sweets:** Kala-jamun, pantooa
   d. **Miscellaneous milk sweets:** Milk agar cake, colostrum pudding
viii. **Refreshing beverages:** Lassi, raabadi, chhachh (Chaas)
ix. **Miscellaneous products:** Kadhi, dahiwada, raita

## 11.4 RASGULLA (SYRUP-FILLED ROLL/SWEETENED CHEESE BALL/SWEET SYRUP CHEESE BALL)

### 11.4.1 Introduction

Among several types of dairy-derived sweets, rasgulla/rosogolla/sweetened cheese ball/syrup-filled ball is one of the most popular sweets made with curdled milk in the South Asian countries like India, Bangladesh, Nepal, Pakistan, and Myanmar (Chanda et al., 2002; Pramanick et al., 2017; Sarkar et al., 2020) (**Figure 11.4**). There are no such functions or festival without sweets. Any type of celebration or guest entertainment, whether local or international, must always include sweets (Haque et al., 2003).

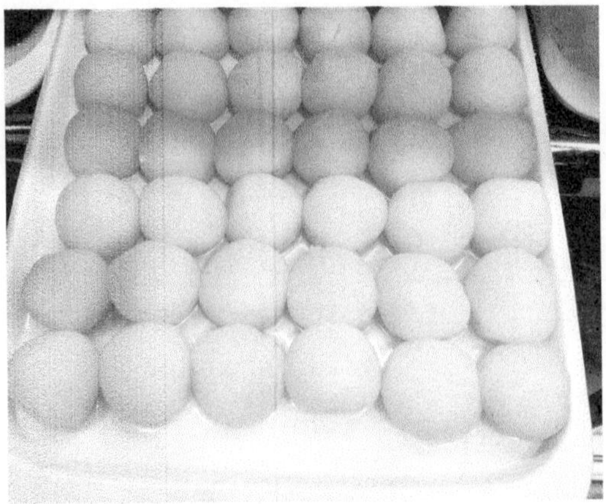

FIGURE 11.4 **Image of rasgulla (sweetened cheese ball).**

### 11.4.2 Nutritional Facts

It is rich in minerals (mainly phosphorus and calcium), fat, protein, and vitamins (vitamin A and D) (Chanda et al., 2002; Sarkar et al., 2020). Rasgulla contains 186 calories per 100 g, of which 153, 17, and 16 calories come from protein, fat, and carbohydrates, respectively (**Table 11.1**) (Sengupta & Bhowal, 2017). Rasgulla is typically produced at home from scratch or from one of the several mixes that are sold commercially. Therefore, the nutritional data may differ greatly (Chanda et al., 2002; Pramanick et al., 2017; Sarkar et al., 2020).

TABLE 11.1
Nutritional Facts of Rasgulla (Made from Cow Milk)

| Components | Amount (%) |
|---|---|
| Moisture | 54.86 |
| Protein | 5.05 |
| Fat | 4.9 |
| Dietary fiber | 0.88 |
| Carbohydrates | 34.35 |

*Source:* Haque et al., 2003; Alam et al., 2020

### 11.4.3 Manufacturing Process

Fresh milk is boiled at its boiling temperature and cooled to about 70°C. A 1% (w/v) solution of lactic acid is mixed gradually into it until the total amount of milk coagulates with an appearance of greenish-yellow hue (Ranganadham et al., 1989; Bandyopadhyay et al., 2008). Then, the coagulated chhana (coagulum) and whey are separated (casein portion) by draining (Katara & Bhargava, 1990). In this case, a muslin cloth can be used. Then, the chhana has to be kneaded and made into balls by rolling. These are cooked in sugar syrup. A rasgulla should be gloopy, mild, and moist and must return to its shape when squeezed (Pal & Roy, 2019). It should not be rubbery or flexible. The manufacturing process for traditional rasgulla is shown in **Figure 11.5.**

It can use rose water while serving, but the amount should be very little and it must be organic or edible type, not any kind of synthetic rose water. It will improve taste and flavor.

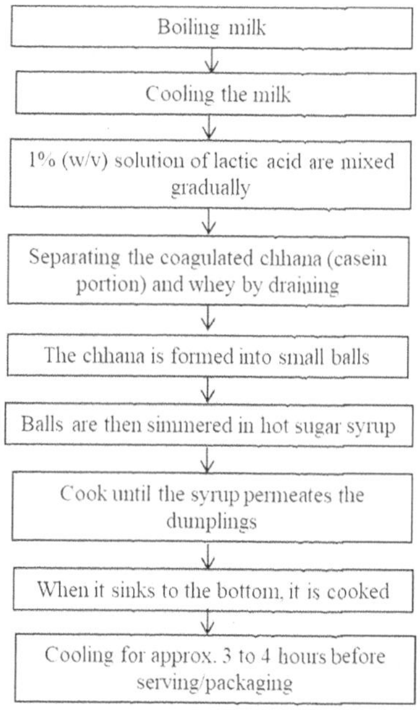


FIGURE 11.5 **General flow diagram for the manufacturing process of rasgulla.**

### 11.4.4 Health Benefits of Rasgulla

Rasgulla contains 186 calories per 100 g portion since it is consumed every day and not just on special occasions or during festivals. Of the total 186 calories, 153 calories are from carbohydrates, which is also 9% of the daily calorie requirement (Bandyopadhyay et al., 2008; Kaur & Goswami, 2020). Due to the rasgulla's low glycemic index, diabetic individuals can easily consume it. The folic acid and thiamine content offer energy and are helpful for brain functioning. The dietary fibers in chhana speed up metabolism (Singh et al., 2015; Sarkar et al., 2021). Rasgulla's main component, milk, contains calcium (Ca) and vitamin D; as a result, eating rasgulla promotes the development of strong teeth, bones, and muscles. Rasgulla is a protein-rich food, as it contains 20% whey protein and 80% casein protein, both of which are found in milk. Chhana contains magnesium (Mg) and potassium (K), which reduce blood pressure and blood sugar levels, respectively. Rasgulla can be eaten shortly after preparation and while still hot to aid in the treatment of different stomach-related illnesses like dysentery (Singh et al., 2015; Sarkar et al., 2021). **Figure 11.6** gives a summary of the health benefits of rasgulla.

## 11.5 CHOMCHOM (SWEETMEATS)

### 11.5.1 Introduction

Chomchom is a common sweet from Bangladesh consisting of homemade cottage cheese named chhana which is cooked into syrup (**Figure 11.7**). Most of the time, it is flavored with lemon juice and cardamom powder. This pleasant item can be present in a few contrasting varieties, with chopped nuts, malai cream, or grated coconut. The very name of Porabari chomchom still bears the old glory of Tangail of Bangladesh. This place is renowned not only as a business center but also as the origin of the famous chomchom. Porabari chomchom is renowned for its burnt brick color and juicy interior that tastes like honey. It is said that the typical burnt brick color came from caramelized sugar. Chomchom is made in a variety of colors such as brick, light pink, light yellow, and white. It is

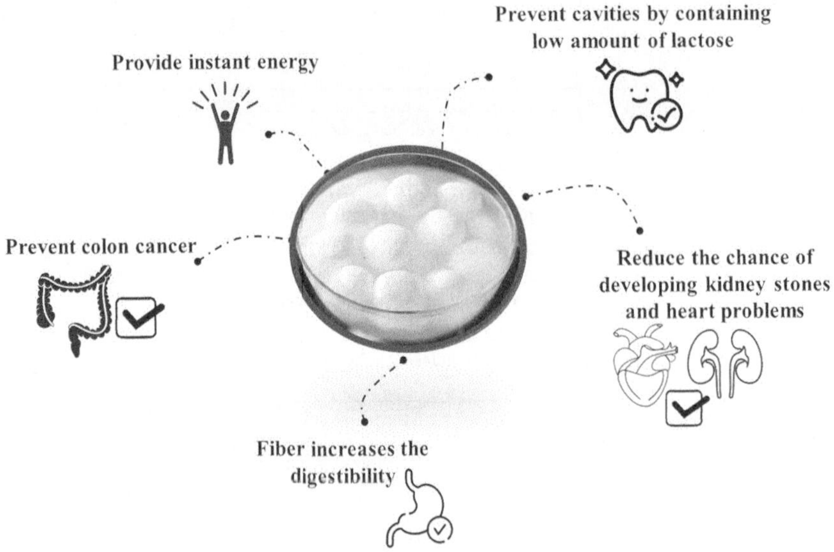


**FIGURE 11.6** **Key potential health benefits of rasgulla.**

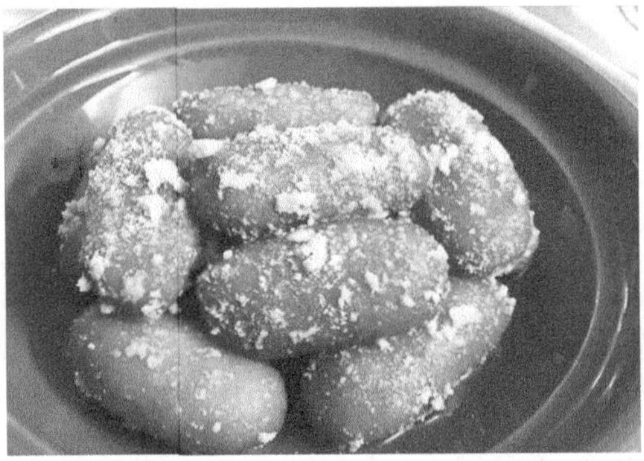

**FIGURE 11.7** **Image of chomchom (sweetmeats).**

made using very thick milk and comes in a variety of styles and forms. Porabari chomchom is well known for its excessive sweetness and unique flavor. Chomchom's flavor is largely influenced by the flavor of Tangail's water. The water of Tangail is the secret that underlies the flavor of chomchom of Porabari (Islam & Basak, 2013).

### 11.5.2 Nutritional Facts

Chomchom is considered a nutritious sweet. It is a nutrient-dense, high-protein meal that is also high in calcium, riboflavin, zinc, magnesium, potassium, phosphorus, and vitamins A, D, and E. **Table 11.2** shows that one chomchom has about 255 calories. Carbohydrates contribute 153 calories, proteins account for 22 calories, and fat accounts for the remaining 81 calories. One Chomchom supplies around 13% of the total daily calorie needs of a regular adult diet of 2000 calories.

**TABLE 11.2**
**Nutritional Facts of Chomchom**

| Components | Amount (%) |
|---|---|
| Moisture | 44.18 |
| Protein | 5.05 |
| Fat | 1.62 |
| Dietary fiber | 0.88 |
| Carbohydrates | 43.93 |
| Calories | 206.50 |

*Source:* Alam et al., 2020

### 11.5.3 Manufacturing Process

Chhana is combined with a little semolina before being formed into little balls. The balls are delicately cooked in ghee or butter oil. Sugar syrup is prepared by heating a mixture of sugar and water. The balls are then cooked in the boiling sugar syrup until the desirable firm body and close texture are formed. Finally, the balls are removed from the syrup and coated with sugar or khoa. The manufacturing process for traditional chomchom is shown in the flow diagram in **Figure 11.8.**

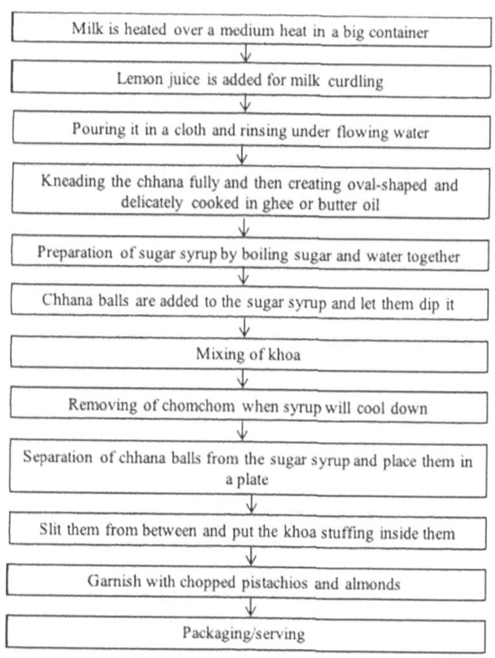


**FIGURE 11.8 The general flow diagram of the manufacturing process of chomchom.**

### 11.5.4 Health Benefits of Chomchom

Chomchom is good source of Ca, P, vitamin $B_1$, and vitamin $B_2$, and has beneficial effects. Calcium makes bones stay strong at all ages, including kids and adults. Phosphorus works closely with calcium to build bones. Vitamin $B_1$ protects nerves, helps in carbohydrate metabolism, prevents heart disease, and helps produce RBCs. Vitamin $B_2$ enables the production of RBCs, which contribute to rising energy levels. This is not good for diabetic individuals or heart disease patients. **Figure 11.9** gives a summary of the health benefits of chomchom.

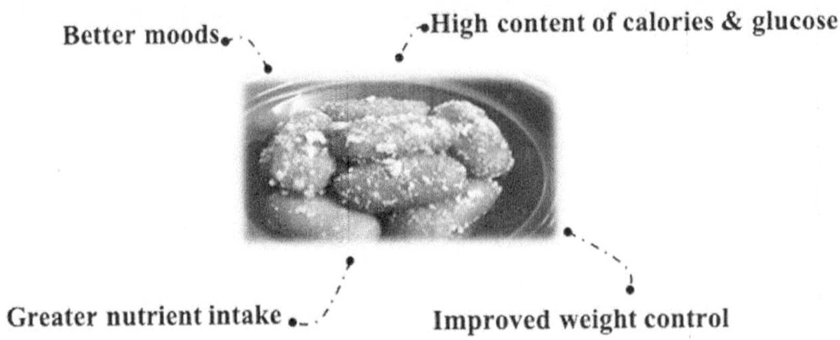
Better moods
High content of calories & glucose
Greater nutrient intake
Improved weight control

FIGURE 11.9 Key potential health benefits of chomchom.

## 11.6 KHEER (RICE PUDDING)

### 11.6.1 Introduction

Kheer, payasa, payasam, or phirni is a heat-desiccated, cereal-based, sweetened, condensed, nutritious Indian dairy dessert (Jha et al., 2013). Kheer is generally made of milk and rice (**Figure 11.10**). Kheer has changed to accommodate regional and individual preferences (Kumar et al., 2011). Kheer is known by different names in different parts of the country, such as "Kheer" in the northwestern region, "Payasam" in the southern region, "Payas" in the Eastern region, "Phirni" in the northern region, and "Kheech" in the Mewar region of Rajasthan (Thompkinson, 1995). Kheer is a semi-solid to fluid product with partially disintegrated cooked rice grains dispersed in viscous liquid comprising soluble starch from rice grains (Jha et al., 2002). It is made by simmering rice in milk while adding sugar or jaggery until the rice starch becomes gelatinous (Gupta et al., 2014). Kheer comprises a sizable number of non-dairy ingredients, such as rice, wheat, sugar, raisins, makhana, coconut powder, flavorings like saffron and cardamom, and dried fruits like almonds and pistachios, in addition to milk (Jha et al., 2013). It is considered a nutritious food for people of all ages

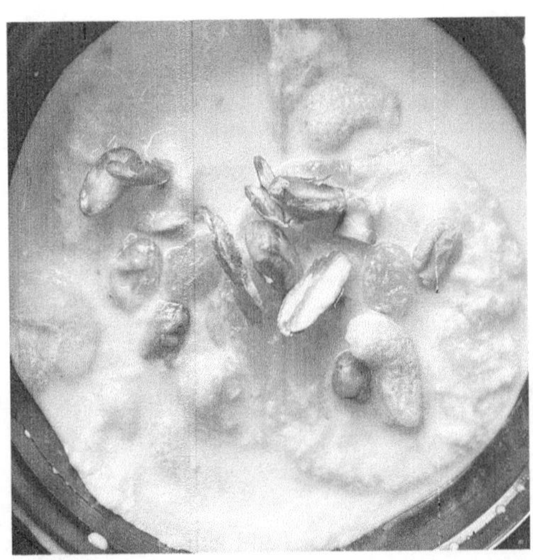

FIGURE 11.10 Image of kheer (rice pudding).

and is characterized by a sweet, nutty, and pleasant flavor that is highly acceptable to the Indian palate. It closely resembles rice pudding, a popular dessert in the United States and in northern and central Europe. As with the other traditional Indian dairy products, kheer also contains considerable fat and sugar (Gautam et al., 2013).

### 11.6.2 Nutritional Facts

Kheer is regarded as a healthy dessert since it includes nutrients from both rice and milk (Kumar et al., 2005). Kheer is therefore considered a diet with a high nutrient density and is utilized as an inexpensive weaning food in many Indian homes (**Table 11.3**) (Kumari & Poonia, 2021).

**TABLE 11.3**
**Nutritional Facts of Kheer**

| Components | Amount (per 50 g) |
|---|---|
| Energy (k cal) | 134.60 |
| Protein (g) | 1.65 |
| Fat (g) | 1.2 |
| Carbohydrates (g) | 19.06 |
| Fiber (g) | 0.02 |
| Iron (mg) | 1.33 |
| Ca (mg) | 37.01 |

*Source:* Singh & Vaidya, 2015

### 11.6.3 Manufacturing Process

Traditional kheer has a dark cream color because rice grains are cooked for a long time (typically takes an hour) in milk. The traditional method of Kheer preparation on an open flame is replaced by a steam kettle. When kheer is prepared in an open pan, i.e., at atmospheric pressure, it becomes a batch process, which limits its mechanized production. For its mechanization, it is necessary to reduce its cooking time, which is usually around 1h in the conventional open-pan process (Kadam et al., 2013). The manufacturing process for traditional kheer is shown in the flow diagram in **Figure 11.11.**

### 11.6.4 Health Benefits of Kheer

Kheer made with rice provides a significant amount of carbohydrates, which promote digestive health and also lessen inflammation. As it is full of carbohydrates, it aids in replenishing the glycogen lost during vigorous exercise. **Figure 11.12** gives a summary of the health benefits of kheer.

## 11.7 GULABJAMUN (ROSE WATER BERRY OR ROSE BERRY DIPPED IN SUGAR SYRUP)

### 11.7.1 Introduction

Gulabjamun is a fried and soaked milk-based South Asian sweet, mainly popular in the Indian subcontinent, notably India, Nepal (where people call it *lalmohan*), Pakistan, the Maldives (*Golab ki Janu*), Bangladesh (as *Gulab jam*), and Myanmar. Along with Mauritius, Fiji, the Malay Peninsula,

Buffalo milk/ cow milk

↓

Standardization (4.5–5.5% fat, 8.5–9% SNF)

↓

Boiling on a non-smoky fire

↓

Rice (good quality) is washed & added to milk (2.5%)

↓

Gentle boiling, thorough stirring & scraping

↓

Sugar (5–7.5%) is added when conc. of milk reaches 1:1.8

↓

Heating & stirring continued until rice is properly cooked & conc. reaches 2–3 times

↓

Powdered cardamom (0.02%) is added at end of heat & garnished with dry fruits

↓

Finally, cooled to 10°C, filled in cups & stored at 6°C

**FIGURE 11.11 General flow diagram for the manufacturing process of kheer.**

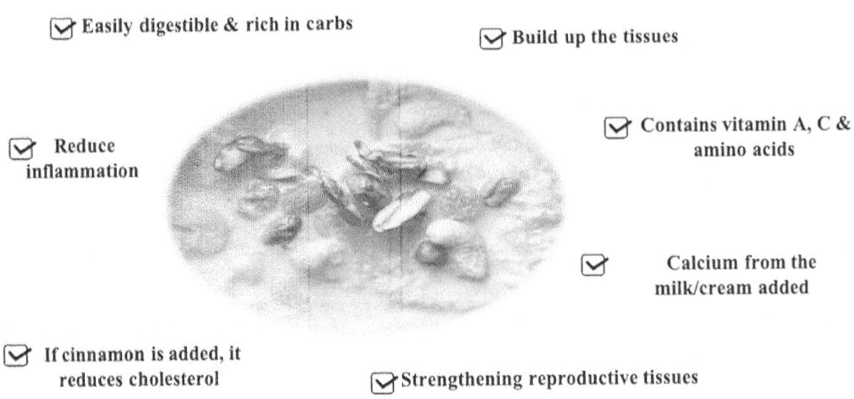


**FIGURE 11.12 Key potential health benefits of kheer.**

Great Britain, South Africa, and the Caribbean republics of Trinidad and Tobago, Guyana, and Suriname, it is also well known in countries with sizable populations of individuals of South Asian heritage (**Figure 11.13**). Gulabjamun are soft, flavorful, berry-sized balls made of milk solids (khoa), flour, and a leaving agent (Chetana et al., 2004). They are immersed in rose-flavored sugar syrup. "*Gulab*" translates to rose in Hindi and "*Jamun*" to berry. So, gulabjamun is berry-sized balls dunked in rose-flavored sugar syrup. It is mainly garnished with dried nuts like almonds and cashews to increase flavor.

### 11.7.2 Nutritional Facts

Gulabjamun is made up of about 43% carbohydrates, 7% protein, and 10% fat (**Table 11.4**). It contains a lot of selenium and biotin. Gulabjamun should be consumed in moderation due to its high calorie, sugar, and saturated fat content. The nutritional composition of gulabjamun is greatly affected by a variety of elements, including khoa composition and quality, component proportion (maida and khoa), frying duration, frying temperature, sugar syrup concentration, and so on.

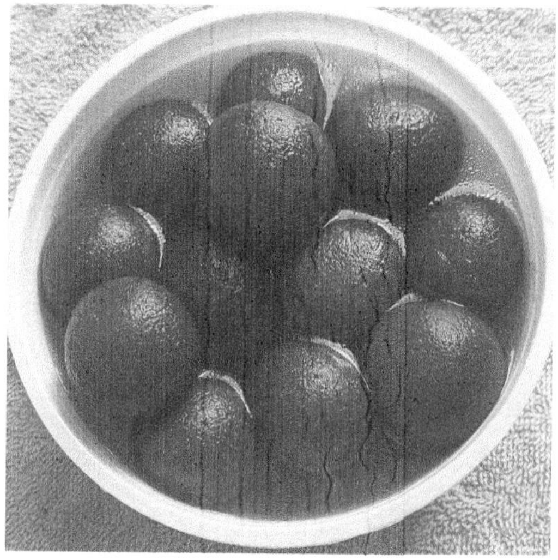

FIGURE 11.13 Image of gulabjamun (rose water berry).

**TABLE 11.4**
**Nutritional Facts of Gulabjamun**

| Components | Amount (%) |
|---|---|
| Moisture | 25.0–35.0 |
| Fat | 8.5–10.5 |
| Proteins | 6.0–7.6 |
| Ash | 0.9–1.0 |
| Lactose | 8.5–11.5 |
| Carbohydrates | 43.0–48.0 |

*Source:* Minhas et al., 1985

### 11.7.3 Manufacturing Process

Khoa is mixed with wheat flour and baking powder and kneaded into a uniform dough. The dough is rolled into small balls and deep fried in ghee or dalda (vegetable ghee) in a shallow pan until the balls acquire a golden-brown color. Sugar is dissolved into water and boiled to make sugar syrup. Fried balls are then placed into the sugar solution and allowed to soak for a few hours before being served. A continuous manufacturing system for gulabjamun has been developed by NDDB (capacity: 10,000 gulabjamun/h). Khoa, wheat flour (*maida*), and other ingredients are mixed in a planetary mixer to get a smooth dough that is portioned by a machine (Kant & Broadwayb, 2017). The portions are converted into balls using a ball forming machine and the balls are deep fat fried in a frying tank at 140°C. The fried balls are placed in a sugar syrup tank (sugar concentration 60%) for 2 h at 60°C to prepare the gulabjamun (Franklin et al., 2014).

The manufacturing process for traditional gulabjamun is shown in the flow diagram in **Figure 11.14.**

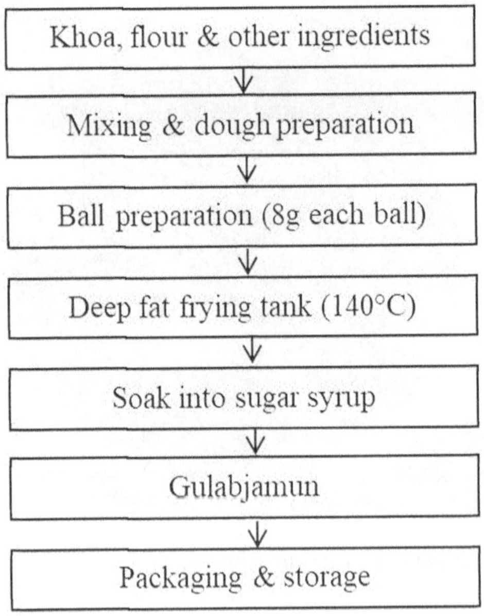


**FIGURE 11.14 The general flow diagram of manufacturing process of gulabjamun.**

### 11.7.4 Health Benefits of Gulabjamun

Gulabjamun is a source of selenium, biotin, calcium, and vitamin A in addition to protein. It should be consumed in moderation as it is high in calories, sugar, and saturated fats. In contrast to the benefits, some of the most prevalent adverse effects of gulabjamun are weight gain, diabetes with elevated blood sugar levels, and mismanaged metabolism. Since gulabjamun is mostly consumed after meals, try to eat a high-fiber, balanced meal to minimize sweet cravings. **Figure 11.15** gives a summary of the health benefits of gulabjamun.

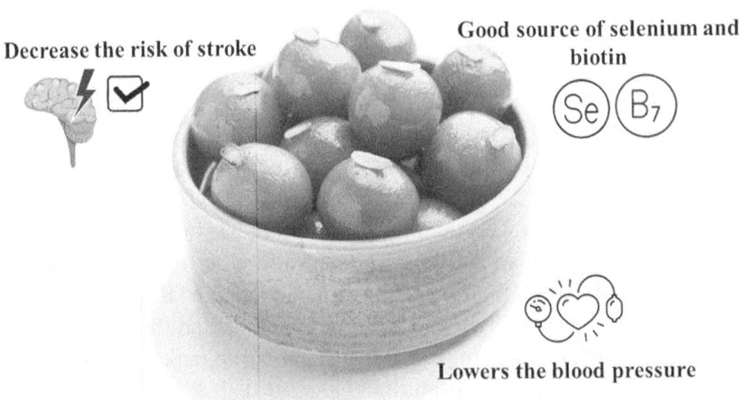
Decrease the risk of stroke
Good source of selenium and biotin
Se
B7
Lowers the blood pressure

**FIGURE 11.15 Key potential health benefits of gulabjamun.**

## 11.8 KACHAGOLLA (RICOTTA CHEESE SWEETS)

### 11.8.1 Introduction

Sweetmeats are well-known, nutritious, delightful foods. Milk sweetmeats have a prominent place from birth to death in every aspect of life on the Indian subcontinent. Everywhere, milk sweetmeats are given at events like birthdays, weddings, funerals, religious festivals, and guest entertainment. Natorer kachagolla is a traditional sweetmeat highly popular in Bangladesh. Despite having the name "*golla*," which in native Bengali languages means "little ball," it does not have the same shape as Roshgolla or other sweetmeat products (**Figure 11.16**). It is made of chhana (cheese curds made from milk) and sugar. It is a mixture of kacha (unripened chhana) and sugar, which is why it is called kachagolla. The history behind the uncovering of kachagolla goes back two and a half centuries, when Natore was ruled by powerful Zamindars. To satisfy Queen Bhabani, who was also known as the "Queen of Natore," the services of Madhusudan Das, a confectioner from the adjacent Lalbazar district, were hired. Modhusudan's 20 workers became ill one day, and the 80 kg of chhana that was stored in his shop and meant for the queen was on the verge of spoiling. He added some sheera to it and continued stirring while it was on heat to prevent the chhana from spoiling. He was shocked to discover that his creation was pretty mouthwatering after tasting it as the syrup quickly disappeared. Thus, it began the kachagolla (Alam et al., 2002; Sen, 1992).

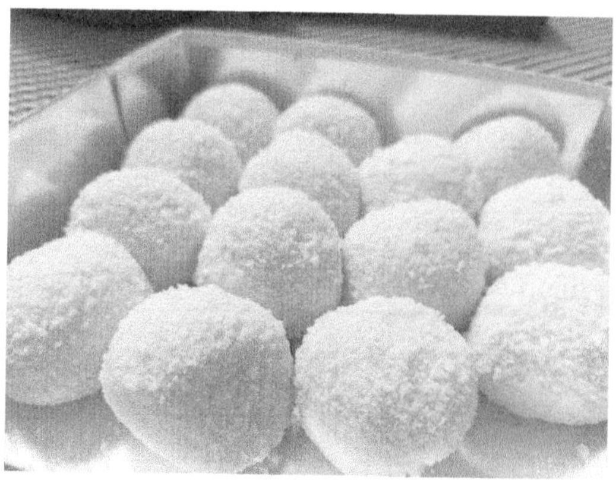

FIGURE 11.16 **Image of kachagolla (ricotta cheese sweets).**

### 11.8.2 Nutritional Facts

Kachagolla is extremely healthy because of its high protein and fat content, minerals (**Table 11.5**), including calcium and phosphorus, and fat-soluble vitamins, particularly vitamins A and D.

**TABLE 11.5**
**Nutritional Facts of Kachagolla**

| Components | Amount (%) |
|---|---|
| Total solid | 62.19 |
| Moisture | 37.18 |
| Fat | 6.60 |
| Proteins | 9.96 |
| Ash | 1.36 |
| Carbohydrate | 43.25 |

*Source:* Alam et al., 2002

### 11.8.3 Manufacturing Process

A little bit of wheat flour, baking powder, and khoa (or chhana) are combined, and the mixture is kneaded into a smooth dough. The manufacturing process for traditional kachagolla is shown in the flow diagram in **Figure 11.17**.

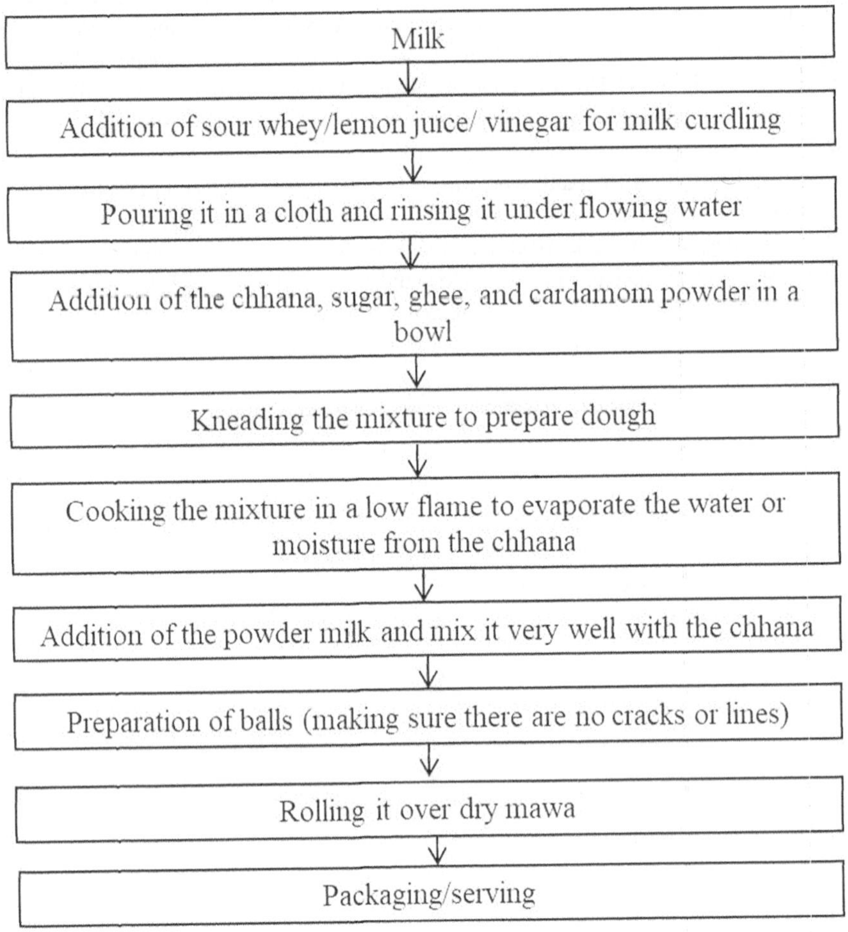


FIGURE 11.17 **General flow diagram of the manufacturing process of kachagolla.**

### 11.8.4 Health Benefits of Kachagolla

Kachagolla, a sweetmeat made from chhana, is exceptionally nutrient dense because of its high levels of protein and fat, as well as its minerals, including calcium and phosphorus, and fat-soluble vitamins, especially vitamin A and D. A schematic presentation of the health benefits of kachagolla (Alam et al., 2002) is shown in **Figure 11.18.**

## 11.9 PEDA (SWEET MADE WITH FULL-FAT MILK AND SUGAR)

### 11.9.1 Introduction

Peda is an indigenous khoa-based, heat-desiccated milk sweet (**Figure 11.19**). A sweet delicacy from the Indian subcontinent is called peda or pera. It came from Mathura in the Indian state of

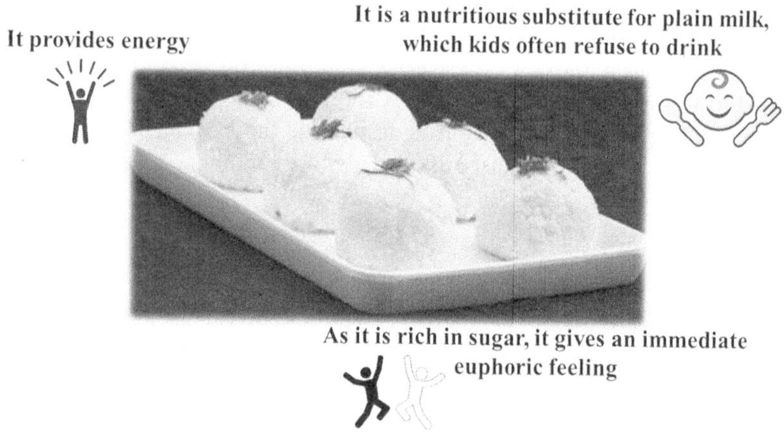
It provides energy
It is a nutritious substitute for plain milk, which kids often refuse to drink
As it is rich in sugar, it gives an immediate euphoric feeling

**FIGURE 11.18** **Key potential health benefits of kachagolla.**

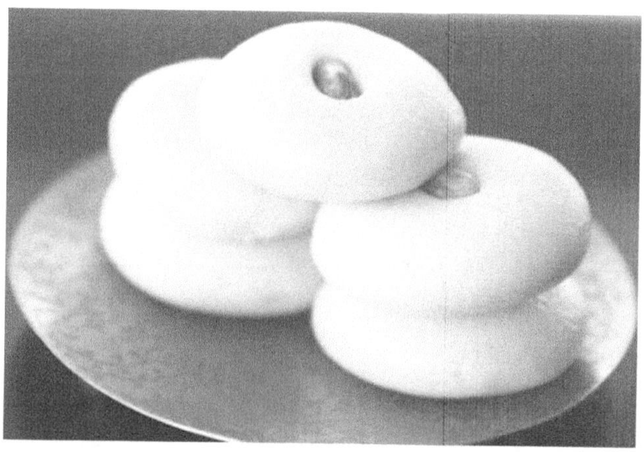

**FIGURE 11.19** **Image of peda (sweet made with full-fat milk and sugar).**

Uttar Pradesh. Mainly it is prepared from khoa (*mawa*), sugar, and traditional flavorings including cardamom seeds, pistachio nuts, and saffron. Since peda contains sugar and has less moisture than khoa, it is of higher quality. It can be anything from creamy white to caramel colored. Peda has religious importance, as they offered in Prassad during the worship of God in the temples (Banjare et al., 2015). Peda is frequently provided to visitors during ceremonial festivities and other events.

### 11.9.2 Types of Peda

i. **Dharwad peda:** The well-known Karnataka dessert “Dharwad peda” is made of sweetened khoa that is caramelized until brown, formed into little balls, and dusted with powdered sugar.
ii. **Thirattupal:** Thirattupal is a popular dish in the states of Tamil Nadu and Kerala and is distinguished by its coarse granular texture. The main ingredients of thirattupal are whole milk and raw sugar. But often slightly sour milk or a little amount of curd is used during the preparation of this sweet to get a granular texture.

iii. **Lalpeda:** It is a popular heat-desiccated traditional dairy product of eastern India, especially Uttar Pradesh and Mathura. Generally, lalpeda is prepared by blending khoa and sugar followed by heat until the characteristic reddish-brown color appears.
iv. **Kesarpeda:** Kesarpeda is the most famous and traditional Indian dessert and it is known for its taste and flavor. Hugely used during festivals in India, it can be made in many flavors like chocolate, vanilla, or even just milk peda without adding any flavor.

### 11.9.3 Nutritional Facts

Peda is nutritional, tasty, and a great source of energy. One peda contains 133 calories. Carbohydrates contribute for 45 calories, proteins account for 22 calories, and fat accounts for the remaining 67 calories (**Table 11.6**). One peda supplies around 7% of the total daily calorie needs of a 2,000-calorie adult diet.

TABLE 11.6
Nutritional Facts of Peda

| Components | Laboratory made (%) | Market samples (%) |
|---|---|---|
| Moisture | 10.20 | 4.2–18.2 |
| Fat | 20.10 | 3.5–25.0 |
| Proteins | 19.00 | 1.4–19.5 |
| Lactose | 18.30 | 4–18.6 |
| Ash | 2.4 | 1.4–3.4 |
| Sucrose | 30.00 | 31.8–61.8 |

### 11.9.4 Manufacturing Process

Khoa and sugar are combined and gently cooked in an indigenous pan until hard balls form (Londhe et al., 2012). After taking the pan from the heat, nuts and flavoring ingredients can be added if anyone likes. The ingredients are then properly combined and formed into balls of the required size (Sukumar, 1980). The manufacturing process for traditional peda is shown in the flow diagram in **Figure 11.20.**

### 11.9.5 Health Benefits of Peda

It comprises around 65 to 70% of the milk components, which include serum proteins, lactose, minerals, and vitamins. One piece has around 82 calories. It enhances skin complexion, happiness, beneficial in depression, boosts energy and digestive strength, and is extremely beneficial for bone and tooth strengthening due to its high calcium content. A schematic presentation for the health benefits of peda is shown in **Figure 11.21**.

## 11.10 BARFI (SWEET CONFECTIONERY)

### 11.10.1 Introduction

Barfi, barfee, or burfi is a sort of indigenous sweet from the Indian subcontinent, made with milk. It is one of the most popular khoa-based indigenous sweets (**Figure 11.22**). Powdered milk and sugar are barfis' essential ingredients. According to market demand, extra additives are typically added in various ratios. In a bowl, the ingredients are heated until the mixture solidifies. Most

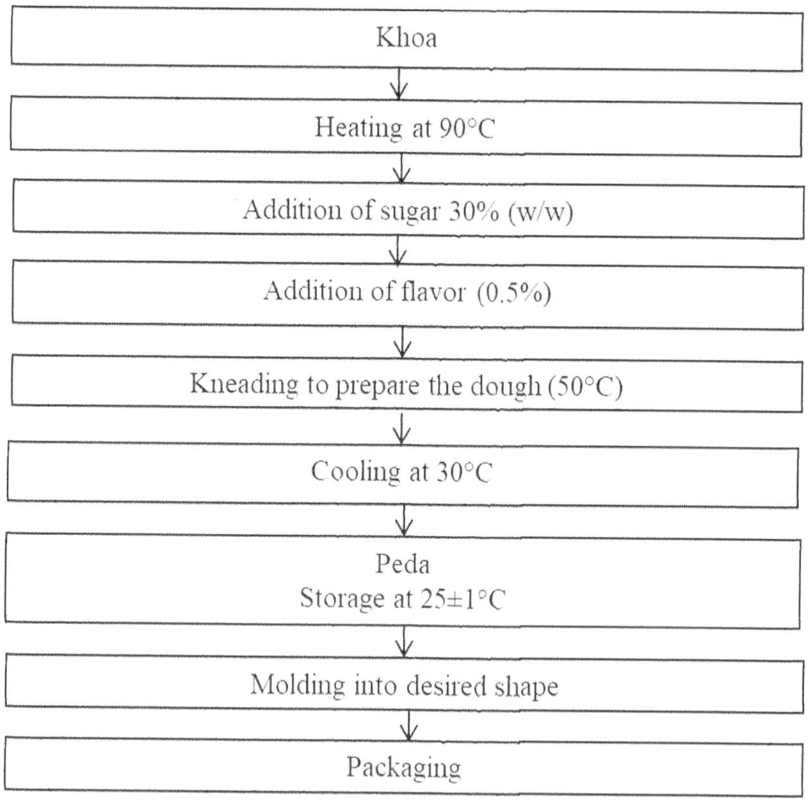


**FIGURE 11.20** **The general flow diagram of the manufacturing process of peda.**

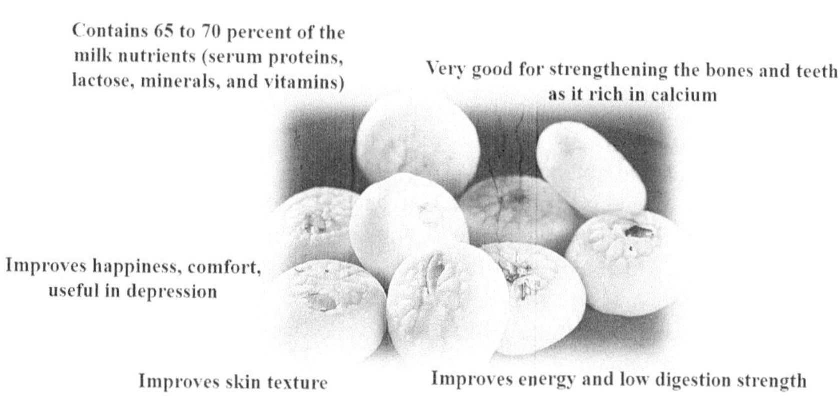


**FIGURE 11.21** **Key potential health benefits of peda.**

frequently, fruits or nuts like cashews, pistachios, or peanuts, as well as spices, enhance the flavor of a barfi (like cardamom or rose water). Barfis typically have a thin layer of vark, a metallic leaf that can be eaten. Typically, they are shaped into square, diamond, or round forms. The dessert is easily altered for both informal and formal occasions. Barfi comes in a variety of colors and

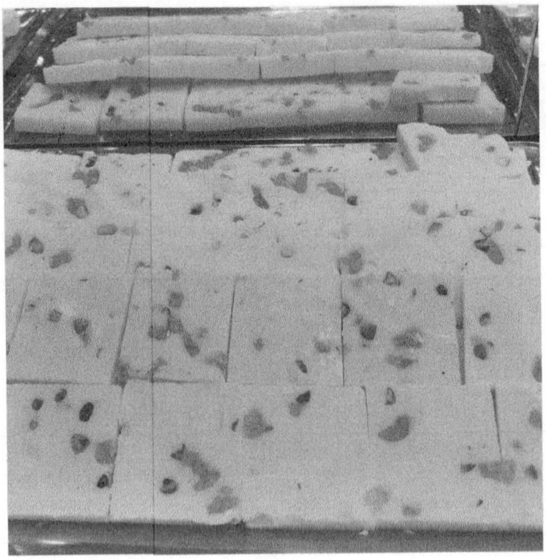

FIGURE 11.22 **Image of barfi (sweet confectionery).**

textures (Sachdeva & Rajorhia, 1982; Ranganadham et al., 2016) along with its variation in its shelf life. The shelf life of barfi can be extended by:

i. **Low moisture content in barfi:** Barfi can be stored for 6 months with low moisture. However, this low moisture content can make the barfi hard, dry, and chewy, which is unacceptable for consumers.
ii. **Addition of antioxidants:** Propyl gallate and dodecyl gallate are used as antioxidants in barfi.
iii. **Packaging in tins:** Barfi can be packed in tins and stored at 30°C ± 10°C for 150 days.
iv. **Hot filling:** Hot filling is necessary to prevent the growth of molds and off-flavor development during storage.

### 11.10.2 Types of Barfi

**Kesribarfi:** Saffron, flattened yellow, round
**Kajubarfi or kajukatli:** Cashew, light tan, diamond
**Pistabarfi:** Forest green, diamond
**Doodhpeda:** Kewra oil and pistachio, flattened, deep tan, round, chocolate barfi
**Badampak:** Rose water and almond, brown, diamond, walnut barfi
**Barfifon or barfifon:** Fig, pink and yellow color
**Gajarbarfi:** Carrot, square, orange color
**Coconut barfi:** Coconut, sugar, and milk, square, yellow color
**Sing barfi:** Peanuts, brown color
**Besanbarfi:** Gram flour, light yellow, diamond
**Ice cream barfi:** Rich vanilla flavor, rectangular, etc.

### 11.10.3 Nutritional Facts

A serving of barfi has 174 calories. Carbohydrates contribute 67 calories, proteins account for 24 calories, and fat accounts for the remaining 82 calories. A single slice of barfi has roughly 9% of the entire daily calorie needs of a 2,000-calorie adult diet. It is nutritional, tasty, and a great source of lactose. carbohydrates, and sucrose (**Table 11.7**).

**TABLE 11.7**
**Nutritional Facts of Barfi**

| Component/parameter | Mawabarfi | Other barfi |
|---|---|---|
| Moisture | 15.0 | 15.0 |
| Lactose | 15.0 | 12.0 |
| Sucrose | 48.0 | 40.0 |
| Acidity % as lactic acid (max) | 0.35 | 0.45 |
| Standard plate count/gm (max) | 30,000 | 30,000 |
| Yeast & molds count/gm (max) | 10 | 10 |

*Source:* Sachdeva & Rajorhia, 1982; Ranganadham et al., 2016

### 11.10.4 Manufacturing Process

There are several methods of production:

i. Manufacture of barfi from buffalo milk
ii. Manufacture of barfi from pre-made khoa
iii. Manufacture of barfi from concentrated milk
iv. Manufacture of barfi from skim milk powder and cream
v. Mechanized production of barfi

To prevent sediments on the surface of the kettle from burning, milk is continuously stirred and scraped while being boiled. Heating is stopped after the substance reaches a semi-solid consistency. Using a flattened wooden ladle, powdered sugar is poured and thoroughly mixed into the khoa at a 30% basis. The mixture is placed on greased trays once it has homogenized into a mass with the desired flow properties. The product must be left a minimum of 4 hours to set. The barfi is then packed and kept at room temperature after being cut with a knife into the desired shapes and sizes. The manufacturing process for traditional barfi is shown in the flow diagram in **Figure 11.23**.

### 11.10.5 Health Benefits of Barfi

Most of the benefits of barfi are similar to those of milk. Like any other dairy product, due to its calcium content, it is excellent for strengthening bones and teeth. It supports a strong immune system, the generation of energy, and the preservation of healthy skin and hair. Additionally, it contains a lot of vitamin D (Sachdeva & Rajorhia, 1982; Ranganadham et al., 2016). A schematic presentation of the health benefits of barfi is shown in **Figure 11.24**.

## 11.11 SANDESH (CHEESE/CHHANA-BASED SWEET)

### 11.11.1 Introduction

Sandesh is a chhana- and sugar-based dessert that is native to the Bengal region in the east of the Indian subcontinent (Poonia, 2015) (**Figure 11.25**). Some recipes of sandesh call for paneer or chhana instead of milk itself. It is a famous Bengali sweet and lightly flavored with cardamom. Some people in Dhaka call it "*Pranahara*" which means "heart-stealer" (Kober et al., 2002, 2003, 2006).

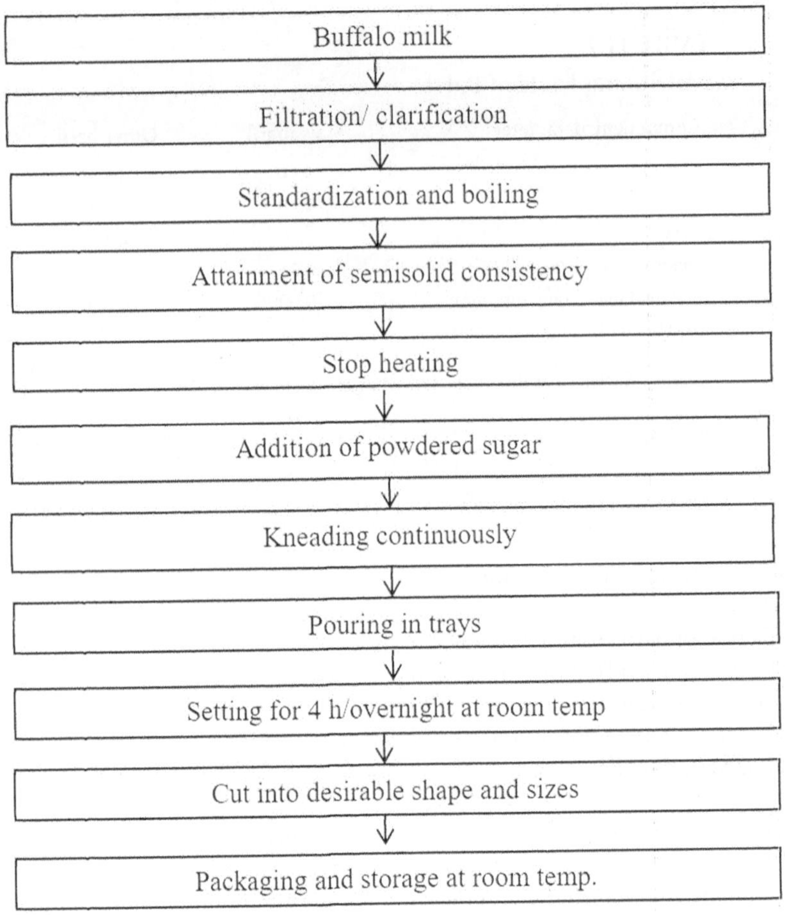


**FIGURE 11.23** General flow diagram of the manufacturing process of barfi.

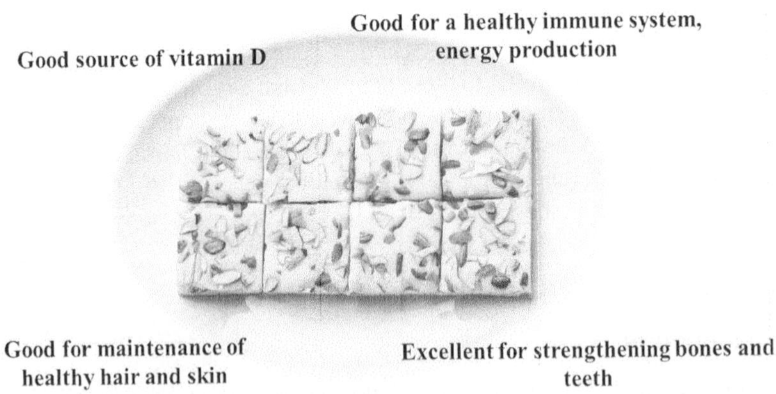


**FIGURE 11.24** Key potential health benefits of barfi.

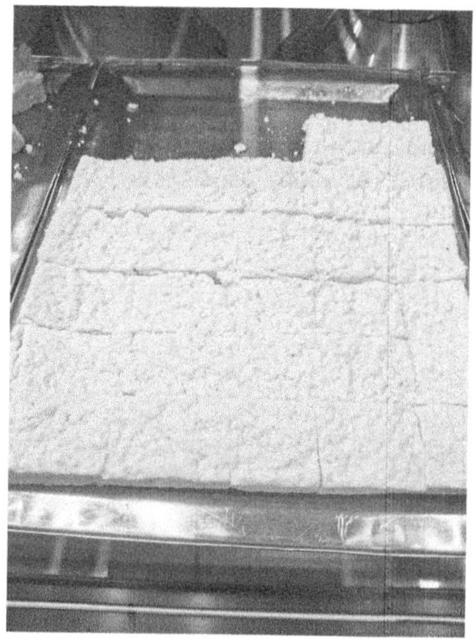

FIGURE 11.25 **Image of sweet sandesh.**

### 11.11.2 Types of Sandesh

Kachagolla's origin is said to be the oldest of the three sandesh kinds (Kober et al., 2002, 2003, 2006).

i. **Raw grade (Kachagolla):** Light and flavorful Indian sweet made using ricotta cheese, cardamom, saffron, and rose water.
ii. **Soft grade (narampak):** It has a characteristic soft cohesive body and smooth texture with small grains.
iii. **Hard grade (karapak):** Its body is hard, seems dry, and it contains little moisture.

#### 11.11.2.1 Difference between Soft-Grade Sandesh and Hard-Grade Sandesh

While hard-grade sandesh has a solid crumbly, coarse, and chewy feel with big grains, soft-grade sandesh has a distinctive soft cohesive body and smooth texture with small grains.

### 11.11.3 Nutritional Facts

It is a delicious, wholesome, nutritious sweetmeat. This popular sweetmeat is liked by most of the people of the Indian subcontinent due to its good flavor and high food value. It can easily be digested. People of all ages like it. It contains a good amount of fat, protein, and other nutrients (**Table 11.8**).

### 11.11.4 Manufacturing Process

Milk is heated to 90–95°C for sandesh production and then cooled to 70°C (Poonia, 2015). To precipitate the milk, a coagulant such as citric acid, calcium lactate (as a solution), lemon juice, or sour whey that has been heated to 70°C is added to the heated milk. The manufacturing process for traditional sandesh is shown in flow diagram in **Figure 11.26**.

### 11.11.5 Health Benefits of Sandesh

Sandesh, a sweetmeat made from chhana, is incredibly nutritive due to its high protein and fat content, as well as its minerals, including calcium and phosphorus, and fat-soluble vitamins, especially

**TABLE 11.8**
**Nutritional Facts of Sandesh**

| Components | Sandesh (soft grade) prepared from cow milk chhana (%) | Sandesh prepared from buffalo milk chhana (%) |
|---|---|---|
| Moisture | 25.5 | 27.14 |
| Fat | 19.89 | 18.42 |
| Protein | 18.48 | 18.71 |
| Ash | 1.66 | 1.90 |
| Sugar | 34.47 | 33.83 |

*Source:* Kober et al., 2002, 2003, 2006

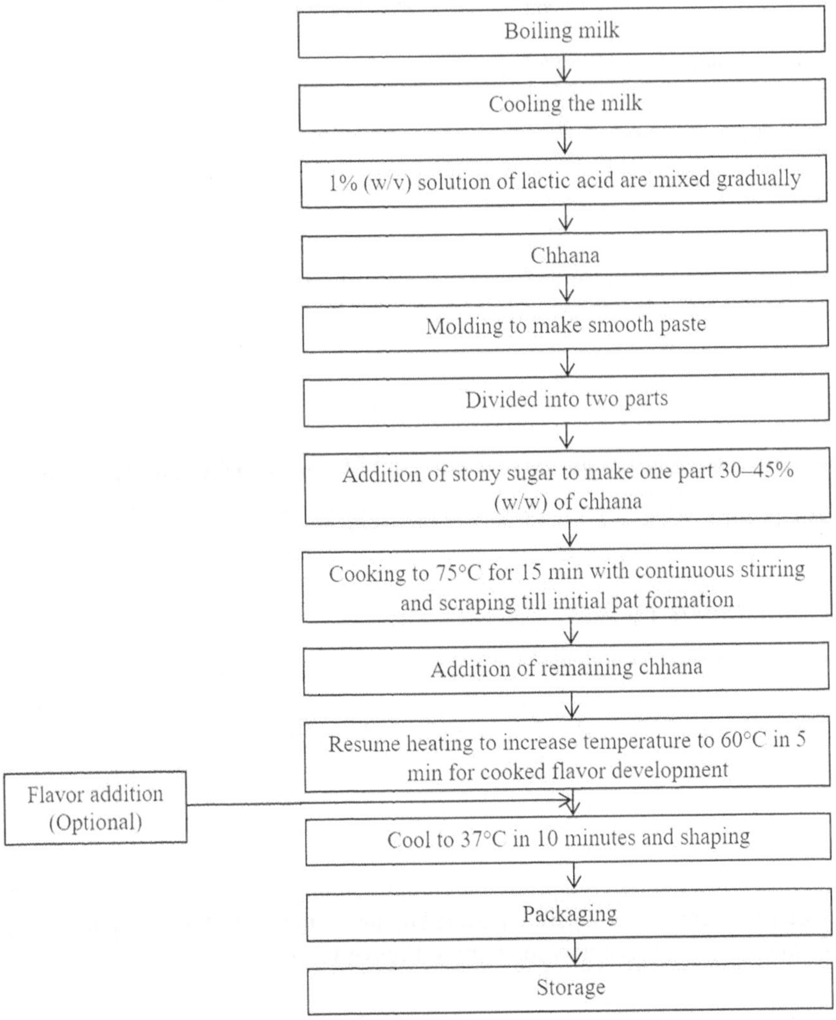


**FIGURE 11.26** **General flow diagram of the manufacturing process of sandesh.**

vitamin A and D. Calcium, potassium, phosphorus, and magnesium assist in weight loss. It's vital to remember that while choosing a diabetic dessert like sandesh, one must adjust the preparation by lowering the sugar content. A schematic presentation for health benefits of sandesh is shown in **Figure 11.27**.

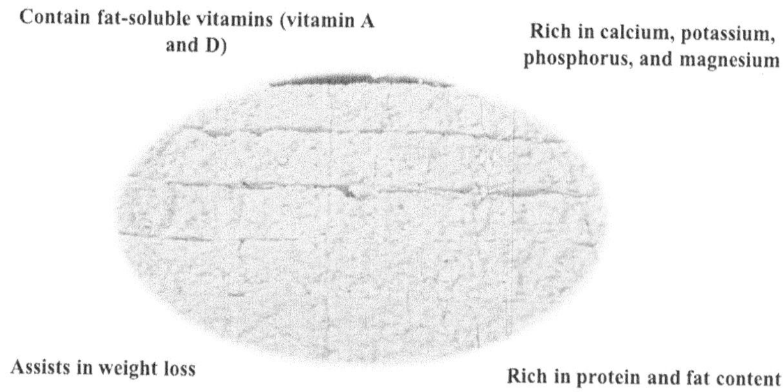


FIGURE 11.27 **Key potential health benefits of sandesh.**

## 11.12 RASMALAI (COTTAGE CHEESE BALLS)

### 11.12.1 Introduction

Rasmalai is a classic South Asian dessert made from chhana that is popular in Bangladesh, Pakistan, and India (Rahman et al., 2003) (**Figure 11.28**). Rasmalai is made of flattened, sweet, cream-to-yellow-colored balls of paneer that have been dipped in malai (clotted cream). Rasmalai is likely to have originated in Eastern India, especially in Orissa and Bangladesh. It is a heat-concentrated milk product containing about 60% total solids, including sugar as the sweetening agent (Sharma et al., 2014). Chhana and rabri are used as base materials for its preparation. Chhana is required for balls

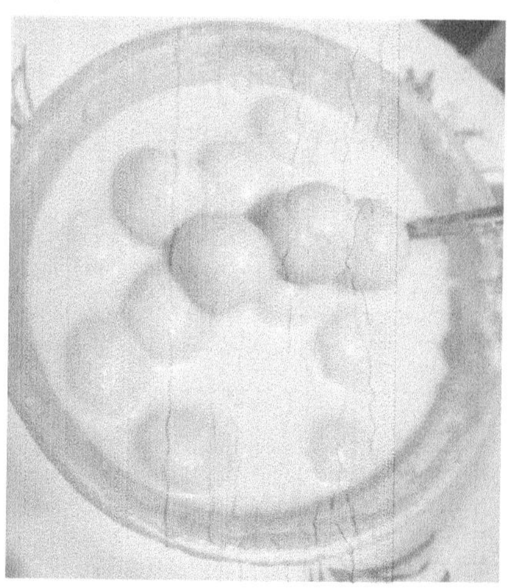

FIGURE 11.28 **Image of sweet rasmalai (cottage cheese balls).**

(*tikki*) and rabri (concentrated milk) is required for dipping these balls before serving. It is popular in northern part of India particularly in Haryana state (Aneja, 1995).

### 11.12.2 Nutritional Facts

Rasmalai is a chhana-based sweetmeat that is highly advised for diabetic people due to its high protein and low sugar content (**Table 11.9**).

**TABLE 11.9**
**Nutritional Facts of Rasmalai**

| Components | Rasmalai prepared from cow milk (%) | Rasmalai prepared from buffalo milk (%) |
|---|---|---|
| Total solids | 46.11 | 54.0 |
| Protein | 6.16 | 8.40 |
| Fat | 7.53 | 12.56 |
| Ash | 0.91 | 1.25 |
| Carbohydrate | 31.49 | 31.80 |

### 11.12.3 Manufacturing Process

Chhana with a small amount of wheat flour is kneaded into smooth dough, portioned, and rolled into balls having a smooth texture free from cracks (Sayedatunnesha et al., 2008). The balls are processed like rasgulla and subsequently stored in thickened milk (to a quarter of its volume by heating) with added sugar. The manufacturing process for traditional rasmalai is shown in a flow diagram in **Figure 11.29.**

### 11.12.4 Defects in Rasmalai

A flaw or irregularity that affects the flavor, body and texture, color, or other properties of rasmalai is referred to as a defect (**Table 11.10**).

**TABLE 11.10**
**Defects, Causes, and Probable Remedies of Rasmalai**

| Defects | Causes | Remedies |
|---|---|---|
| Hard, chewy, and rubbery | Late staining | Quickly stain to feel creamy.<br>Keep chhana covered with cheese cloth until it is ready to be cooked. |
| Sour taste | Improper washing | Wash properly to remove lemon and vinegar. |
| Cracking | Squeezed lightly | For creamy feel, squeeze it tightly. |

### 11.12.5 Health Benefits of Rasmalai

Rasmalai supplies the most essential elements like calcium, protein, minerals, vitamin B, and phosphorus, along with numerous other essential major and minor substances (Karthikeyan & Dhanalakshmi, 2010). Even diabetics can consume low-sugar or no-sugar rasmalai once in a while, and it depends on their blood sugar levels (Tiwari & Grewal, 1999). A schematic presentation for the health benefits of rasmalai is shown in **Figure 11.30**.

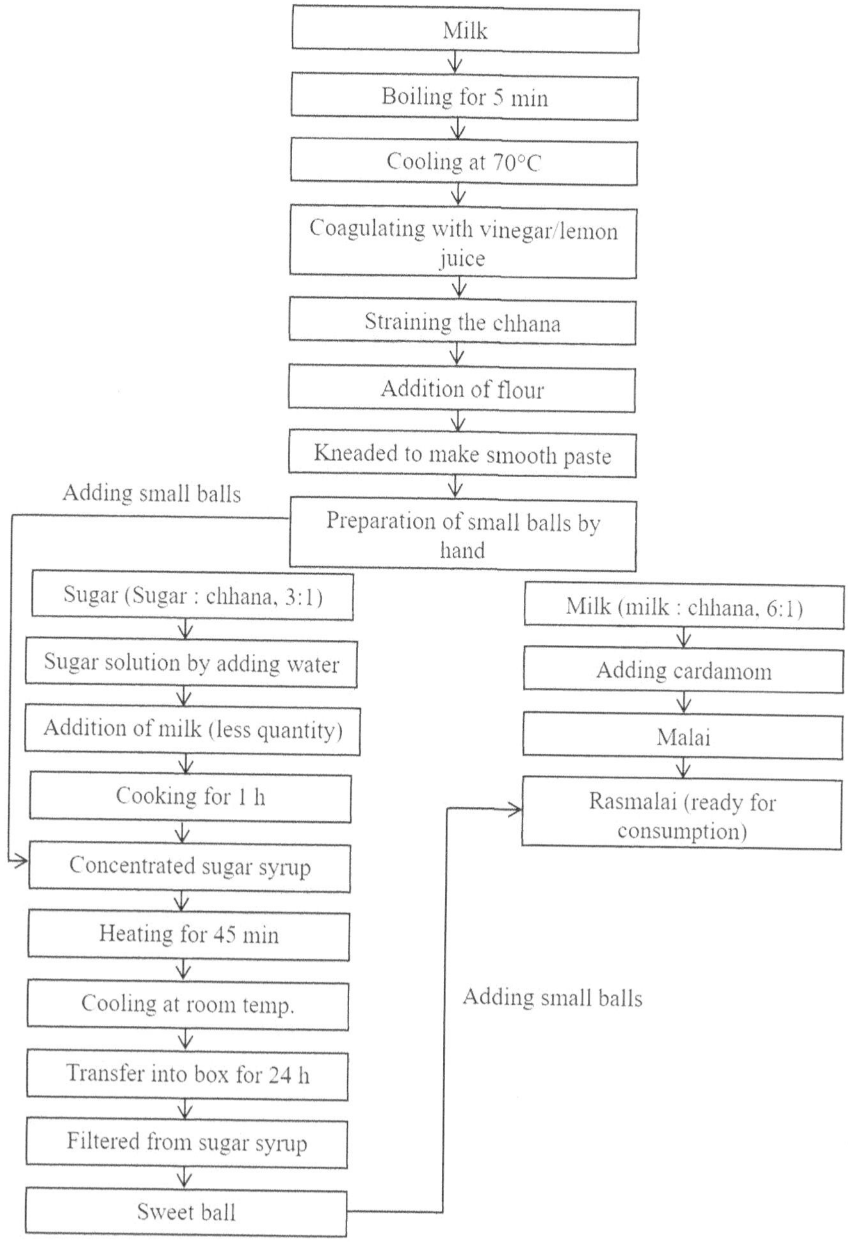


**FIGURE 11.29** **General flow diagram of the manufacturing process of rasmalai.**

## 11.13 BUTTERMILK

### 11.13.1 Introduction

Buttermilk is the byproduct of the butter making process, made from pasteurized cream by fat globule agglomeration (**Figure 11.31**). Depending on the conditions of butter production, it contains the majority of the components of the milk fat globule membrane (MFGM) and only trace levels of triglycerides (Sakkas et al., 2022; Ali, 2019). Sweet buttermilk is the most common variety of commercial buttermilk, with a non-acidic pH that is suitable for the majority of food formulae (Sakkas et al., 2022; Ali, 2019).

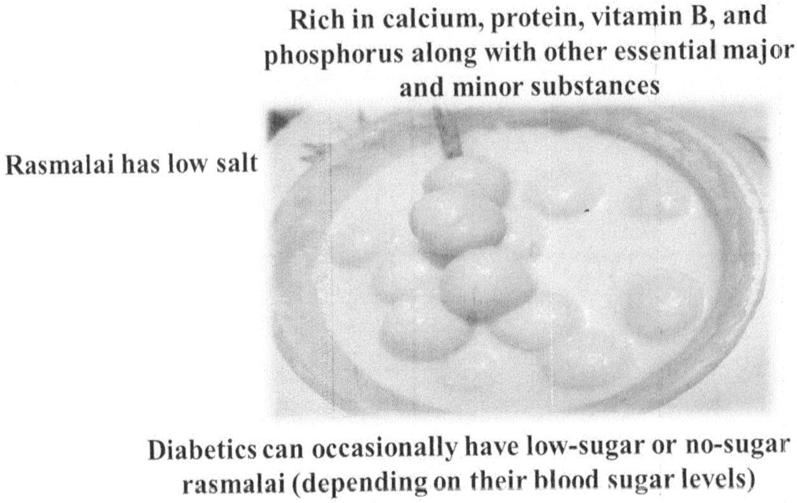


FIGURE 11.30 **Key potential health benefits of rasmalai.**

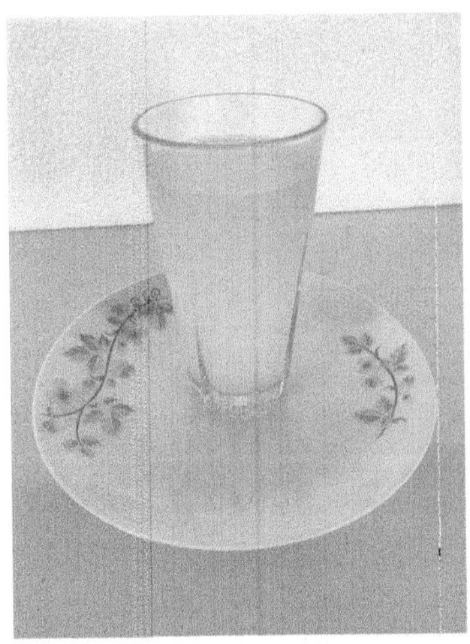

FIGURE 11.31 **Image of buttermilk.**

### 11.13.2 Nutritional Facts

In terms of gross composition, sweet buttermilk is similar to skim milk and contains primarily the non-fat components of churned cream, such as caseins, serum/whey proteins, lactose, and minerals (Sakkas et al., 2022; Ali, 2019). The season of the year and butter making method significantly impact the chemical components of buttermilk. In addition to lactose and proteins from skim milk, it also contains proteins and phospholipids from the membrane of milk fat globules (**Table 11.11**).

### 11.13.3 Manufacturing Process

Buttermilk was historically the freshly separated serum used to make butter on farms after churning cream was ripened with lactic acid bacteria that are present in nature. It occasionally had little butter particles in it. Buttermilk is a byproduct of the butter making process in industrial settings.

**TABLE 11.11**
**Nutritional Components of Traditional and Cultured Buttermilk**

| Components (%) | Traditional buttermilk | Cultured buttermilk |
|---|---|---|
| Total solids | 7–10 | 8–10 |
| Fat | 0.3–1.0 | 0–2.5 |
| Lactose | 3.5–4.9 | 4.8–5.8 |
| Protein | 2.66–3.75 | 3.4–3.8 |
| Phospholipids | 0.075–0.25 | ND |
| Conjugated linoleic acid (mg/100 g) | ND | 0.6 (0.1 in yogurt) |
| Minerals | 0.6–0.75 | 0.6–0.9 |

ND, not done

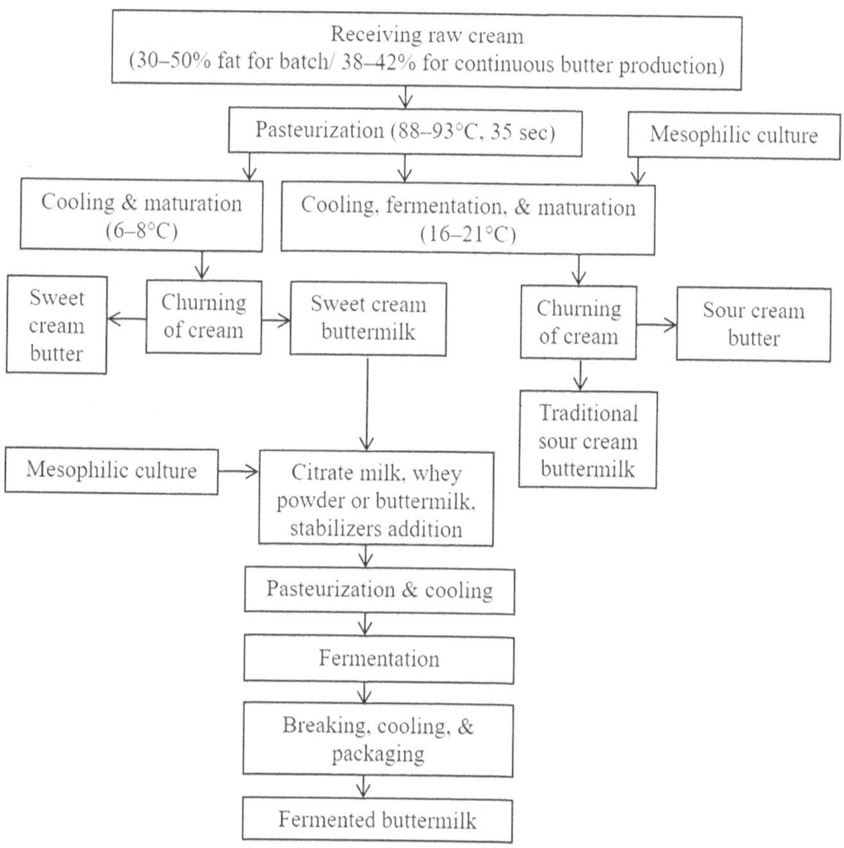


**FIGURE 11.32** **General flow diagram of the manufacturing process of conventional buttermilk.**

Buttermilk can be produced using either sour cream or sweet cream, depending on the processing circumstances. Its qualities are determined by the type of cream used to make butter. By using mesophilic lactic acid bacteria, sweet cream buttermilk can be transformed into fermented buttermilk. The manufacturing process for traditional buttermilk is shown in flow diagram form in **Figure 11.32.**

### 11.13.4 Health Benefits of Buttermilk

Protein, which is necessary to develop strong muscles, skin, and bones, is abundant in buttermilk. The majority of commercial buttermilk is also fortified with additional vitamins and minerals, like vitamin A and vitamin D. Milk peptides have shown their ability to achieve lower blood pressure in several medical trials (Ali, 2019). **Figure 11.33** illustrates the health benefits of buttermilk.

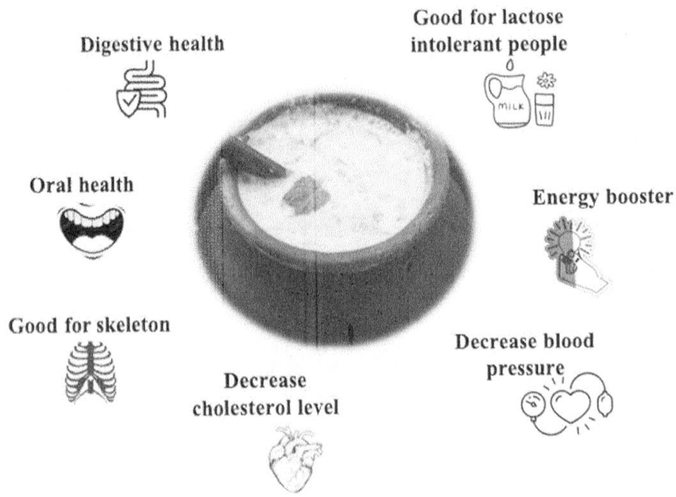


FIGURE 11.33 **Key potential health benefits of buttermilk.**

## 11.14 LABAN (FERMENTED MILK)

### 11.14.1 Introduction

Laban is a healthy traditional fermented milk product that is widely consumed globally, including in Arabic countries (**Figure 11.34**). With the use of chosen bacterial strains and a systematic procedure, several of these conventional items have been produced industrially. In Tunisia and other Arab

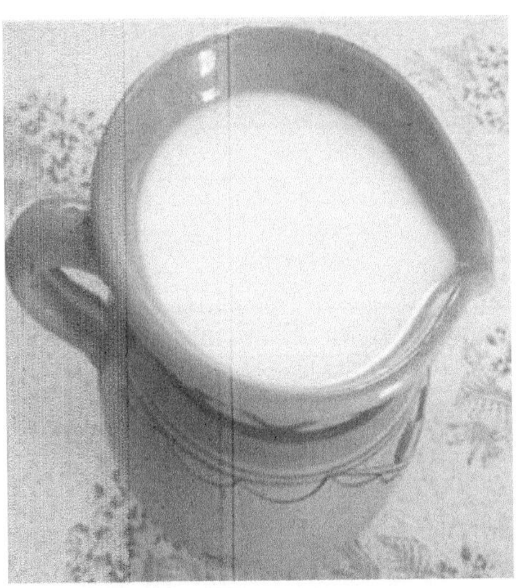

FIGURE 11.34 **Image of laban.**

nations, laban is a fermented milk product that is traditionally made from cow's milk (Samet-Bali et al., 2012). It's also called the Arabic version of yogurt.

### 11.14.2 Nutritional Facts

Nutritional facts of Tunisian laban is illustrated in **Table 11.12.**

**TABLE 11.12**
**Nutritional Facts of Tunisian Laban**

| Components | Amount (%) |
|---|---|
| Total solids | 7.05–7.40 |
| Protein | 1.86–2.56 |
| Fat | 1.48–3.50 |
| Lactose | 1.90–2.59 |

*Source:* Samet-Bali et al., 2012

### 11.14.3 Manufacturing Process

Both large industrial manufacturers and small, artisanal producers use diverse production methods to produce laban. Traditional producers mainly use artisanal starters, consisting of a mixed culture of an unknown number of undefined and indigenous thermophilic strains. This process produces a variety of products with common flavors that are generally appreciated by consumers (Béal & Chammas, 2012). By combining chosen starters with well-defined qualities and employing a consistent technique, the laban is commercially produced. The manufacturing process for traditional laban is shown in a flow diagram in **Figure 11.35**.

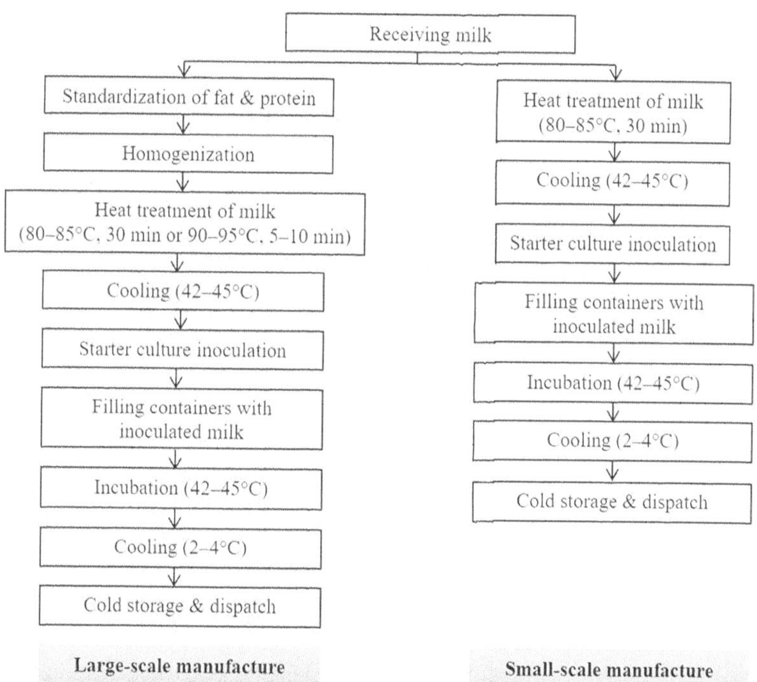


**FIGURE 11.35 General flow diagram of the manufacturing process of laban (large-scale and small-scale production).**

### 11.14.4 Health Benefits of Laban

The health advantages of eating yogurt are also present for laban. It has a lot of vitamins, proteins, calcium, and other nutrients. Consuming laban is better than any other soft drink popular in the market as it improves digestion, bones, and the immune system (**Figure 11.36**).

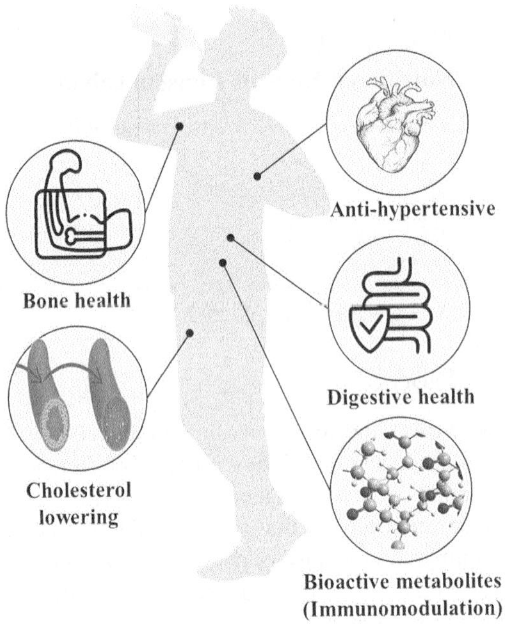


FIGURE 11.36 **Key potential health benefits of laban.**

## 11.15 LASSI (YOGURT DRINK)

### 11.15.1 Introduction

As mostly known, lassi is a Punjabi drink, which is mostly consumed after a meal. It is a yogurt-based beverage that originated in the Indian subcontinent (**Figure 11.37**). It is an excellent beverage to hydrate and improve body digestion as well as a great food source. Since lassi is produced from

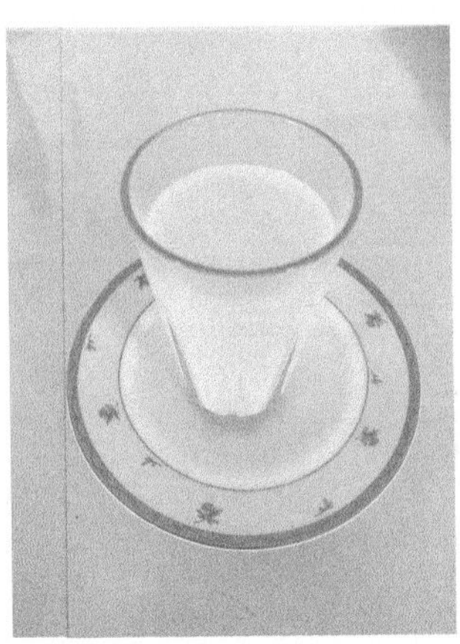

FIGURE 11.37 **Image of lassi.**

yogurt or dahi and is said to be very beneficial for our stomach, it is a sound and regular treatment for stomach swelling. In addition, lassi eliminates the body's excessive levels of cholesterol.

### 11.15.2 Nutritional Facts

Lassi is a delightful drink for individuals of all ages. It has a high nutritious value in relation to its cost. Lassi is high in minerals such as calcium, vitamin D, and phosphorus (**Table 11.13**). It has the potential to give more nutrients and health advantages than other beverages.

**TABLE 11.13**
**Nutritional Facts of Lassi**

| Components | Amount (%) |
|---|---|
| Water | 96.2 |
| Fat | 0.8 |
| Protein | 1.29 |
| Lactose | 1.2 |
| Lactic acid | 0.44 |
| Ash | 0.4 |
| Calcium | 0.6 |
| Phosphorus | 0.04 |

### 11.15.3 Manufacturing Process

A fermented milk beverage known as lassi is produced by growing specific lactic acid bacteria in the warmed milk and then sweetening it with sugar. In the summer, people drink it as a cold, pleasant beverage. It is made by agitating the curd and breaking it up into small pieces. Sugar, water, and flavoring are optional. The manufacturing process for traditional lassi is shown in flow diagram in **Figure 11.38**.

### 11.15.4 Health Benefits of Lassi

Being a probiotic drink, lassi helps in the improvement of correct microbes and controls the pathogenic microorganisms in the gut. Probiotic microorganisms increase the functionality of lassi, while the integration of antioxidant-rich fruit juice boosts the final product's value by adding powerful antioxidant properties (Mule et al., 2018). Lassi offers several health advantages, including the ability to enhance digestion, boost immunity, improve bone health, skin care, blood pressure control, weight management, and general well-being. It is widely acknowledged that consuming probiotics helps to maintain and develop a healthy gut microbiota. There is strong evidence that these probiotics can be used to prevent and cure conditions like lactose intolerance, high blood pressure, cholesterol, and numerous gastrointestinal issues such as Crohn's disease, peptic ulcers, infections, looseness of the bowels, etc. Probiotics additionally are hostile to cancer-causing agents and improve the immune system (Padghan et al., 2015). **Figure 11.39** illustrates the health benefits of lassi.

## 11.16 OPPORTUNITIES AND CHALLENGES IN GLOBAL TRADITIONAL DAIRY FOODS

Global traditional dairy foods have several opportunities and challenges at the production, nutritional, and health attribute levels (**Figure 11.40**).

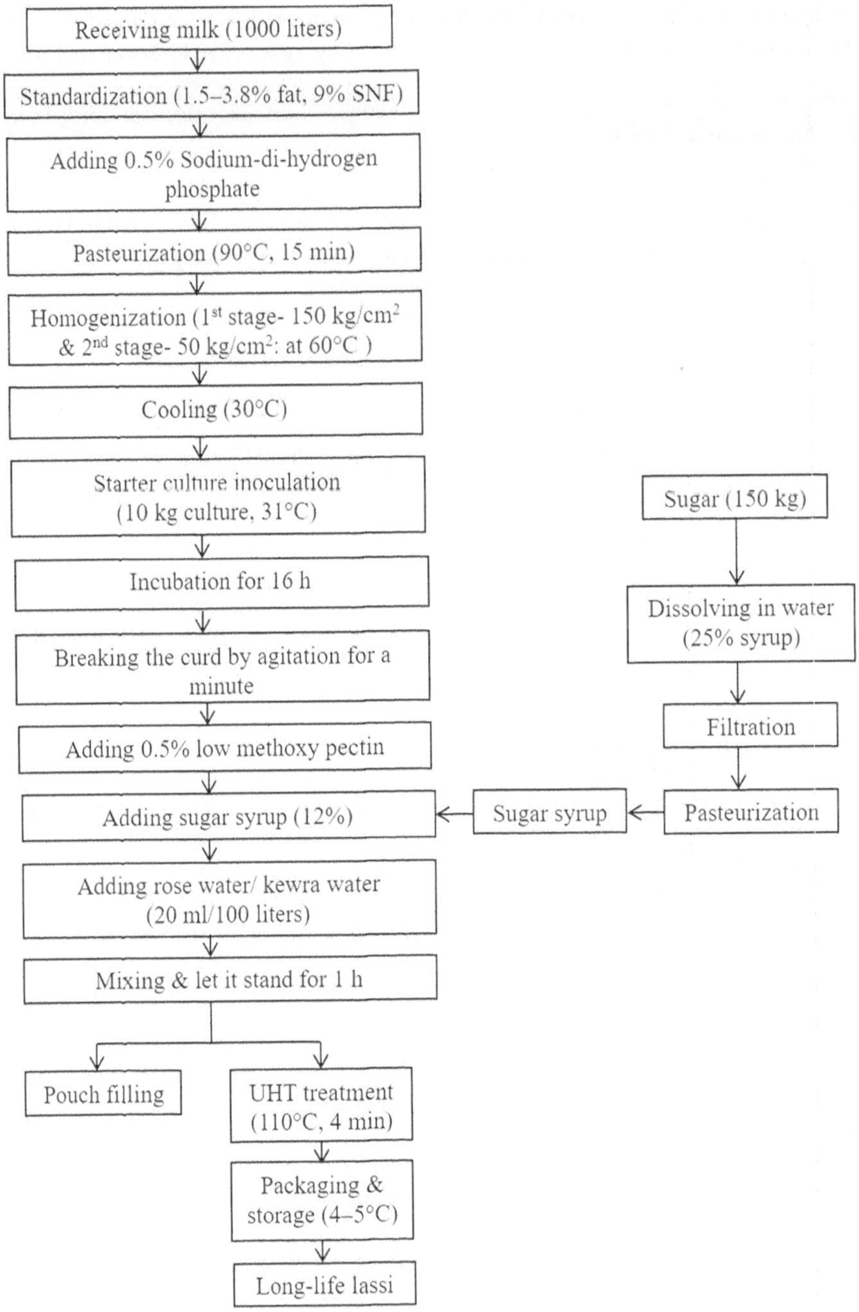


FIGURE 11.38 **The general flow diagram of the manufacturing process of lassi (yogurt-based beverage).**

## 11.17 TRADITIONAL DAIRY FOOD INNOVATIONS

The diversity of people and their need for novel and convenient dairy products, coupled with technology improvements, are driving the innovations in indigenous dairy products. Dairy products are regarded as healthy food choices globally, rather than being favored only in a particular area. The availability

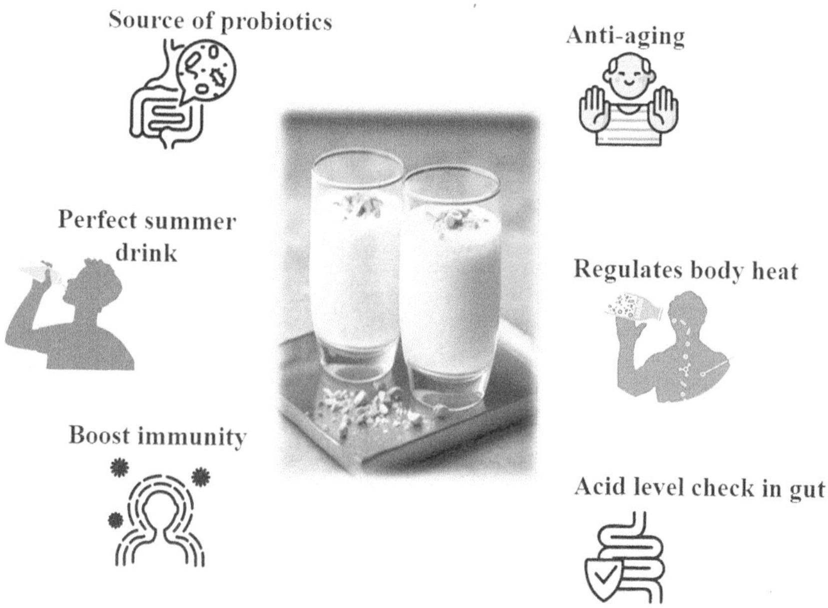


FIGURE 11.39 **Key potential health benefits of lassi.**

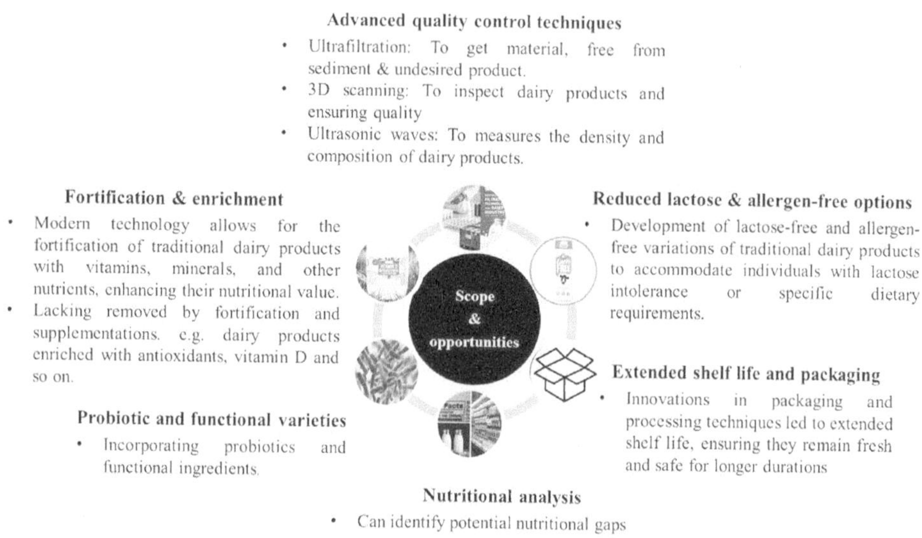


FIGURE 11.40 **Future opportunities/scope and challenges of traditional dairy foods.** The global traditional dairy foods face several opportunities and challenges at the production, nutritional, and health attribute levels.

of fortified dairy products, their convenient packaging systems, and easy transportation have led to their global popularity. Due to their favorable nutritional and health aspects, customers are embracing low-sugar, allergy-free, fiber-enriched confections. Thus, new varieties are emerging as time goes on. **Figure 11.41** illustrates traditional dairy food innovations from production to nutritional and health attributes.

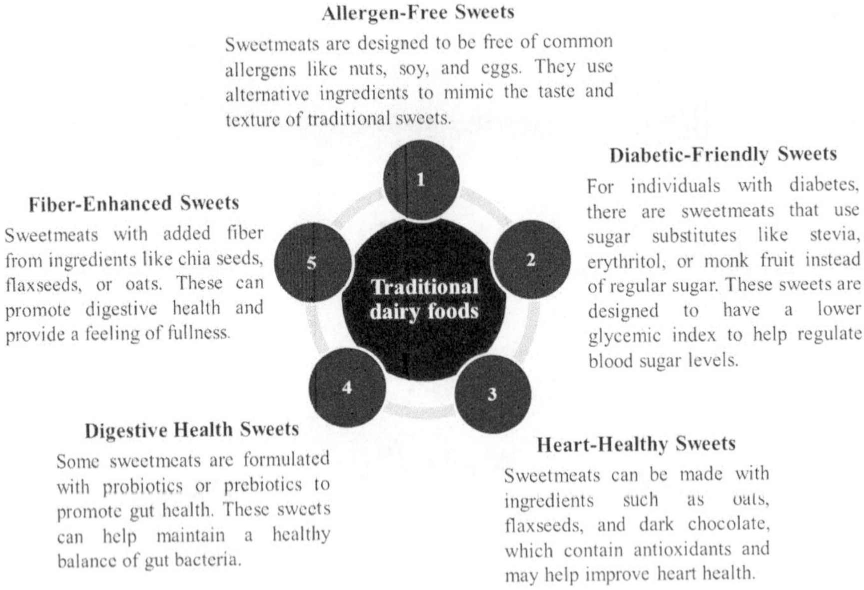


**FIGURE 11.41 Traditional dairy foods innovations from production to nutritional and health attributes.**

## 11.18 CONCLUSIONS

Traditional dairy foods are an integral part of our food basket. It is a frequent belief that using mechanical production methods causes the traditional quality of locally produced milk products to decline. Innovations in these items' processing methods can help solve this issue. It will also be beneficial to scale up the production of intermediate primary products. Elite brands for traditional dairy products must be developed through a marketing network and efficient communication. Since a huge number of people routinely consume traditional dairy products, adding value to these goods will not only improve health but also increase profits for dairy farmers and processors. There has been a lot of research done on technological advancements in the market for conventional dairy products. But for a variety of reasons, the dairy industry has not embraced many of these technologies. To fully realize their potential, work must be done quickly on the process development, design optimization, shelf-life enhancement, and packaging of traditional dairy products. On the other hand, businesses should assist by offering backup assistance for commercial production trials and market acceptability studies for the produced items. Since traditional dairy products are essential to the rich dairy legacy, one must nurture and improve them through innovations. For traditional dairy foods, an effort should be made to create a uniform method of preparation. It is important to look into the functionality of traditional dairy products.

## REFERENCES

Alam, M., Huq, A. K. O., Jahan, I., & Ahmed, E. (2020). Calorie density and nutrient content of commonly consumed sweetmeats of jashore district in Bangladesh. *EPRA International Journal of Multidisciplinary Research*, 174–179.

Alam, S. M. R. R., Rahman, A. K. M. A., Mannan, A., & Shams-ud-Din, M. (2002). Quality attributes of Kachhagolla—A delicious indigenous milk product of Bangladesh. *Pakistan Journal of Biological Sciences*, *5*, 725–727.

Ali, A. H. (2019). Current knowledge of buttermilk: Composition, applications in the food industry, nutritional and beneficial health characteristics. *International Journal of Dairy Technology*, *72*(2), 169–182.

Aneja, R. P. (1995). *The technology of traditional milk products in India, dairying in India*. 26th Dairy Industry Conference, Vigyan Bhawan.

Bandyopadhyay, M., Chakraborty, R., & Raychaudhuri, U. (2008). Effect of carrot on quality improvement of sweet syrupy cheese ball (Rasgulla). *International Journal of Dairy Technology, 61*(3), 290–299.

Banjare, K., Kumar, M., Goel, B. K., & Uprit, S. (2015). Studies on chemical, textural and sensory characteristics of market and laboratory peda samples manufactured in Raipur City of Chhattisgarh. *Oriental Journal of Chemistry, 31*(1), 231–238.

Béal, C., & Chammas, G. (2012). Production of laban. In Y. H. Hui (Ed.), *Handbook of animal-based fermented food and beverage technology* (2nd ed., pp. 181–212). CRC Press.

Chanda, T., Islam, M. N., Debnath, G. K., Kober, A. K. M. H., & Chanda, G. C. (2002). Preparation of rosogolla from different proportionate mixture of cow's milk and soy-milk curd. *Bangladesh Journal of Veterinary and Animal Sciences, 31*, 99–106.

Chetana, R., Manohar, B., & Reddy Yella Reddy, S. (2004). Process optimization of Gulabjamun, an Indian traditional sweet, using sugar substitutes. *European Food Research and Technology, 219*(4), 386–392.

Franklin, M. E. E., Pushpadass, H. A., Ravindra Menon, R., Rao, K. J., & Nath, B. S. (2014). Modeling the heat and mass transfer during frying of gulab jamun. *Journal of Food Processing and Preservation, 38*(4), 1939–1947.

Gautam, A., Jha, A., & Singh, R. (2013). Sensory and textural properties of chhana kheer made with three artificial sweeteners. *International Journal of Dairy Technology, 66*(1), 109–118.

Gupta, K., Verma, M., Jain, P., & Jain, M. (2014). Process optimization for producing cowpea added instant kheer mix using response surface methodology. *Journal of Nutrition Health and Food Engineering, 1*(5), 00030.

Haque, A., Alam, M. J., Hasanuzzaman, M., Islam, M. N., & Azad, M. A. (2003). Comparison of rasogolla made from fresh cow milk, fresh buffalo milk and mixture of cow and buffalo milk. *Pakistan Journal of Nutrition, 2*, 296–299.

Islam, M. S., & Basak, S. (2013). Study on sweetmeat processing in Bangladesh. *The International Journal of Engineering Science, 2*, 46–54.

Jha, A., Patel, A. A., Singh, R. R. B. (2002). Physio-chemical properties of instant kheer mix. *Le Lait, 82*(4), 501–513.

Jha, A., Tripathi, A. D., Alam, T., & Yadav, R. (2013). Process optimization for manufacture of pearl millet-based dairy dessert by using response surface methodology (RSM). *Journal of Food Science and Technology, 50*(2), 367–373.

Kadam, S., Gulati, T., & Datta, A. K. (2013). Optimization of process parameters for continuous kheer-making machine. *LWT-Food Science and Technology, 51*(1), 94–103.

Kant, R., & Broadwayb, A. A. (2017). Enhancement of functional properties of Gulabjamun by soya fortified milk. *The Pharma Innovation, 6*(3, Part B), 94.

Karthikeyan, N., & Dhanalakshmi, B. (2010). Hygienic quality of Indian sweet milk products from different sources. *Bangladesh Journal of Microbiology, 27*(2), 32–37.

Katara, R. V., & Bhargava, V. N. (1990). Production of rasogolla from cow milk containing different levels of soymilk. *Asian Journal of Dairy Research, 9*(4), 175–180.

Kaur, G., & Goswami, T. K. (2020). Effect of stevia level on chemical, microbiological, and sensory properties of dairy dessert (rasgulla) at different storage periods and temperatures. *Journal of Food Processing and Preservation, 44*(1), e14293.

Kober, A. K. M. H., Islam, M. N., & Amin, M. R. (2003). Effects of cardamom on shelf life of sandesh (milk sweet) at room temperature. *Bangladesh Veterinarian, 20*(1), 64–71.

Kober, A. K. M. H., Islam, M. N., & Debnath, G. K. (2002). Physical, chemical and microbiological qualities of sandesh (milk sweet). *The Bangladesh Veterinarian, 19*, 23–28.

Kober, A. K. M. H., Islam, M. N., & Hassan, M. N. (2006). Effects of cardamom (Elettaria cardamomum) as preservative of sandesh (chana sweet). *Bangladesh Veterinary Journal, 23*, 42–46.

Kumar, A. J., Singh, R. R. B., Patil, G. R., & Patel, A. A. (2005). Effect of temperature on moisture desorption isotherms of kheer. *LWT-Food Science and Technology, 38*(3), 303–310.

Kumar, H., Sharma, D., Palaha, R., Sharma, P., & Sonkusale, S. (2011). Isolation of Escherichia Coli from indigenous sweet milk products in relation to public health sold at sweet-meat shops of Jalandhar city, India. *Internet Journal of Food Safety, 13*, 332–335.

Kumari, A., & Poonia, A. (2021). Process optimization for the manufacture of red rice (Oryza sativa L.) kheer. *Indian Journal of Dairy Science, 74*(5).

Londhe, G., Pal, D., & Raju, P. N. (2012). Effect of packaging techniques on shelf life of brown peda, a milk-based confection. *LWT-Food Science and Technology, 47*(1), 117–125.

Minhas, K. S., Rangi, A. S., & Sidhu, J. S. (1985). Indigenous milk products. II. Effect of recipe on the chemical composition of gulabjamun. *Journal of Food Science and Technology (Mysore)*, *22*(4), 244–247.

Mule, S. M., Jadhav, S. R., Kadam, S. S., Dandekar, V. S., & Ramod, S. S. (2018). Low fat lassi prepared by incorporation of lemon grass (Cymbopogon citratus L.) extract. *Asian Journal of Dairy and Food Research*, *37*(1), 22–25.

Padghan, P. V., Mann, B., Rajeshkumar, R. S., & Kumar, A. (2015). Studies on bio-functional activity of traditional Lassi. *Indian Journal of Traditional Knowledge*, *14*(1), 124–131.

Pal, N., & Roy, S. (2019). Mint Rasgulla: A sweet with medicinal value. *Parana Journal of Science and Education*, *5*(6), 28–32.

Poonia, A. (2015). Developments in the manufacture and preservation of sandesh: A review. *Asian Journal of Dairy and Food Research*, *34*(3), 173–179.

Pramanick, P., Roy, A., Roy, S., & Mitra, A. (2017). Value addition to Rasgulla (a traditional Indian Sweet) through Tulsi (Ocimum sanctum) leaf extract. *Parana Journal of Science and Education*, *3*, 9–15.

Rahman, S. M. R., Islam, M. Z., Alam, M. M., & Mannan, A. K. M. A. (2003). Manufacture of rassomalai and its quality attributes: An indigenous milk sweetmeat of Bangladesh. *Pakistan Journal of Nutrition*, *2*(5), 300–304.

Ranganadham, M., Rao, M. S., Rao, M. R., & Rao, B. V. R. (1989). Studies on preparation of chhana from buffalo milk and its suitability for rasogolla manufacture. *Indian Journal of Dairy Science*, *42*(4), 810–816.

Ranganadham, M., Satish Kumar, M. H., Devraja, H. C., & Garg, F. C. (2016). *Traditional dairy products*. ICAR E-Course Book.

Sachdeva, S., & Rajorhia, G. S. (1982). Studies on the technology and shelf life of Burfi. *Indian Journal of Dairy Science*, *35*(6), 513–517.

Sakkas, L., Evageliou, V., Igoumenidis, P. E., & Moatsou, G. (2022). Properties of sweet buttermilk released from the churning of cream separated from sheep or cow milk or sheep cheese whey: Effect of heat treatment and storage of cream. *Foods*, *11*(3), 465.

Samet-Bali, O., Ayadi, M. A., & Attia, H. (2012). Development of fermented milk "Leben" made from spontaneous fermented cow's milk. *African Journal of Biotechnology*, *11*(8), 1829–1837.

Sarkar, T., Salauddin, M., & Chakraborty, R. (2021). Rasgulla-the ethnic Indian sweetmeat delicacy and its evolutionary journey through contemporary research. *Journal of Ethnic Foods*, *8*, 1–14.

Sarkar, T., Salauddin, M., Hazra, S. K., & Chakraborty, R. (2020). The impact of raw and differently dried pineapple (Ananas comosus) fortification on the vitamins, organic acid and carotene profile of dairy rasgulla (sweetened cheese ball). *Heliyon*, *6*(10), e05233.

Sayedatunnesha, W. A., Islam, M., Islam, M., & Hossain, M. A. (2008). Comparative study of the quality of rasomalai manufactured from cow and buffalo milk. *Bangladesh Journal of Animal Science*, *37*(1), 57–63.

Sen, D. C. (1992). Studied on kachhagolla a delicious milk sweetmeat of Bengal. Kachhagolla, a type of sandesh. *Indian Dairyman*, *44*, 249–251.

Sengupta, S., & Bhowal, J. (2017). Studies on preparation of dietetic rasgulla (cheese ball) from edible quality flours and antioxidant rich vegetable oils. *LWT-Food Science and Technology*, *86*, 473–482.

Sharma, S. P., Kapoor, C. M., Khanna, S., Rani, M., Bishnoi, S., & Ahlawat, S. S. (2014). Technological aspects of indigenous chhana based rasmalai. *Haryana Vet*, *53*(2), 124–126.

Singh, A., & Vaidya, M. (2015). Traditional weaning foods and practices in Jabalpur district with reference to prevalence of malnutrition. *Journal of Dairying, Foods & Home Sciences*, *34*(1), 32–38.

Singh, S. P., Thakur, S. N., & Chandra, R. (2015). Studies on preparation of rasogolla from blend of cow milk and soya milk. *Journal of Pharmaceutical Innovation*, *2*, 6–9.

Sukumar, D. (1980). *Outlines of dairy technology*. Oxford University Press.

Thompkinson, D. K. (1995). Dairy Industry in India-A Scenario. *Indian Food Industry*, *14*, 17–17.

Tiwari, R. P., & Grewal, J. S. (1999). Studies on the effect of preservatives on the keeping quality of rasmalai. *Journal of Food Science and Technology*, *36*(1), 84–87.

# 12 UN's SDGs in the Dairy Sector (Contributions and Opportunities)

## 12.1 LEARNING OBJECTIVES

By the end of the chapter, the reader will be able to:

- Understand how to prepare the dairy sector to assist in attaining the United Nations' sustainable development goals (SDGs).
- Identify and prioritize factors that are more substantial for dairying in the global context.

Approximately 240 million individuals worldwide gain their livelihood from the dairy sector. The dairy industry holds the potential to contribute to the attainment of the SDGs in several ways: (i) Household: boosted direct consumption of balanced food; female empowerment and gender impartiality (ii) Rural community: creating jobs; making more products and services available; helping small dairy farmers make more money and be more productive. (iii) National economy: contribute to the government's revenue generation and stimulate the economy by engaging in international trade, leading to job creation and overall growth. (iv) Global: ensuring an adequate and reliable supply of milk and dairy products; promoting dairy systems that are environmentally friendly and can withstand challenges; making sure that food markets are working correctly.

## 12.2 INTRODUCTION

In 2022, global raw milk production reached 935.9 million tons, which is 1.1% higher than in 2021 (The Dairy News Global, 2023). But the global dairy industry still faces several challenges regarding its carbon footprint (or greenhouse gas footprint), consumption, nutrition, and sustainability (Granato et al., 2022). The United Nations' (UN) sustainable development goals (SDGs) state that by 2030, food processors, governing bodies, and consumers should take action regarding food consumption and production models to reduce the production of byproducts and side-streams and increase their circularity by creating more inventive and healthier dairy foods. Dairy foods have traditionally been produced without bioactive ingredients to improve consumer health and well-being. It is crucial to develop integrated strategies that reflect the "farm-to-fork" strategy to meet sustainability goals, lower the carbon footprint, and reformulate dairy goods to make them more nutrient dense (Granato et al., 2022).

DOI: 10.1201/9781003397786-12

## 12.3 HOW THE DAIRY SECTOR CONTRIBUTES TO THE UN'S SDGs

To ensure a more sustainable future for the planet and its inhabitants, the UN has established 17 SDGs. The UN estimates that there are currently 7.6 billion people on earth, and that number will increase to 9.8 billion by 2050, primarily due to population growth in developing nations. Because there are so many people on the planet, the UN's SDGs can aid in resolving significant global concerns (Granato et al., 2022).

### 12.3.1 The Dairy Industry Assumes Responsibility

In 2016, the International Dairy Federation (IDF) and the Food and Agriculture Organization (FAO) of the UN made a joint agreement called the Rotterdam Declaration. This agreement focuses on how the dairy industry helps in the development of the planet. The declaration says that the worldwide dairy industry is dedicated to achieving the UN's SDGS (Bhat et al., 2022). According to the statement, the dairy industry provides the global population with wholesome and secure food. The declaration also emphasizes the dairy sector's social and economic importance, especially in developing countries, where approximately 80 million women are employed in milk production. This industry supports 240 million employees worldwide. This means around 240 million people's livelihoods are supported by the worldwide dairy industry. The FAO has acknowledged that the dairy industry has a rightful place in an ecological future by signing the Rotterdam Declaration. The majority of the UN's SDGs apply to the efforts made by the dairy industry. The dairy sector can solve four SDGs: poverty reduction (SDG1), zero hunger (SDG2), good health and well-being (SDG3), and gender equality (SDG5) (**Figure 12.1**).

### 12.3.2 Poverty Reduction (SDG1)

Milk and dairy foods help to eradicate hunger and poverty (**Figure 12.1**). Worldwide, there are about 120 million dairy cattle farms. The majority of these farms are small and located in developing and

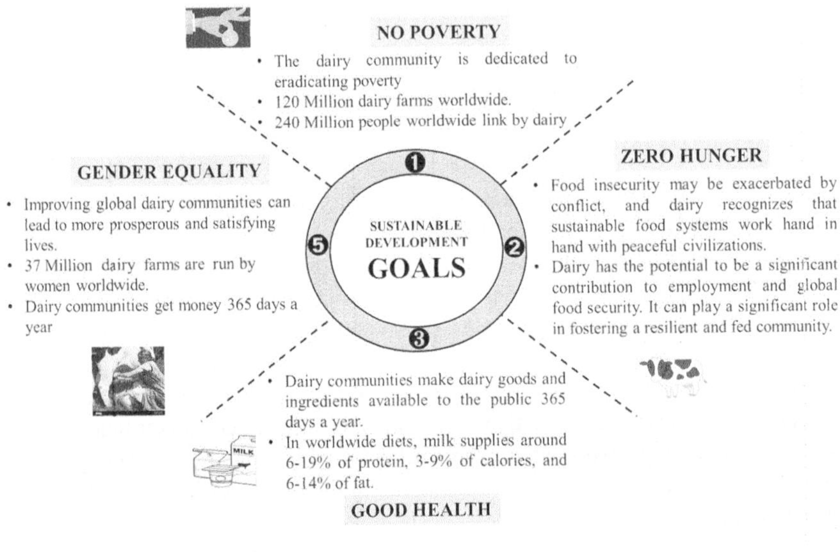

NO POVERTY
• The dairy community is dedicated to eradicating poverty
• 120 Million dairy farms worldwide.
• 240 Million people worldwide link by dairy
ZERO HUNGER
• Food insecurity may be exacerbated by conflict, and dairy recognizes that sustainable food systems work hand in hand with peaceful civilizations.
• Dairy has the potential to be a significant contribution to employment and global food security. It can play a significant role in fostering a resilient and fed community.
GENDER EQUALITY
• Improving global dairy communities can lead to more prosperous and satisfying lives.
• 37 Million dairy farms are run by women worldwide.
• Dairy communities get money 365 days a year
SUSTAINABLE DEVELOPMENT GOALS
1
2
3
5
• Dairy communities make dairy goods and ingredients available to the public 365 days a year.
• In worldwide diets, milk supplies around 6-19% of protein, 3-9% of calories, and 6-14% of fat.
MILK
GOOD HEALTH


**FIGURE 12.1 The dairy industry's contribution to the accomplishment of the UN's SDGs.** The dairy sector can solve four SDGs: poverty reduction (SDG1), zero hunger (SDG2), good health and well-being (SDG3), and gender equality (SDG5).

underdeveloped countries. Two or three cows are owned by the small family-run farms in this area, which serve as the foundation of their regular income. The cows provide milk, and some of it is sold to nearby markets. The money earned from selling milk is used to provide food for people living in the countryside. The dairy industry provides employment for many people in every step of the process, from taking care of the cows to making the finished products that are sold in supermarkets. The dairy industry employs almost 240 million people worldwide, as was already mentioned. Consequently, the dairy industry is playing a significant role in the fight against global poverty (Granato et al., 2022).

### 12.3.3 Zero Hunger (SDG2)

Many rural households in underdeveloped nations can combat hunger with a few cows. The family consumes a share of the milk that the cows make each day (**Figure 12.1**). As a result, the family's regular source of nourishment is milk. Milk is a nutritious food full of nutrients that contribute to satiety and are crucial to the family's general nutrition. Many families in developing countries can significantly reduce their hunger by having one or two cows (Granato et al., 2022; Kober et al., 2014; Dhar et al., 2018).

### 12.3.4 Good Health and Well-being (SDG3)

Milk and dairy foods contribute to the health of people around the world. Milk and dairy foods contain important proteins, vitamins, and minerals that both children and adults need. These nutrients are crucial for children's development as well as for the formation and maintenance of the body's essential organs, including the bones, muscles, brain, and others. Dairy foods also help prevent several of the various lifestyle diseases that primarily appear in industrialized countries. Dairy foods have been linked to a lower risk of type 2 diabetes and osteoporosis, according to numerous scientific studies. Therefore, dairy foods also have a beneficial effect in the long term and can advantageously be included in a healthy and varied diet (Granato et al., 2022) (**Figure 12.1**).

### 12.3.5 Gender Equality (SDG5)

The production of milk in developing nations enables women to achieve greater equality and self-reliance. In rural areas, it is typically women who handle the family's cows and are primarily responsible for milk production. The women also make sure that the cows get water and feed and that they are milked. Additionally, they sell the excess milk on the local market. Thus, the women get an income that allows them to buy the most necessary things for the family. In male-dominated developing countries, by doing their jobs as dairy farmers, women get room to maneuver, both socially and economically. Overall, it advances gender equality and the empowerment of women (Granato et al., 2022) (**Figure 12.1**).

## 12.4 FURTHER OPPORTUNITIES FOR THE DAIRY SECTOR

Adopting a sustainable, "state-of-the-art" strategy is essential for success along the whole production and supply chain of the dairy industry. In this sense, it is crucial to comprehend major sustainability indicators and issues from a global perspective. A few important elements to be measured include appropriate design, the use of cutting-edge technologies, the adoption of life cycle analysis, upgrades, and optimization of the complete manufacturing process. Additionally, the requirements of the producers, consumers, and reliant industries must be properly considered. However, considerations for the area's economics, social security, and ecology should not be underestimated. Precise planning is essential, both on and off the farm, especially when circular economy policies must be considered.

By 2067, it is anticipated that there will be 10.5 billion people on the planet, up from 7.6 billion, while the amount of arable land per person will fall by 25%. It is anticipated that the difference in arable land per capita will widen as a result of the uneven population growth. Increased population density boosts urbanization as well, which has typically led to greater personal income and greater demand for dairy products. Climate change is expected to drive changes in the regions where dairy production takes place. Oceanic impacts have less of a calming influence on the effects of climate change in the northern hemisphere, where 86% of the world's milk is produced. In response to climate change, dairy production will be moved to regions with a more reliable water supply and long enough growing seasons.

Dairy farms will need to be profitable and sustainable to meet the rising demand in the face of these difficulties (Kober et al., 2014; Dhar et al., 2018). Dairy farmers in 2067 will meet the world's needs for essential nutrients by adopting modern technologies and practices that provide improved cow health and longevity, profitable dairy farms, and sustainable agriculture. According to the author, dairy farmers will embrace techniques for controlling the microbiomes of cows' digestive tracts and other bodily systems to enhance their health and well-being. They also expect that the management of a cow's epigenome, which regulates longer-term reactions to the environment, will receive increased focus.

Consolidation, modernization, and specialization will boost output and safety in the dairy business. Global commerce will have a significant impact on profitability, and larger dairy farms will continue to employ automation more extensively to cut costs. Dairy cattle lines that are healthier, produce milk more effectively and are more disease and heat resistant will result from advancements in genetic selection. The author predicts a change from just exporting surpluses to creating products with added value that are catered to certain tastes and cultures.

In the coming 50 years, feeding an increasing global population will be difficult, and it is predicted that the dairy industry will overcome this obstacle by utilizing knowledge and technology to improve dairy cows and create more productive, sustainable dairy farms. Our vision is that dairying in the future will reflect sustainable growth that benefits animals, agroecosystems, and humankind through the production of key nutrients for human consumption.

In 2067, there will be roughly 10.4 billion people on the planet, with 81% of them living in either Africa or Asia. The amount of arable land per person that can be used to grow food will drop to 0.15 hectares. The temperature will increase in the tropical and temperate zones, especially in the northern hemisphere, and this will push growing seasons and dairy farming away from arid areas and into more northern latitudes. Because it delivers key nutrients more effectively than many other agricultural systems, dairy consumption will rise. Additionally, dairy farming will be modernized in developing nations, and the amount of milk produced per cow will double in those with highly developed dairy farming systems.

The key to dairy farms' sustainability will be their financial success. Genetic improvements will include the importance of the coding genome and associated noncoding epigenome of cattle and of microbiomes of dairy cattle and farmsteads. The scale of farms will grow, and there will be more lateral integration in the housing and administration of dairy cattle at various ages and phases of production. Much of the manual labor on farms will be replaced by integrated sensors, robotics, and automation. Epigenome and microbiome management will be integrated into standard herd management. The health of cows will also be improved, and natural behaviors will be allowed to be expressed due to innovations in dairy facilities. Herds will be seen as superorganisms, and research on herds as observational units will improve the agroecology and sustainability of dairy farms as well as the productivity, health, and well-being of dairy cattle. Advanced technologies and methods will be employed by dairy farmers in 2067 to ensure they can meet the global demand for crucial nutrients. Their main objective is to ensure the well-being and longevity of cows, manage profitable farms, and incorporate sustainable techniques in animal agriculture.

## 12.5 OPPORTUNITIES AND CHALLENGES IN THE GLOBAL DAIRY SECTOR

The global dairy sector faces several opportunities and challenges at the producer, processor, retailer, and ecological levels (Deloitte, 2016, 2017; Bojovic & McGregor, 2023; Bhat et al., 2022) (**Figure 12.2**).

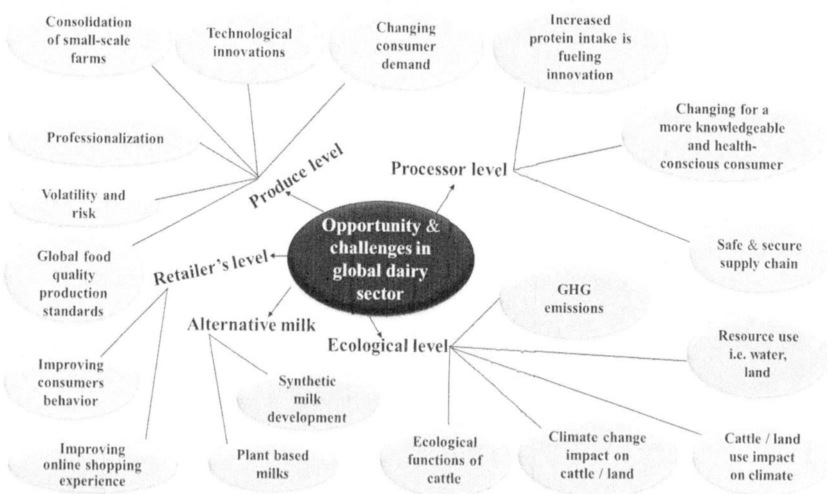


**FIGURE 12.2 Future scope and challenges in the global dairy sector.**

### 12.5.1 Producer Level

#### 12.5.1.1 Professionalization in the Global Dairy Sector

Running dairying on a "professional" (and in some cases industrial) basis has been ordinary for some time in several countries around the globe. Regardless of scale, developing technologies and better farm management techniques will become more important on dairy farms all over the world in the years to come (Kober et al., 2014; Dhar et al., 2018). Successful farmers will need to focus on the following few aspects to grow their enterprise sustainably and profitably: (i) Take advantage of new technologies. These include recording and improvement, genomic evaluation methods, together with the development of statistical, bio-informatics, computational, and geographical information system technologies. (ii) Complement technology with suitable processes. (iii) Enhance commercial skills.

#### 12.5.1.2 Volatility and Risk in the Global Dairy Sector

Volatility is a way of life in the dairy industry. Dairy farmers must contend not just with fluctuating milk prices but also with input costs, animal health, and weather conditions. For long-term success, both managing volatility at the farm level and managing volatility at the processor level, having efficient strategies to manage this volatility are essential.

#### 12.5.1.3 Improving Consumer Education and Health Consciousness in the Global Dairy Industry

Consumers are now more aware of their nutritional choices for the aging population, rising rates of obesity and diabetes in the globe, including developed countries, and increased research on the relationship between diet and health. This has increased consumer demand for "clean label" products and healthy alternatives. Customers are becoming more and more interested in protein due to the wide range of health advantages it offers, from weight loss, satiety, and healthy aging to muscle building and exercise recovery. Profiting from this development, many dairy companies have increased the protein content of their products with supplementing their products with extra protein. Focusing on two crucial areas will be necessary to present this point of view: (i) health and wellness and (ii) the demand for a "clean label" (Sexton et al., 2019).

The global dairy sector faces several opportunities and challenges at the producer, processor, retailer, and ecological levels.

### 12.5.2 Processor Level

#### 12.5.2.1 Changing for a More Knowledgeable and Health-Conscious Consumer in the Global Dairy Industry

In this scenario, the most successful firms will be those that are able to reduce the quantity of additives utilized in their products and substantiate their health benefits through scientific research. From this perspective, three key aspects must be addressed: (i) the demand for organic products, (ii) the demand for genetic modification (GM)-free products, and (iii) the requirement for transparency.

#### 12.5.2.2 Innovation in the Global Dairy Sector

From this perspective, several key aspects must be addressed: (i) innovation to drive margins, (ii) downstream collaboration, (iii) global innovation, and (iv) building an innovation network (Deloitte, 2017).

#### 12.5.2.3 Increased Protein Intake is Fueling Innovation in the World's Dairy Industry

Dairy protein consumption has increased in recent years, owing to rising income in emerging markets, an increase in "gym culture," and a shift toward foods with functional benefits. The global protein market is expected to grow at a 6% compound annual growth rate (CAGR) through 2018. Dairy proteins are frequently regarded as the "gold standard" in protein by consumers due to their complete amino acid profile, easy digestibility, and satiety benefits, and they are increasingly used for fitness and weight management. Dairy companies are capitalizing on this trend by adding value to proteins for use in a wide range of applications. From this perspective, there are few key aspects to focus on: (i) Expansion in the sports nutrition market. (ii) Healthy aging: In order to avoid sarcopenia (loss of muscle mass), senior customers are also exhibiting interest in dairy-based nutrition products, giving rise to the "healthy aging" category. In response to these trends, some sports nutrition businesses have introduced new products focused toward elderly clients. The elderly populations in many high-income countries make this a potentially valuable sector, even if breaking into this market will be challenging due to marketing difficulties. (iii) Clinical nutrition: Dairy constituents like casein and whey proteins, which are frequently used in medications and therapies for malnutrition, give another opportunity for the dairy business in the expanding clinical nutrition market. Clinical nutrition is a branch of medicine that seeks to identify and treat medical disorders in humans caused by an improper or insufficient diet, or by diseases that render the body unable to handle the nutrients provided by the normal diet (Iriondo-DeHond et al., 2018). The worldwide clinical nutrition market was worth $38.1 billion in 2020 and is expected to reach $54.5 billion by 2028, growing at a 4.5% CAGR from 2021 to 2028 (Verified Market Research, 2023). A variety of demographic trends are contributing to this growth, including an aging population, an increase in products for premature babies, an increase in products to treat malnutrition, and an increase in the incidence of lifestyle-related diseases.

#### 12.5.2.4 Safe and Secure Supply Chain in the Global Dairy Sector

Safety and supply security are major concerns in the dairy industry, where short shelf lives and many suppliers increase the possibility of product deficiencies. From this perspective, the focus needs to be on blockchain technology and adjusting to the new environment (Boz, 2021; Campi et al., 2021).

### 12.5.3 Retailer Level

Retailers must use technology and data more effectively to adapt to changing consumption patterns and provide consumers with the food they want, when and where they want it. From this point, attention must be paid to the demand for local produce, continued recessionary behavior, personal shopping experience, online and mobile/convenience store growth, and leveraging data to target consumers (Deloitte, 2016).

### 12.5.4 Ecological Level

#### 12.5.4.1 Global Warming

The severity of climate change effects is anticipated to be greater in the southern hemisphere as opposed to the northern hemisphere, as indicated by scientists. Greenhouse gas emissions and food waste are major sources of concern. The livestock industry is said to be responsible for 18% of all greenhouse gas emissions in $CO_2$ terms, which is greater than the amount produced by the total transportation system, according to a FAO (2006) report titled "Livestock's Long Shadow" (Rotz, 2018). However, implementing sustainable practices can save input costs and enhance brand recognition among customers. From this perspective, attention must be given to three crucial elements: (i) growing demand to "become green," (ii) new technologies and applications, and (iii) Marketing a "green" image (IDF, 2022).

It is mostly created through burp that happens naturally while cattle digest feed. Other emissions arise during manure excretion and storage

#### 12.5.4.2 Enteric Methane ($CH_4$) Production

Methane makes up about 16% of total world gas emissions and is the second most important greenhouse gas (GHG). Its atmospheric warming activity is 23 times higher than that of $CO_2$. The animal digestive tract is the main source of methane (28% of global $CH_4$ emissions) (IDF, 2022) (**Figure 12.3**).

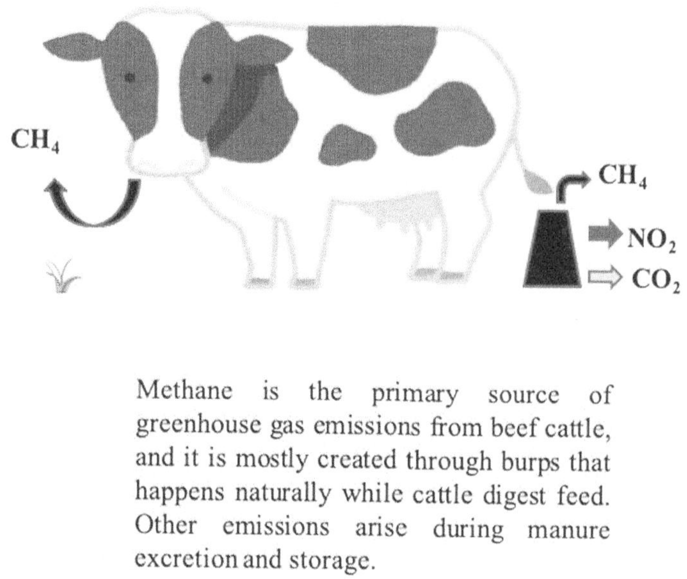


FIGURE 12.3 **Methane is the primary source of greenhouse gas emissions from cattle.**

#### 12.5.4.3 Effect of Global Warming on Livestock Production

Nutrition stress is the largest indirect effect. Natural pasture has a lower nutritional value and lower tiller density (tropically adapted $C_4$ grasses). In comparison to $C_3$ grasses, $C_4$ has high fiber content, reduced digestibility, and higher methane production (IDF, 2022).

#### 12.5.4.4 Adaptation

Due to global warming, animals will have to adapt to higher temperatures, lower nutritional value of grasses, and expansion of diseases. Balancing genotypes with the production environment is crucial. The question is how to measure adaptation and how to select for it. However, more research is required on adaptation.

## 12.6 CONCLUSIONS

The global dairy industry wants to contribute to the resolution of some of the world's most pressing issues. For the benefit of the entire world's population, the dairy sector has accepted responsibility for this and pledged, through the Rotterdam Declaration, to make milk and dairy products even more sustainable. To summarize, fulfilling traditional and evolving dairy demands will require producers, processors, and retailers to provide consumers with nutritious, safe, convenient, and cost-effective options. The "datafication" of agriculture must be used by producers to increase output sustainably. There are still many ongoing sustainability problems throughout the entire process of manufacturing and delivering products. This has shown the need to create new and effective technology solutions, like new ways of processing and preserving food, models for predicting things, analyzing the entire lifespan of something, using computers to think like humans, connecting things through the internet, and making things digital. It is very important that these new ideas and improvements help to satisfy the needs of the people who buy products, make products, and work in the dairy industry. Processors must employ technology to create new goods while also ensuring that their supply chains and production processes are as safe and secure as possible. Retailers must utilize technology and data more effectively to adjust to shifting consumer habits and give customers access to the food they want, when and where they want it. Additionally, actors throughout the value chain will need to put in more effort to keep the trust of a customer base that is becoming more affluent and demanding. To summarize, challenges facing the global dairy sector include low production levels, global warming, adaptation, and enteric methane production. The global dairy sector has good opportunities including an increase in demand, production environments, recording and improvement, and genomics. Finally, in light of the SDGs and the global dairy sector situation, more research is needed, specifically more nutritious dairy foods with added ingredients (innovative and healthy functional dairy foods) that may improve consumer health/aging and the impact of dairying on the environment, society, and regional/global markets (Bhat et al., 2022).

## REFERENCES

Bhat, R., Di Pasquale, J., Bánkuti, F. I., Siqueira, T. T., Shine, P., & Murphy, M. D. (2022). Global dairy sector: Trends, prospects, and challenges. *Sustainability*, *14*(7), 4193.

Bojovic, M., & McGregor, A. (2023). A review of megatrends in the global dairy sector: What are the socioecological implications? *Agriculture and Human Values*, *40*, 373–394.

Boz, Z. (2021). Moving food processing to industry 4.0 and beyond. *Food Technology Magazine*, *75*(6), 1–6.

Campi, M., Duenas, M., & Fagiolo, G. (2021). Specialization in food production affects global food security and food systems sustainability, 141. World Development, Article 105411.

Deloitte. (2016). *The consumer goods forum, health and wellness progress report 2016*. Deloitte Touche Tohmatsu Ltd.

Deloitte. (2017). *Global dairy sector-trends and opportunities*. Deloitte Touche Tohmatsu Ltd.

Dhar, A., Amin, U. S., & Kober, A. K. M. H. (2018). Dairy industry in Bangladesh: Challenge and prospectus. In *15th international scientific conference 2018* (p. 174). CVASU (Abstr-12).

FAO. (2006). *Livestock's long shadow*. UN Food & Agriculture 2006 report.

Granato, D., Carocho, M., Barros, L., Zabetakis, I., Mocan, A., Tsoupras, A., Cruz, A. G., & Pimentel, T. C. (2022). Implementation of sustainable development goals in the dairy sector: Perspectives on the use of agro-industrial side-streams to design functional foods. *Trends in Food Science & Technology, 124*, 128–139.

IDF. (2022). The IDF global carbon footprint standard for the dairy sector. In International Dairy Federation (Ed.), *Bulletin of the IDF No 520/2022*. IDF.

Iriondo-DeHond, M., Miguel, E., & Del Castillo, M. D. (2018). Food byproducts as sustainable ingredients for innovative and healthy dairy foods. *Nutrients, 10*(10), 1358. https://doi.org/10.3390/nu10101358.

Kober, A. K. M. H., Bari, M. S., Nath, B. K., & Chakma, J. (2014). Small scale dairy cattle management in hilly district of Bangladesh. *Advances in Agriculture, Sciences and Engineering Research, 4*(1), 1445–1452.

Rotz, C. A. (2018). Modeling greenhouse gas emissions from dairy farms. *Journal of Dairy Science, 101*(7), 6675–6690.

Sexton, A. E., Garnett, T., & Lorimer, J. (2019). Framing the future of food: The contested promises of alternative proteins. *Environment and Planning E: Nature and Space, 2*(1), 47–72.

The Dairy News Global. (2023). *Global milk production reached 935.9 million tons in 2022*. https://dairynews.today/global/news/mirovoe-proizvodstvo-moloka-v-2022-godu-dostiglo-935-9-mln-tonn.html.

Verified Market Research. (2023). *Clinical nutrition products market size and forecast*. www.verifiedmarket-research.com/product/clinical-nutrition-products-market/.

# Index

Note: Page numbers in *italics* indicate a figure and page numbers in **bold** indicate a table on the corresponding page.

## T



## U



## V



## W

## X



## Y



## Z